Herd/Flock Health and Medicine for the Exotic Animal Practitioner

Editor

SHANGZHE XIE

VETERINARY CLINICS OF NORTH AMERICA: EXOTIC ANIMAL PRACTICE

www.vetexotic.theclinics.com

Consulting Editor
JÖRG MAYER

September 2021 • Volume 24 • Number 3

ELSEVIER

1600 John F. Kennedy Boulevard • Suite 1800 • Philadelphia, Pennsylvania, 19103-2899
http://www.vetexotic.theclinics.com

VETERINARY CLINICS OF NORTH AMERICA: EXOTIC ANIMAL PRACTICE Volume 24, Number 3
September 2021 ISSN 1094-9194, ISBN-13: 978-0-323-79620-0

Editor: Stacy Eastman
Developmental Editor: Axell Ivan Jade M. Purificacion

Veterinary Clinics of North America: Exotic Animal Practice (ISSN 1094-9194) is published in January, May, and September by Elsevier, Inc., 360 Park Avenue South, New York, NY 10010-1710. Subscription prices are $290.00 per year for US individuals, $687.00 per year for US institutions, $100.00 per year for US students and residents, $338.00 per year for Canadian individuals, $735.00 per year for Canadian institutions, $352.00 per year for international individuals, $735.00 per year for international institutions, $100.00 per year Canadian students/residents, and $165.00 per year for international students/residents. To receive student/resident rate, orders must be accompanied by name of affiliated institution, date of term, and the *signature* of program/residency coordinator on institution letterhead. Orders will be billed at individual rate until proof of status is received. Foreign air speed delivery is included in all *Clinics* subscription prices. All prices are subject to change without notice. **POSTMASTER:** Send address changes to *Veterinary Clinics of North America: Exotic Animal Practice*, Elsevier Health Sciences Division, Subscription Customer Service, 3251 Riverport Lane, Maryland Heights, MO 63043. **Customer Service: Telephone: 1-800-654-2452** (U.S. and Canada); **1-314-447-8871** (outside U.S. and Canada). **Fax: 1-314-447-8029. E-mail: journalscustomerservice-usa@elsevier.com (for print support); journalsonlinesupport-usa@elsevier.com (for online support).**

Reprints. For copies of 100 or more of articles in this publication, please contact the Commercial Reprints Department, Elsevier Inc., 360 Park Avenue South, New York, New York 10010-1710. Tel.: 212-633-3874; Fax: 212-633-3820; E-mail: reprints@elsevier.com.

Veterinary Clinics of North America: Exotic Animal Practice is covered in *MEDLINE/PubMed (Index Medicus).*

Contributors

CONSULTING EDITOR

JÖRG MAYER, Dr med vet, MSc
Diplomate, American Board of Veterinary Practitioners (Exotic Companion Mammals); Diplomate, European College of Zoological Medicine (Small Mammals); Diplomate, American College of Zoological Medicine; Associate Professor of Zoological Medicine, Department of Small Animal Medicine and Surgery, University of Georgia College of Veterinary Medicine, Athens, Georgia, USA

EDITOR

SHANGZHE XIE, BSc/BVMS, MVS (Conservation Medicine), PhD
Diplomate, American Board of Veterinary Practitioners (Avian Practice); Assistant Director, Department of Conservation, Research and Veterinary Services, Jurong Bird Park, Wildlife Reserves Singapore, Singapore

AUTHORS

HAMISH BARON, BVSc (Hons), FANZCVS (Avian Medicine & Surgery)
The Unusual Pet Vets, Frankston, Victoria, Australia

JUAN CORNEJO, BSc(Bio), PhD
Assistant Vice President, Attractions Development, Mandai Park Development Pte. Ltd, Singapore, Singapore

LORENZO CROSTA, DVM, PhD, GP Cert (ExAP), FNOVI (Avian and Zoo Medicine)
Diplomate, European College of Zoological Medicine; EBVS European Veterinary Specialist in Zoo Health Management, Associate Professor of Avian and Zoological Medicine, Faculty of Science, Director, Sydney School of Veterinary Science, The University of Sydney, Avian, Reptile and Exotic Pet Hospital, Camden, New South Wales, Australia

ZHI JIAN KELVIN LIM, BSc/BVMS, MPH-VPH, MS
Diplomate, American College of Veterinary Preventive Medicine; Director, Veterinary Health Management, National Parks Board, Singapore, Singapore

KIM LE, BSc, BVSc, MVS
Diplomate, American Board of Veterinary Practitioners (Exotic Companion Mammal); Bulger Veterinary Hospital, Lawrence, Massachusetts, USA

AMBER LEE, BVSc
Diplomate, American Board of Veterinary Practitioners (AVIAN PRACTICE); The Unusual Pet Vets, Frankston, Werribee, Victoria, Australia

JOSHUA LLINAS, BVSc (Hons), MVS, BSc (Hons)
The Unusual Pet Vets, Jindalee, Queensland, Australia

DAVID J. MCLELLAND, BSc(Vet), BVSc, DVSc, MANZCVS (Zoo Medicine)
Diplomate, American College of Zoological Medicine; Diplomate, European College of Zoological Medicine (Zoo Health Management); Veterinarian, Zoos South Australia, Adelaide, Australia

JENNIFER M. MCLELLAND, BVSc (Hons), MVSc (Avian and Wildlife Health), MANZCVS (Avian), MVS (Conservation Medicine)
Veterinarian, Zoos South Australia, Adelaide, Australia

DANIELE PETRINI, DVM, MSc, GPCert (ExAP), SPACS
Medicina e Chirurgia Degli Animali Non Convenzionali, Segretario

ELLEN K. RASIDI, BBiomedSc, BSc(Vet) (Hons), BVSc
Veterinarian, Conservation, Research and Veterinary Services, Jurong Bird Park, Wildlife Reserves Singapore, Singapore, Singapore

SHIVANANDEN SAWMY, BSc (Hons) Biol, BVM&S (Edinburgh, UK), Cert AVP Zoological Medicine (UK), MRCVS
Royal College of Veterinary Surgeons Advanced Practitioner in Zoological Medicine, Clinical Veterinary Registrar, Faculty of Science, Avian, Reptile and Exotic Pet Hospital, Sydney School of Veterinary Science, The University of Sydney, New South Wales, Australia

JOANNE SHEEN, BVMS, CertZooMed
Diplomate, American Board of Veterinary Practitioners (Exotic Companion Mammal); Sydney Exotics and Rabbit Vets, North Shore Veterinary Specialist Hospital, Sydney, New South Wales, Australia

SHANE CRAIG SIMPSON, BVSc (Hons), GCM(VP), CMAVA
Veterinarian, The Unusual Pet Vets, Frankston, Victoria, Australia

MICHELLE SUTHERLAND, BVM&S, BSc (Hons), MANZCVS (Avian Health), CertAVP (ZooMed)
Diplomate, American Board of Veterinary Practitioners (Avian Practice); The Unusual Pet Vets, Frankston, Victoria, Australia

TRENT CHARLES VAN ZANTEN, BSc (Hons), DVM
Veterinarian, Conservation, Research and Veterinary Services, Wildlife Reserves Singapore, Singapore

SHANGZHE XIE, BSc/BVMS, MVS (Conservation Medicine), PhD
Diplomate, American Board of Veterinary Practitioners (Avian Practice); Assistant Director, Department of Conservation, Research and Veterinary Services, Jurong Bird Park, Wildlife Reserves Singapore, Singapore

SHIRLEY YEO LLIZO, VMD
Director of Animal Health, Topeka Zoo & Conservation Centerm, Topeka, Kansas, USA

Contents

Against a backdrop of climate change and epidemics, the exotic animal veterinarian is well positioned to detect emerging and exotic disease threats, prevent and control zoonotic diseases, and identify antimicrobial resistance. Within the traditional context of animal and public health, epidemiology has had a focus on veterinary preventive health and in disease investigation and control particularly in food animal and safety application. The understanding of preventive health management and veterinary epidemiology expands the repertoire of the clinical veterinarian to advise and implement and evaluate group animal health programs and biosecurity measures as well as conduct disease investigations.

When treatment is required for a herd/flock health concern, a range of factors must be considered to determine the preferred treatment strategy. If a group treatment strategy is pursued, considerations to optimize the likelihood of safe and effective group treatment include taxon-specific pharmacokinetics/pharmacodynamics, the formulation of prescribed medication, the type and amount of food, the number and type of water sources, enclosure design, size and demography of the group, weather conditions, and health status of individuals in the group. In addition, antimicrobial stewardship principles and relevant legislation/regulation must be at the forefront of decision making.

There are many intersecting aspects to the avicultural management of a captive flock. Extensive knowledge of the natural history of the species kept is key to fulfilling the environmental, social, nutritional, and behavioral requirements of the birds, whether in a mixed- or sole-species aviary. Species compatibility with the environment, climate, and other co-occupants plays a role as well, as does hygiene, good avicultural management, and veterinary involvement and consultation. In understanding and meeting these requirements, optimal health can be maintained through the reduction or elimination of stressors and the maintenance of normal physiologic function.

VETERINARY CLINICS OF NORTH AMERICA: EXOTIC ANIMAL PRACTICE

SERIES OF RELATED INTEREST

Veterinary Clinics of North America: Small Animal Practice
Available at: https://www.vetsmall.theclinics.com/

THE CLINICS ARE NOW AVAILABLE ONLINE!
Access your subscription at:
www.theclinics.com

Preface
Birds of a Feather Flock Together

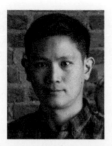

Shangzhe Xie, BSc/BVMS, MVS (Conservation Medicine), PhD,
Diplomate ABVP (Avian Practice)
Editor

As exotic animal medicine progresses, the demand from clients owning large groups of exotic animals, whether due to their personal or business interests, will increase. Most exotic animal practitioners have good training and fundamentals in small animal medicine, which focuses on the individual patient. Herd and flock medicine requires a different approach, with many principles derived from production animal medicine. Furthermore, as the level of veterinary medicine and standard of care for exotic animals increase, antemortem diagnoses and individualized medication/treatment regimens can allow for earlier diagnoses of disease in a herd/flock, leading to better treatment outcomes.

A series of publications from 1991 to 2001 laid down basic principles for avian flock medicine and health management targeted at aviculturists. Many of these principles are timeless and apply across different taxonomic groups, but with the advancement of the exotic animal industry, some of the principles may require updating. Other current publications on the topic focus on farm/production animals or shelter medicine, which are fields where many of the same principles can be extrapolated to exotic animal herd/flock medicine, but where there are also many aspects that may not apply. The topics covered in this special issue bring together knowledge that already exists in the mélange of veterinary medicine to guide exotic animal practitioners who may be called upon to provide advice on the management of herds/flocks of exotic animals and/or manage outbreaks of diseases in them.

The articles combine the approaches and advances in small animal, farm/production animal, and exotic animal medicine to enable exotic animal practitioners to manage herd/flock health and practice herd/flock medicine to a higher standard. Other than the introductory article summarizing the principles of herd/flock medicine based on epidemiological principles and the article discussing therapeutic options for treatment of herds/flocks, the other articles cover the principles of managing herds/flocks of birds, exotic companion mammals, and reptiles/amphibians in health and disease.

Vet Clin Exot Anim 24 (2021) ix–x
https://doi.org/10.1016/j.cvex.2021.06.002
1094-9194/21/© 2021 Elsevier Inc. All rights reserved.

vetexotic.theclinics.com

The concluding articles discuss the management of reproduction and disease prevention programs of herds/flocks of exotic pets.

Shangzhe Xie, BSc/BVMS, MVS (Conservation Medicine), PhD, DABVP (Avian Practice)
Conservation
Research and Veterinary Department
Wildlife Reserves Singapore
80 Mandai Lake Road
Singapore 729826

E-mail address:
shangzhe.xie@wrs.com.sg

Application of Epidemiology and Principles of Herd/Flock Health for the Exotic Animal Veterinarian

Zhi Jian Kelvin Lim, BSc/BVMS, MPH-VPH, MS, DACVPM[a],*,
Shangzhe Xie, BSc/BVMS, MVS (Conservation Medicine), PhD, DABVP (Avian Practice)[b]

KEYWORDS

• Epidemiology • Exotic pets • Biosecurity • Herd health • Flock health

KEY POINTS

- There is a role for the exotic animal veterinarian to detect emerging and exotic disease threats, prevent and control zoonotic diseases, and identify antimicrobial resistance.
- The understanding of preventive health management and veterinary epidemiology expands the repertoire of the clinical veterinarian to advise and implement group animal health programs, implement and evaluate biosecurity measures, and conduct disease investigations.
- Preventive health management programs should be developed based on evidence-based studies and critical evaluation and interpretation of tests that allow targeted management of risk factors and disease.

INTRODUCTION

Exotic pets are animals that are nonnative to a region or nondomesticated.[1] Exotic pets are becoming increasingly popular companion animals, and the global trade in these animals is significantly large[2] as demonstrated in the United States and China. Pet ownership is on the rise in the United States, and there have been significant increases in exotic pets such as backyard poultry and lizards, with more than 13% of US households now owning exotic pets as well.[3] The United States imported nearly 1.5 billion live nondomestic animals between 2000 and 2006, of which 92% were destined for commercial sale as pets.[4] As per the annual report on China's pet market

[a] National Parks Board, Singapore, 1 Cluny Road, Singapore 259569; [b] Conservation, Research and Veterinary Department, Wildlife Reserves Singapore, 80 Mandai Lake Road, Singapore 729826
* Corresponding author.
E-mail address: kelvin_lim@nparks.gov.sg

Vet Clin Exot Anim 24 (2021) 495–507
https://doi.org/10.1016/j.cvex.2021.04.001
1094-9194/21/© 2021 Elsevier Inc. All rights reserved.

published by Goumin (China's largest pet Web site), 36% of 73 million Chinese pet owners keep reptiles and rodents. Nondomestic animal species are generally allowed to be bred or traded, as long as these activities comply with the international regulations, for example, the requirements of the Convention on International Trade in Endangered Species of Wild Fauna and Flora. Animal health requirements are also required to be complied with as laid out in national, regional, and international texts, for example, the World Organization of Animal Health (OIE) Terrestrial Animal Health Code or the Aquatic Animal Health Code. According to Bush and colleagues'[5] study on global trade in exotic pets from 2006 to 2012, birds are the most species-rich and abundant reported in trade, reptiles were the second most abundant, and mammals were the least abundant. There is acknowledgment that exotic animals, similar to dogs and cats, will become an integral part of owners' lives and the human-animal bond can be beneficial.[6]

However, the keeping and trade of exotic pets, including wildlife, have also introduced and produced multiple opportunities for interactions of disease transmission that has had an adverse impact on animal and public health, and threatened biodiversity, and the health of livestock and ecosystems.[7] Furthermore, exotic pets tend to have complex needs relating to their natural diet, environment, and behavior.[8] The clinical veterinarian would need to understand these needs in the process of diagnosis and treatment of the animal. Epidemiology has traditionally been used in the context of public health, food safety, production animal medicine, and companion animal clinical medicine. However, the aspects of epidemiology relating to outbreak investigations, evaluation and interpretation of tests, and study of disease are relevant to the exotic animal practitioner for the reasons stated. The understanding of the principles of veterinary epidemiology and preventive health management would allow the clinical veterinarian to understand how to advise, implement, and evaluate herd health programs and biosecurity measures as well as conduct disease investigations in exotic pet populations.[9]

This article explains the significance and role and of veterinary epidemiology and herd health management, using diseases associated with exotic pets as examples. This article is also written against a backdrop of coronavirus disease 2019 (COVID-19) pandemic when there is growing public awareness of COVID-19 with disease risks associated with wild animals and exotic pets.[10] Although the article will not discuss the ethics, regulations, and policies related to the keeping of exotic pets, the application of veterinary epidemiology and herd health management can minimize the disease risks from and to these exotic animals.

EMERGING AND EXOTIC DISEASE DETECTIONS

There is a role for the exotic animal veterinarian to exercise epidemiologic principles to identify and detect emerging and exotic disease threats. Emerging exotic diseases are transboundary in nature and threaten animal populations, especially if there is an existing susceptible wild population.[11] Rabbit hemorrhagic disease (RHD) was first identified in China in 1984,[12] and it subsequently spread across continents to Europe, Canada, and New Zealand. Veterinarians play a significant role in encouraging owners to allow not only clinical assessments but also where necessary, postmortem and histopathological examination, as part of active investigations into histories of acute to peracute deaths of rabbits in households, all of which form part of the early warning system for RHD.[13] Chytridiomycosis, caused by *Batrachochytrium dendrobatidis* (Bd) is spreading in various parts of the world, including Australia, Central and North America, Europe, and Asia, causing devastating decline in various amphibian populations.[14] The veterinarian, cognizant that this is a possible differential, should not only take a thorough history and perform a dermatologic examination but also evaluate the population of kept amphibians when evaluating any case of amphibian skin disease.[15] Veterinarians would also need to stay abreast of emerging trends such as beekeeping and bee diseases such as foulbrood (*Melissococcus plutonius* and *Paenibacillus larvae*) and go beyond being a prescriber of medications to looking at population health, risk factors, and explore integrated management options when dealing with bee diseases.[16]

In most countries, there are requirements for notifiable disease reporting systems at national and international levels. Notifying the authorities of a disease should not be viewed merely as a legal requirement and bureaucratic exercise, but as an opportunity for veterinarians, versed in epidemiology and herd health management, to be involved in the overall disease investigation process. With the growing trade of animals, including exotic pets, these animals may also pose an increased risk of zoonotic disease infections. Zoonotic diseases are estimated to comprise 75% of emerging infectious diseases,[17] and a significant number are associated with exotic pets or wildlife species.[18] Epidemiologic investigations confirmed that the first community-acquired cases of monkeypox in humans in the United States were from the infected prairie dogs, which had been in contact with imported African rodents.[11] There have also been several instances of human outbreaks of samonellosis associated with hedgehogs in various countries.[19-21]

COMBATING ANTIMICROBIAL RESISTANCE

The veterinarian will face several challenges in determining appropriate antimicrobial treatments for exotic pets, for which guidelines may not be readily available. Yet, household pets are a source of infections of multidrug resistant bacteria such as methicillin-resistant *Staphylococcus aureus* and extended-spectrum beta-lactamase-producing *Escherichia coli*.[22] The application of epidemiology could inform the antimicrobial options and approach to be applied. Proper epidemiologic investigation, together with the clinical diagnosis of bacterial infections, allows the appropriate antibiotic to be used via the appropriate route, dose, and duration for the individual animal or population to minimize the chances of antimicrobial resistance becoming a problem in the long term.[23]

KEY CONCEPTS OF EPIDEMIOLOGY

Veterinary epidemiology is the study of disease in animal populations and the determinants or factors that determine their occurrence and spread.[24] The fundamental tenet of veterinary epidemiology and the importance of herd/flock health is that disease does not occur in isolation in a population but is more likely to follow patterns.[25] Thus, in epidemiology, the focus is on the population, as opposed to the individual. The origin of the word epidemiology refers to the Greek words *epi* meaning on or upon, *demos* meaning people, and *logos* meaning the study of.[24] Although the term epidemiology is used in human populations, epizootiology for the studies in animal populations, and epizootics for outbreaks in animal populations, we would now refer to epidemiology and epidemics for most purposes.[9] Applying epidemiologic principles to traditional clinical practice shifts the paradigm from one focused on treating clinically ill animals to one designed to support group health programs as well as the prevention and control of diseases. The epidemiologic revolution in preventive veterinary medicine perhaps started when the 4 preventive veterinary medical crises in livestock reflected the need for identification and assessment of disease determinants and causal factors.[26] These crises comprise (1) problem herds remaining after lengthy livestock disease management campaigns, (2) demands on authorities to document the burden of disease and disease control, (3) lack of appropriate research or control approaches for prevalent and emerging production diseases of unknown etiologies, and (4) inability of veterinarians and livestock producers to adapt economically and scientifically viable methods to livestock production.[26] The exotic animal veterinarian, arguably, would face similar challenges and would have to be just as involved in the management of husbandry, nutrition, and epidemiology of disease in the population as the livestock veterinarian.

This application of epidemiology in clinical practice, clinical epidemiology, could be defined as the use of epidemiologic methods to questions directly relevant to the practice of medicine in the care of individual animals or at the herd/flock level.[9] Traditional clinical veterinary medicine has been associated with the use of subjective approaches based on experience,[27] whereas clinical epidemiologic approaches and tools would allow veterinarians to apply experiential knowledge, theirs and others', and medical literature to their decision making[9]; this allows the veterinary practitioner to explore population health issues such as frequency/occurrence of disease, disease risk factors, causation or transmission pathways of the disease, and the interpretation of diagnostic tests.[28] Traditional veterinarians may extrapolate from individual-animal diagnosis and medicines, whereas the veterinarian with epidemiologic background can make herd or flock decisions by making comparisons of treatments and nontreatments across populations or subpopulations. The latter group of veterinarians can also determine whether trials are warranted and assess if their patients require interventions at the individual or herd level. Given the generally less scientific literature associated with exotic animal medicine, veterinarians with epidemiologic skills are better placed to differentiate various sources of scientific facts such as those from anecdotal accounts and case studies; this is also part of the foundation of evidence-based medicine, which is to use epidemiologic insights with the application of research, clinical and public health experiences, and findings in clinical practice.[29]

ASSESSING CAUSATION

Disease can be explained using 3 different conceptual models—the deterministic sufficient cause model, the causal-web model with indirect and direct causes, and the probabilistic model of causation.[30] A commonly used model for understanding the multifactorial disease, including infectious and noninfectious ones, is that of the sufficient cause or causal pie model.[31] The sufficient cause model would allow the veterinarian to apply interventions to remove or reduce factors needed to cause the disease.[32] The components of the sufficient cause can be a combination of the factors relating to the triad of the host, agent, or environmental factors.[32] Managing these factors would allow the practitioner to manage disease beyond the traditional clinical management of individual patients. By increasing the disease resistance of the individual and population, the severity and impact of disease can be reduced or ruled out during the hypothesis generation process.[25] Disease control in rabbitries against rabbit hemorrhagic disease virus (RHDV) relies mainly on vaccinations to boost the immunity of rabbits.[33] Standard vaccination protocols for canine distemper and rabies have also been established for ferrets.[34] Pathogens that lack host specificity, such as chytrid disease, which affect amphibians including frogs and newts, would require the veterinarian to consider more intensive control, prevention, and elimination/eradication efforts.[35] Managing and adjusting environmental factors would reduce the likelihood of diseased incursion and establishment. Environmental factors can include feed contamination, overcrowding, and the presence of carriers or vectors of pathogens.[36] For example, investigation of disease patterns in a bird population affected by avian mycobacteriosis revealed that risk factors include history of housing with a bird affected by intestinal tract mycobacterial disease, increased movement among enclosures, history of the bird being imported from outside the existing collection, exposure to mycobacteriosis at a young age, exposure to the same bird species, and exposure within small enclosures.[37,38] The veterinarian could work with the owner to identify these risk factors and allow the owner to make husbandry changes that will avoid or mitigate disease.

BIOSECURITY

Biosecurity is frequently regarded as the foundation of disease and risk factor prevention and control programs.[39] Biosecurity, defined in the OIE Terrestrial Animal Code, refers to "a set of management and physical measures designed to reduce the risk of introduction, establishment and spread of animal diseases, infections or infestations to, from and within an animal population."[40] When dealing with a population of animals, biosecurity is incorporated into daily activities to protect the population. Biosecurity is composed of bioexclusion, biomanagement, and biocontainment.[41] Bioexclusion and biocontainment are frequently associated with external biosecurity to keep pathogens out of the animal population and to avoid the spread of pathogens between these populations, respectively.[39,41] In contrast, biomanagement is associated with internal biosecurity and is focused on limiting the spread of pathogens within the specific animal population.[39,41] The appropriate application of biosecurity measures, together with other preventive measures such as vaccination and good animal husbandry practices, should reduce the need for subsequent treatment. Unfortunately, the Internet age has opened the doors to both legal and illegal online trade of exotic pets that brought challenges to implementing biosecurity measures and controlling disease transmission.[42] It has been hypothesized that chytrid disease was introduced via commercial collectors who had unknowingly been in contact with imported frogs or pet owners who released these animals to the wild as a consequence of disinterest or inability to keep these animals.[43] The veterinarian can inform practical biosecurity steps to ensure that the exotic pets are purchased from known sources, transported hygienically and safely, and quarantined in separate facilities for a designated period of time coupled with close health monitoring and management of these animals.

QUARANTINE/ISOLATION

Quarantine is a specific disease management process that refers to the separation and restriction of individuals possibly exposed to a disease to determine if these individuals will become diseased. Isolation, another disease management tool, refers to the separation of infected or diseased individuals from the healthy population.[44] There have been development and evolution of procedures to prevent the entry of such exotic pathogens for animals and diseases of public health concern. However, these procedures are frequently understudied for exotic animals. There have been detections of exotic bacterial pathogens that highlight the significance of isolation and quarantine, for example, *Edwardsiella tarda* and *Edwardsiella ictaluri* from imported ornamental fish in Australia.[45] Considering the scale of ornamental fish imported into Australia, and the poorly documented disease translocation risks associated with the trade, it has been argued that more aggressive import policies are warranted to meet their appropriate level of protection (ALOP).[46] ALOP is referred to as "the level of protection deemed appropriate by the Member establishing a sanitary or phytosanitary measure to protect human, animal or plant health within its territory."[47] Members of the World Trade Organization can decide their acceptable risk to protect their human, animal, and plant life from relevant hazards.

DISEASE OUTBREAK INVESTIGATION IN EXOTIC PETS

When a veterinarian comes across a case, the immediate goal would be to take active steps to minimize suffering to the animal and improve the health of the animal. Exotic animals likely live in pairs or groups. Thus, one of the immediate goals should also be to take steps to minimize health issues to the rest of the population. Actions can often be taken to resolve the problem even before the specific cause is identified. Descriptive epidemiology can be practiced to answer the questions to who, what, where, and when, addressing the animal, place, and time factors.[9]

Define the Problem: Individual Incident or Population Problem and Who, Where, and When?

An outbreak is defined by the OIE as the occurrence of one or more cases in an epidemiologic unit.[40] An epidemiologic unit is a group of animals that are related epidemiologically, for example, space or time, which allows them to share the same likelihood of exposure to a disease.[40] In the investigation of an outbreak of Newcastle disease in parrots in Michigan, Indiana, Illinois, and Texas, following reports from a pet store owner and veterinarian, epidemiologic investigations led to the conclusion that the outbreak was part of single source of introduction and outbreak, which informed subsequent interventions.[48] Early identification and quick implementation of planned interventions can reduce the duration and severity of an outbreak. At the start of the investigation, the veterinarian will need to determine the problem. As part of the outbreak investigation process, hypothesis generation would be needed as well as case definition and case classification. Case definition is used to actively search for more cases beyond the early cases and the ones that presented themselves, whereas case classifications, for example, suspect, probable, and confirmed, are used to reflect the degree of certainty regarding diagnosis.[24] After developing the case definition and classification, the veterinarian can subsequently determine the extent of the problem in the population and identify possible risk factors.[9] Thus the case definition and classification becomes important early in the outbreak investigation as defined by animal, place, and time to facilitate rapid case detection and reporting. In an outbreak setting, the case definition generally starts as deliberately sensitive to enable case detection but then becomes more specific as data become evident; these data could be as simple as birds within a study population with histopathologic evidence of avian mycobacterial infection[37] to a set of more complicated criteria in the event of a novel or emerging disease. Case definitions can be used in nonoutbreak settings, for example, biosurveillance programs, and generally do not need to adhere to the triangulation purposes of animal, time, and place. An example of use of case definition in a nonoutbreak setting was the publication by the United Kingdom's Animal and Plant Health Agency of a case definition based on the current scientific knowledge of severe acute respiratory syndrome coronavirus 2 (SARS-CoV-2) infection in animals based on whether the animal was a felid, canid, or mustelid, and if it were exhibiting a set of clinical signs, the ruling out of common diagnoses and confirmed contact with a suspect or known human case of COVID-19 within 3 weeks of developing clinical signs.[49]

After it has been assessed that an outbreak has occurred, as part of the descriptive epidemiologic process, the following steps would be to determine WHAT is the problem, WHO is ill and what are the characteristics, WHEN did the affected animals become ill, WHERE are the affected animals located, and HOW MANY are affected.[9,24]

The amount of information that can be extracted varies depending on the exotic animal species and owner, but the clinician should aim to collect as much available information on the diseased animals, including their relevant health information and potential risk factors. It is necessary to determine the spatial impact of the disease through the mapping of the index case and recorded movements using traceback and traceforward processes, to other secondary or tertiary locations. The temporal pattern of the disease can provide clues to the origin of disease, for example, through a histogram of cases per day to demonstrate the epidemic curve[9,24]; this will allow the veterinarian to determine the disease transmission dynamics of the outbreak. At the same time, the veterinarian could infer whether the disease is endemic in the population or if it is an epidemic or sporadic occurrence. In brief, endemic refers to a steady state of usual or constant occurrence of a disease in the population, epidemic refers to a sudden increase in the number of cases of a disease in a population, and sporadic refers to a scenario in which cases occur irregularly and haphazardly.[24]

Hypothesis Generation About Key Determinants

After data are collected, data are organized and summarized to generate hypotheses. This generation of hypotheses is an exploratory data collection about all possible sources of the outbreak and is critical in identifying commonalities among the cases, which will allow the development of a list of possible exposures.[9,24] The development and affirmation of epidemiology to establish causes of health-related events is a topic of frequent discussion and iteration.[50] Investigators could consider Mill's canons to infer causal relationships[51] and refer to Henle-Koch postulates for infectious diseases.[52] With the increase of chronic diseases being a key issue in health management, Hill criteria and Evans criteria follows thereafter with a new set of postulates to address the problems with the Henle-Koch postulates.[52,53] Several rounds of data collection and analyses could be required for complex and unknown herd issues.

IDENTIFYING AND TESTING HYPOTHESES, INCLUDING DISEASE RISK FACTORS

Epidemiologic studies such as cross-sectional, case-control, and cohort studies have been used frequently to identify disease risk factors and test hypotheses in various food and companion animal establishments.[54] These studies can be used in exotic animal medicine as well. These risk factors can be husbandry or management related or environmental in nature and are frequently assessed through these epidemiologic studies and calculating odds ratios or risk ratios and 95% confidence intervals (CIs).[36]

Cross-sectional studies are frequently used to assess the prevalence of a disease, assess the susceptibility of different animals to the disease, and evaluate management practices as risk or protective factors against a disease.[9,25] In a study of serpentovirus infections in captive snakes,[55] the authors found that the infection was more commonly associated in pythons and boas when compared with other snake families such as colubrids. At the same time, divergent serpentoviruses were detected in different snake families and older snakes were more likely to be infected than younger snakes, which suggests the affinity of different serpentoviruses toward snakes of different families and age-related risk of infections.[55] These studies can also provide evidence for public health messaging and assisting the exotic animal practitioner in explaining the need for preventive and veterinary treatments for owners' pets. Kupsch and colleagues[56] reported a disease prevalence of more than 90% of zoonotic dermatophyte Trichophyton benhamiae in symptomatic and asymptomatic guinea pigs from pet shops in Berlin, Germany, of which 9% showed visible tinea symptoms.

Case-control studies are well suited for outbreak events and involve comparison studies between cases (diseased animals) and matched controls (nondiseased animals).[9,25] d-Ovidio and Santoro[57] conducted a case-control study of orodental diseases (ODD) and dermatologic disorders (DD) in pet rabbits. The study provided evidence of a strong association between the 2 diseases, and rabbits diagnosed with ODD were 63 times (odds ratio [OR], 63.75; 95% CI, 23.9–170.2; $P<.0001$) more likely to be diagnosed with DD when compared with rabbits with ODD.[57] In a different case-control study, Pilny and colleagues[58] uncovered 2 significant risk factors for the development of atherosclerosis in pet psittacine birds, which are positive immunohistochemical staining for Chlamydophila psittaci antigens in blood vessels and high plasma cholesterol concentrations; this provides evidence for the veterinarian to make an informed decision on the methods of prevention of atherosclerosis in birds, including reduction in weight and nutritional imbalances.[58]

Cohort studies involve the following of a selected population or group of animals to determine if they present disease. This process is typically costly and time consuming but is useful to calculate incidence[9,25]; it may also provide evidence to rule out risk factors. Huynh and colleagues[59] conducted a retrospective cohort study of gastrointestinal stasis in pet rabbits in an exotic animal referral practice in England over a 5-year period, and they have concluded that there was no sex, seasonal, or breed predisposition to the disease. Such studies have also been useful to study disease associations and human-animal bonds between pet owners and pets. Zirngibl and colleagues[60] analyzed a large German birth cohort study to assess the association between pet ownership in the first year of life and the development of atopic dermatitis during the first and second years of life. The logistic regression model showed that keeping any pets was protective against the development of atopic dermatitis after adjusting for confounders (OR, 0.71; 95% CI, 0.55–0.92). The same study showed that ownership of small furred pets (hamsters, rabbits, and guinea pigs) also showed a borderline protective effect for the first year (OR, 0.37; 95% CI, 0.13–1.01).[60] A cohort study can also be conducted among animal handlers that would allow the practitioner to provide informed recommendations in the handling of exotic pets. During an outbreak of psittacosis in a bird park in Japan, a cohort study was conducted among park staff and students to determine the risk factors for psittacosis infection.[61] The study confirmed that entering the staff building where ill birds were maintained without proper isolation and quarantine measures was associated with an almost 4-fold increase in the risk of psittacosis infection, relative to not entering (relative risk, 3.61; 95% CI, 1.03–12.60).[61]

DIAGNOSTIC TESTING

When it comes to exotic pets, it is tempting to apply various diagnostic tests on a patient because of availability. It is certainly true that "the worst approach to diagnostics is to perform every conceivable test on a patient, in the hope that something will show up."[9] Diagnostics to be used should be fit for purpose, and results should always be interpreted within the context of clinical and epidemiologic information. Understanding the diagnostic tests and their limitations would also aid the clinician in making evidence-based decisions as several diseases can produce antibodies that cross-react for different tests. There are existing enzyme-linked immunosorbent assay tests for RHDV, but antibodies to nonpathogenic rabbit caliciviruses, which are not OIE-notifiable, would cross-react in serologic tests for RHDV.[62] It has also been demonstrated that cross-reactivity occurs between Borrelia burgdorferi (causative agent of Lyme disease) and leptospiral serovars,[63] and clinicians will need to evaluate the clinical picture. Clinicians also need a good understanding of the test characteristics, that is, diagnostic sensitivity, which is the likelihood of a positive test result in diseased patient, and diagnostic specificity, the likelihood of a negative test result in nondiseased patient.[64] Skerratt and colleagues[65] presented the use of quantitative polymerase chain reaction, a more sensitive test method for the screening of amphibians for chytridiomycosis, especially to minimize the risk of disease introduction during translocation events. Histopathology, as a more specific test, is still relevant, especially to confirm the diagnosis because of the risk of contamination of samples.[65] Pooled sampling strategy is attractive to reduce the cost of testing and improve the efficiency of testing. However, the veterinarian should refer to literature as pooled diagnostic sensitivity could be lower than that of individual animal testing. Johnson and colleagues[66] demonstrate that a pooled sampling strategy for megalocytivirus infectious spleen and kidney necrosis virus in ornamental fish is still useful in specific circumstances, for example, when the prevalence is greater than 10% or to use as a screening test to identify populations with high disease prevalence.

HERD/FLOCK HEALTH MANAGEMENT PROGRAM

In production animal medicine, veterinarians work with farmers to use and analyze information from various sources to design herd health prevention, management, and control programs to improve the health of the animals, increase productivity, and maximize profits from the animals.[67] In exotic animal medicine, whereas productivity and economic considerations may not be as critical unless it is a breeding colony, the secondary objectives of improvement of the overall health and welfare of animals are equally crucial. The herd health program would comprise the elements of establishing production and risk reduction targets; developing, using, and interpreting data gathered from various sources; implementing a plan of action; and monitoring and evaluating progress[67]; this would require epidemiologic insights to change the focus from the individual animal to the population.

The 3 requirements of a successful health management program are arguably a progressive animal owner, an animal health and production data and information system, and an enthusiastic and competent veterinarian.[67] The attitude and aptitude of the animal owner to desire and implement a successful health management program would go a long way. Exotic pet owners should be information-oriented people who recognize the need to keep and use animal health and production records and are interested in and recognize that production, nutrition, health management, and veterinary support are interrelated and have many interactions.[67] As part of the management of the herds or flocks of exotic animals, it is important to monitor and have accurate assessments of health and disease at the population level. The assessments should come in the simplest data recording system practicable be it electronic records cage cards, which allow the animal owner and veterinarian to analyze the data quickly and provide early warnings of deviations of performance and health of their animals.[68] The final piece to this would then be the exotic animal practitioner. After developing competence and confidence in clinical skills with exotic pets, they can provide advice to pet owners by integrating preventive health management, biosecurity advice, and disease mitigation to clinical consults.[69] The efforts of these veterinarians would then be directed toward not only the individual case management but also the animal enterprise.

SUMMARY

The management of disease in exotic pets not only requires the veterinarian to have a sound understanding of the disease in the species of concern but also the application of veterinary epidemiology and principles of animal population health to be able to understand the disease situation in the exotic pet population, the risk factors, and how to minimize and prevent the risk of disease incursion and spread. Knowledge of epidemiology and population health would also aid the veterinarian in conducting disease investigations and developing biosecurity plans for the exotic pet enterprise. As each outbreak, exotic animal operations, and management system differs, the attending veterinarian must be able to adapt these principles and knowledge to each specific situation.

DISCLOSURE

The authors have nothing to disclose.

ACKNOWLEDGMENTS

The authors would like to thank Dr Charlene Fernandez from the Animal & Veterinary Service for assisting to review the manuscript. This study is supported by National Parks Board and Wildlife Reserves Singapore.

REFERENCES

1. Warwick C, Steedman C, Jessop M, et al. Exotic pet suitability: Understanding some problems and using a labeling system to aid animal welfare, environment, and consumer protection. J Vet Behav 2018;26:17–26.
2. Smith KM, Smith KF, D'Auria JP. Exotic pets: health and safety issues for children and parents. J Pediatr Heal Care 2012;26(2):e2–6.
3. American Veterinary Medical Association. AVMA pet ownership and demographics sourcebook: 2017-2018 edition. Schaumburg: Am Vet Med Assoc; 2018. p. 247.
4. Smith KF, Behrens M, Schloegel LM, et al. Reducing the risks of the wildlife trade. Science 2009;324(5927):594–5.
5. Bush ER, Baker SE, Macdonald DW. Global trade in exotic pets 2006-2012. Conserv Biol 2014;28(3):663–76.
6. Hess L. Exotic animals: appropriately owned pets or inappropriately kept problems? J Avian Med Surg 2011;25(1):50–6.
7. Karesh WB, Cook RA, Bennett EL, et al. Wildlife trade and global disease emergence. Emerg Infect Dis 2005;11(7):1000–2.
8. Marston HD, Dixon DM, Knisely JM, et al. Antimicrobial resistance. JAMA 2016; 316(11):1193–204.
9. Smith RD. Veterinary clinical epidemiology: from patient to population. Florida: CRC Press; 2019.
10. Loeb J. Covid-19 wake-up call for exotic pet trade. Vet Rec 2020;186:432.
11. Guarner J, Johnson BJ, Paddock CD, et al. Monkeypox transmission and pathogenesis in prairie dogs. Emerg Infect Dis 2004;10(3):426–31.
12. Liu SJ, Xue HP, Pu BQ, et al. A new viral disease in rabbits. Anim Husb Vet Med 1984;16(6):253–5.

13. Harcourt-Brown N, Silkstone M, Whitbread TJ, et al. RHDV2 epidemic in U.K. pet rabbits. Part 1: clinical features, gross post mortem and histopathological findings. J Small Anim Pract 2020;61(7):419–27.
14. Swei A, Rowley JJL, Rödder D, et al. Is chytridiomycosis an emerging infectious disease in Asia? PLoS One 2011;6(8):e23179.
15. Palmeiro BS, Roberts H. Clinical approach to dermatologic disease in exotic animals. Vet Clin Exot Anim Pract 2013;16(3):523–77.
16. Neff EP. Veterinarians meet honey bees in the U.S. Lab Anim (NY) 2019;48(5): 125–6.
17. Taylor LH, Latham SM, Woolhouse ME. Risk factors for human disease emergence. Philos Trans R Soc Lond B Biol Sci 2001;356(1411):983–9.
18. Jones KE, Patel NG, Levy MA, et al. Global trends in emerging infectious diseases. Nature 2008;451(7181):990–3.
19. Handeland K, Refsum T, Johansen BS, et al. Prevalence of Salmonella Typhimurium infection in Norwegian hedgehog populations associated with two human disease outbreaks. Epidemiol Infect 2002;128(3):523–7.
20. Craig C, Styliadis S, Woodward D, et al. African pygmy hedgehog–associated Salmonella tilene in Canada. Can Commun Dis Rep 1997;23(17):129.
21. Centers for Disease Control and Prevention (CDC). African pygmy hedgehog-associated salmonellosis–Washington, 1994. MMWR Morb Mortal Wkly Rep 1995;44(24):462.
22. Damborg P, Broens EM, Chomel BB, et al. Bacterial zoonoses transmitted by household pets: state-of-the-art and future perspectives for targeted research and policy actions. J Comp Pathol 2016;155(Supplement 1):S27–40.
23. Lloyd DH, Page SW. Antimicrobial stewardship in veterinary medicine. In: Schwarz S, Cavaco LM, Shen J, editors. ASM Press; 2018. p. 675–97.
24. Thrusfield M. Veterinary epidemiology. Cambridge, USA: Black Well Science Ltd; 2005. p. 225–8.
25. Dohoo IR, Martin W, Stryhn HE. Veterinary epidemiologic research. Prince Edward Island, Canada: AVC Inc; 2003.
26. Schwabe C. The current epidemiological revolution in veterinary medicine. Part I. Prev Vet Med 1982;1(1):5–15.
27. Grufferman S, Kimm SY. Clinical epidemiology defined. N Engl J Med 1984;311 8: 541–2.
28. Fletcher GS. Clinical epidemiology: the essentials. Philadelphia: Lippincott Williams & Wilkins; 2019.
29. Jenicek M. Epidemiology, evidenced-based medicine, and evidence-based public health. J Epidemiol 1997;7(4):187–97.
30. Martin W. Linking causal concepts, study design, analysis and inference in support of one epidemiology for population health. Prev Vet Med 2008;86(3):270–88.
31. Rothman KJ. Causes. Am J Epidemiol 1976;104(6):587–92.
32. Rothman KJ, Greenland S. Causation and causal inference in epidemiology. Am J Public Health 2005;95(S1):S144–50.
33. Abrantes J, Van Der Loo W, Le Pendu J, et al. Rabbit haemorrhagic disease (RHD) and rabbit haemorrhagic disease virus (RHDV): a review. Vet Res 2012; 43(1):12.
34. Quesenberry KE, de Matos R. Basic approach to veterinary care of ferrets. In: Ferrets, rabbit, and rodents. Elsevier Inc; 2020. p. 13–26.
35. Loeb J. Keeping the U.K.'s newts free from chytrid fungi. Vet Rec 2019;184(12): 366–7.

36. Robertson ID. Disease control, prevention and on-farm biosecurity: the role of veterinary epidemiology. Engineering 2020;6(1):20–5.
37. Witte CL, Hungerford LL, Papendick R, et al. Investigation of factors predicting disease among zoo birds exposed to avian mycobacteriosis. J Am Vet Med Assoc 2010;236(2):211–8.
38. Witte CL, Hungerford LL, Papendick R, et al. Investigation of characteristics and factors associated with avian mycobacteriosis in zoo birds. J Vet Diagn Investig 2008;20(2):186–96.
39. Dewulf J, Immerseel F. General principles of biosecurity in animal production and veterinary medicine. Biosecur Anim Prod Vet Med Princ Pract 2019;63–76.
40. World Organisation for Animal Health (OIE). Terrestrial animal health code. 28th Edition 2019. Available at: https://www.oie.int/standard-setting/terrestrial-code/access-online/. Accessed November 19, 2020.
41. Pudenz CC, Schulz LL, Tonsor GT. Adoption of secure pork supply plan biosecurity by U.S. Swine producers. Front Vet Sci 2019;6:146.
42. Derraik JGB, Phillips S. Online trade poses a threat to biosecurity in New Zealand. Biol Invasions 2010;12(6):1477–80.
43. Waldman B, Van de Wolfshaar KE, Klena JD, et al. Chytridiomycosis in New Zealand frogs. Surveillance 2001;28(3):9–11.
44. Oberholtzer K, Sivitz L, Mack A, et al. Learning from SARS: Preparing for the next disease outbreak: workshop summary. Washington, DC: National Academies Press; 2004.
45. Humphrey JD, Lancaster C, Gudkovs N, et al. Exotic bacterial pathogens Edwardsiella tarda and Edwardsiella ictaluri from imported ornamental fish Betta splendens and Puntius conchonius, respectively: isolation and quarantine significance. Aust Vet J 1986;63(11):369–71.
46. Whittington RJ, Chong R. Global trade in ornamental fish from an Australian perspective: the case for revised import risk analysis and management strategies. Prev Vet Med 2007;81(1–3):92–116.
47. WTO. The WTO agreement on the application of sanitary and phytosanitary measures SPS agreement 1995. Available at: https://www.wto.org/english/tratop_e/sps_e/spsagr_e.htm.
48. Bruning-Fann C, Kaneene J, Heamon J. Investigation of an outbreak of velogenic viscerotropic Newcastle disease in pet birds in Michigan, Indiana, Illinois, and Texas. J Am Vet Med Assoc 1993;201:1709–14.
49. APHA Briefing Note 09/21. SARS-CoV-2 in animals–case definition, testing and international reporting obligations 2020. Available at: apha.defra.gov.uk/documents/ov/Briefing-Note-0921.pdf.
50. Barreto ML. Epidemiologists and causation in an intricate world. Emerg Themes Epidemiol 2005;2(1):3.
51. John ML. A Dictionary of epidemiology. New York: Oxford University Press; 2001.
52. Evans AS. Causation and disease: the Henle-Koch postulates revisited. Yale J Biol Med 1976;49(2):175.
53. Hill AB. The environment and disease: association or causation? J R Soc Med 2015;108(1):32–7.
54. Peeler EJ, Taylor NG. The application of epidemiology in aquatic animal health -opportunities and challenges. Vet Res 2011;42(1):1–15.
55. Hoon-Hanks LL, Ossiboff RJ, Bartolini P, et al. Longitudinal and Cross-Sectional Sampling of Serpentovirus (Nidovirus) Infection in Captive Snakes Reveals High Prevalence, Persistent Infection, and Increased Mortality in Pythons and

Divergent Serpentovirus Infection in Boas and Colubrids. Front Vet Sci 2019; 6:338.

56. Kupsch C, Berlin M, Gräser Y. Dermophytes and guinea pigs: an underestimated danger? Hautarzt 2017;68(10):827.

57. d'Ovidio D, Santoro D. Orodental diseases and dermatological disorders are highly associated in pet rabbits: a case–control study. Vet Dermatol 2013; 24(5):531, e125.

58. Pilny AA, Quesenberry KE, Bartick-Sedrish TE, et al. Evaluation of Chlamydophila psittaci infection and other risk factors for atherosclerosis in pet psittacine birds. J Am Vet Med Assoc 2012;240(12):1474–80.

59. Huynh M, Vilmouth S, Gonzalez MS, et al. Retrospective cohort study of gastro-intestinal stasis in pet rabbits. Vet Rec 2014;175(9):225.

60. Zirngibl A, Franke K, Gehring U, et al. Exposure to pets and atopic dermatitis during the first two years of life. A cohort study. Pediatr Allergy Immunol 2002;13(6): 394–401.

61. Matsui T, Nakashima K, Ohyama T, et al. An outbreak of psittacosis in a bird park in Japan. Epidemiol Infect 2008;136(4):492–5.

62. Liu J, Kerr PJ, Strive T. A sensitive and specific blocking ELISA for the detection of rabbit calicivirus RCV-A1 antibodies. Virol J 2012;9:182.

63. Shin SJ, Chang YF, Jacobson RH, et al. Cross-reactivity between B. burgdorferi and other spirochetes affects specificity of serotests for detection of antibodies to the Lyme disease agent in dogs. Vet Microbiol 1993;36(1–2):161–74.

64. Gardner IA, Hietala S, Boyce WM. Validity of using serological tests for diagnosis of diseases in wild animals. Rev Sci Tech Int Des Epizoot 1996;15(1):323–36.

65. Skerratt LF, Mendez D, McDonald KR, et al. Validation of diagnostic tests in wildlife: the case of chytridiomycosis in wild amphibians. J Herpetol 2011;45(4): 444–50.

66. Johnson SJ, Hick PM, Robinson AP, et al. The impact of pooling samples on surveillance sensitivity for the megalocytivirus Infectious spleen and kidney necrosis virus. Transbound Emerg Dis 2019;66(6):2318–28.

67. Radostits OM. Principles of health management of food-producing animals. Rados OM Herd Heal. 3rd Edition. Philadelphia: WB Saunders Company; 2001.

68. Gidenne T, Savietto D, Goby JP, et al. A referencing system to analyze performances of French organic rabbit farms. Org Agric 2020.

69. da Silva JC, Noordhuizen JPTM, Vagneur M, et al. Veterinary dairy herd health management in Europe Constraints and perspectives. Vet Q 2006;28(1):23–32.

Therapeutics in Herd/Flock Medicine

David J. McLelland, BSc(Vet), BVSc, DVSc, MANZCVS (Zoo Medicine), Dipl ACZM, Dipl ECZM (Zoo Health Management)*,
Jennifer M. McLelland, BVSc (Hons), MVSc (Avian and Wildlife Health), MANZCVS (Avian), MVS (Conservation Medicine)

KEYWORDS

- Therapeutics • Flock treatment • Group treatment • In-feed • In-water
- Pharmacology • Exotic pet

KEY POINTS

- When treatment is indicated for a herd/flock health issue, the relative merits of a group treatment versus individual dosing should be considered.
- Group treatments involve additional variables that influence the pharmacology, and hence the safety and effectiveness, of a medication compared with individual dosing.
- Administration of medication in feed or in water tends to result in lower plasma drug concentrations and should be reserved for highly susceptible pathogens.
- Where evidence is lacking, veterinarians should adopt a science-based approach, drawing on clinical experience and expert opinion, to make informed decisions for their patients.

INTRODUCTION

A range of medications may be indicated for the management of health concerns affecting a group of animals. Medications used for such purposes include antiparasitic, antimicrobial, and antifungal drugs and nutritional supplements.

Broadly, there are 2 approaches for delivering medication to a group of animals:

1. Individual dosing, where the group is considered as a collection of individuals for the purposes of administering medication and doses are delivered directly to those individuals.
2. Group treatment, where the medication for the group as a whole is delivered in a single treatment. In most cases this is achieved by mixing medication in feed or in water. Other routes of administration that may be used for group treatment

The authors have nothing to disclose.
Zoos South Australia, Frome Road, Adelaide, SA 5000, Australia
* Corresponding author.
E-mail address: dmclelland@zoossa.com.au

Vet Clin Exot Anim 24 (2021) 509–520
https://doi.org/10.1016/j.cvex.2021.04.002
1094-9194/21/© 2021 Elsevier Inc. All rights reserved.

include nebulization, spraying or dusting of enclosures/substrates, and immersion/ bath treatments for aquatic species.

Among exotic pets and zoo animals, avian flocks and aquatic species (fish, marine invertebrates, and, in some situations, amphibians) will most commonly be considered for group treatments. In zoo settings, ungulate herds may be administered group treatments, especially to aid in the control of endoparasites. Other mammalian taxa, reptiles, and most amphibians in most exotic pet or zoo settings are generally better suited to individual dosing wherein treatment of a herd/flock is required. Group treatment regimens established for laboratory and production animals may be adaptable to applicable exotic pet or zoo taxa.

Health concerns that are limited to an individual animal within a herd/flock typically do not warrant treatment of the group as a whole. Such cases are appropriately managed by targeting that individual for treatment while maintaining it within the group or by separating the animal from the group to facilitate appropriate care.

Regardless of the taxon requiring treatment in a herd/flock situation, the indication for that treatment, or the medication to be administered, the principles outlined in this article are applicable.

PHARMACOLOGIC CONSIDERATIONS FOR HERD/FLOCK TREATMENTS

There is an expanding body of literature on the pharmacokinetics (PK) and pharmacodynamics (PD) of a wide range of medications, predominantly based on individual dosing, in exotic pets and zoo animals, yet substantial gaps in knowledge remain for many drugs in many species. Where studies have been performed for a given drug or species, variables including age, sex, reproductive status, body condition, and body temperature (especially for ectotherms) are infrequently investigated. PK/PD studies typically use healthy individuals, yet animals affected by treatment-relevant diseases or comorbidities may have clinically significant differences in PK/PD profiles. Hence there is often some degree of uncertainty of the safety and effectiveness of medications administered to individual exotic pets and zoo animals.

The challenge of predicting safety and effectiveness of treatment is only exacerbated with a group treatment approach. The treatment of herds/flocks in feed or water adds multiple additional variables that can influence the PK/PD of the medications being administered. These characteristics of the herd/flock situation may include, but are not limited to, group size and structure, group social dynamics, species diversity, enclosure characteristics, diet and its presentation, type and number of food stations and water sources, the extent to which species derive water from their food or freestanding water, climatic conditions, and variability in health status of individuals. How these variables influence the PK/PD of the drug administered may be inconsistent across individuals within the group.

Studies examining the safety, effectiveness, and/or PK/PD of in-feed and in-water medications have generally been performed under controlled conditions, typically indoors, with low numbers of healthy animals per group. The validity of such studies for field situations that may involve large herd/flock sizes, mixed species, complex naturalistic enclosures, outdoor conditions, and/or unhealthy animals (that may consume less food/water and/or metabolize drug different from healthy individuals) should be critically evaluated.

Administration of antimicrobials in feed generally results in lower plasma drug concentrations than complete doses delivered orally or parenterally to an individual.[1] In-feed medication should be reserved for the treatment of highly susceptible pathogens.[1]

Administering medication in drinking water often results in low plasma concentrations (owing to factors that may include poor acceptance or frequent consumption of small volumes of medicated water) that may be subtherapeutic and, in the case of infectious/parasitic disease, promote drug resistance.[1,2] In-water medication is only recommended when there is an evidence base for therapeutic efficacy.[1] In-water medication can result in significantly different plasma concentrations in different species when administered at the same concentration, even under identical conditions.[2–5] The concentration of in-water medication does not necessarily correlate with plasma drug concentrations. Increasing concentrations of in-water enrofloxacin from 90 to 3000 mg/L administered to African gray parrots (*Psittacus erithacus*) resulted in at most a 2-fold increase in plasma concentration; a reduction in plasma concentrations occurred with higher in-water concentrations due to reduced acceptance and/or altered drinking patterns of the medicated water.[4]

Formularies

Dosing regimens for in-feed and in-water medication, and other routes of delivery applicable to herd/flock treatment, have been published.[6–11] Some formularies report dosages without citations, with the reader reliant on the expert opinion and experience of the investigators. Others do report references for the dosing regimens listed; however, those references may themselves be sources that do not cite the evidence base for the dosage. Some in-feed or in-water protocols are reported based on the safe and/or effective use of the drug in personal experiences and case reports. Relatively few reported dosage regimens are supported by studies investigating the PK/PD, safety, and/or efficacy of medication provided in water or in feed to exotic pets and zoo animals.[12]

THE EVIDENCE BASE FOR HERD AND FLOCK TREATMENTS IN SPECIFIC TAXA

It is beyond the scope of this article to review all studies investigating group treatments for all species applicable to exotic pets and zoo animals. A selection of publications investigating the group treatment of birds and rodents is discussed in the following sections. The provision of appropriate therapy to fish and invertebrates has been comprehensively reviewed.[10,11,13,14]

The studies discussed in this article include many that are commonly referenced in formularies and/or illustrate some of the challenges of in-water and in-feed medications. Most studies reported here have been conducted under controlled conditions, often using healthy animals housed separately or in pairs. Deployment of these protocols in larger groups in less controlled environments may give different results. Unless indicated otherwise, no adverse effects were reported to the medications administered.

Birds

Doxycycline

The compliance, safety, and/or efficacy of doxycycline in water and in feed have been evaluated in a range of avian species under controlled conditions.[5,15–20]

Multiple studies have reported that doxycycline concentrations greater than or equal to 400 mg/L in drinking water are generally required to achieve plasma concentrations likely to be therapeutic for the treatment of *Chlamydia psittaci* or spiral bacteria in psittacines, and 800 mg/L is generally recommended.[5,15] Powers and colleagues[19] reported that plasma concentrations considered therapeutic were achieved in healthy cockatiels (*Nymphicus hollandicus*) with 280 mg/L doxycycline in drinking water over

45 days. Flammer and colleagues[5] reported significant differences in plasma concentrations between multiple psittacine species administered doxycycline 800 mg/L in water under identical conditions, demonstrating the pitfalls of extrapolating dosing protocols across even closely related species. In-water doxycycline 500 mg/L for 45 days maintained therapeutic plasma concentrations and successfully eliminated C psittaci infection in fruit doves (various species) housed in individual cages.[18]

A hulled seed mix coated with sunflower oil and mixed thoroughly with the content of doxycycline capsules to give a concentration of 300 mg doxycycline per kg oiled seed maintained plasma concentrations considered to be therapeutic in healthy budgerigars (Melopsittacus undulatus) when fed exclusively over a 42-day period.[17] Doxycycline 1000 mg/kg mash feed resulted in high plasma concentrations and adverse signs consistent with toxicity within 3 days in healthy cockatiels, whereas 500 mg/kg oiled hulled seed maintained plasma concentrations considered safe and therapeutic.[19] A low-fat pellet diet combined in a cement mixing machine with doxycycline powder (from capsules) suspended in soybean oil at 300 mg/kg feed maintained plasma concentrations considered to be therapeutic when fed exclusively to healthy cockatiels over a 47-day period.[16]

Fluoroquinolones
Broiler chickens were dosed with 10 mg/kg enrofloxacin or 5 mg/kg danofloxacin in drinking water based on daily water consumption rates, giving in-water concentrations of 25 to 36 mg/L and 12 to 18 mg/L, respectively.[21] Plasma concentrations for both drugs after in-water administration were comparable to those after direct oral administration; tissue concentrations were consistently higher than plasma, with enrofloxacin expected to have higher therapeutic efficacy.[21]

Enrofloxacin administered in water at concentrations of 90 to 3000 mg/L to healthy African gray parrots, housed in controlled indoor conditions in pairs, suggested that 190 mg/L gave plasma concentrations effective only against highly susceptible bacteria, with little benefit offered by increasing concentrations and high concentrations (1500–3000 mg/L) associated with adverse effects.[4] A mixed-species group of healthy psittacine birds housed in pairs provided with 200 mg/L in-water enrofloxacin made using an injectable formulation also resulted in plasma concentrations that would be effective only against highly susceptible bacteria.[2]

Plasma concentrations measured in healthy sandhill cranes (Grus canadensis), housed singly or in pairs, provided with 50 mg/L in-water enrofloxacin (based on recommendations for commercial poultry) remained below therapeutic concentrations.[3]

Other antibacterial medications
Ampicillin (2000 mg/L), erythromycin (1000 mg/L), and doxycycline (500 mg/L) in drinking water for 5 days significantly reduced morbidity associated with experimental infection with Streptococcus bovis in individually housed Columba livia; morbidity with in-water enrofloxacin (150 mg/L) and trimethoprim (200 mg/L) was not significantly different from that in nonmedicated controls.[22] These results for in-water erythromycin are in contrast to the findings of Vanhaecke and colleagues[23] who reported that erythromycin in drinking water (1000 mg/L) resulted in barely detectable plasma concentrations after 24 hours in C livia, similar to a previous study in chickens, and concluded that in-water erythromycin was an inappropriate method for treatment.

In-water amoxicillin 1500 mg/L for 5 days to healthy C livia housed individually in controlled conditions gave plasma concentrations greater than the minimum inhibitory concentration (MIC) for S. bovis for several hours at least twice each day following periods of more frequent drinking and significantly reduced morbidity associated with experimental S bovis infection.[24]

Antifungal medications

A commercially available in-water formulation of amphotericin B (at the label dosage of 100 mg/L) suppressed but did not eliminate Macrorhabdus ornithogaster from a group of 16 naturally infected budgerigars, housed together; of 11 birds that stopped shedding with 20 days of treatment, 4 were shedding again 3 weeks later.[25] In a retrospective study, 23 naturally infected budgerigars and cockatiels were treated by owners within their respective variably sized flocks with 100 mg/L in-water amphotericin B for 28 days, resulting in 52% (12 of 23) testing polymerase chain reaction-negative on feces 10 to 14 days posttreatment; in 16 additional cases effectiveness was not improved by concurrent amphotericin B 100 mg/kg by mouth twice a day for the initial 10 days of in-water treatment.[26] Reduced effectiveness of treatment may be attributable to subtherapeutic concentration at the infection site or infection with resistant strains of M. ornithogaster.[25]

Nystatin 3,500,000 IU/L in drinking water for 48 hours and then 2,000,000 IU/L for 28 days successfully controlled an outbreak of M ornithogaster in a large breeding colony of budgerigars; postmortem examination of 3 birds after 15 days had no histologic evidence of infection.[27] However, strain variation in the susceptibility of M ornithogaster to nystatin is likely.[28]

Healthy cockatiels administered fluconazole 100 mg/L in drinking water for 8 days under laboratory conditions gave plasma concentrations with favorable time above MIC and AUC:MIC ratio for strains of Candida albicans.[29]

Itraconazole-medicated seed (200 mg/kg oiled seed) offered to Gouldian finches (Chloebia gouldiae) for 40 to 100 days gave plasma and skin concentrations greater than the levels considered therapeutic with no clinical or histologic evidence of toxicity.[30]

Antiparasitic medications

Metronidazole (200 mg/L) in drinking water for 5 days resolved clinical signs associated with Trichomonas gallinae in a group of canaries (Serinus canaria), although clinical signs returned a month later; individual treatment with metronidazole 20 mg/kg by mouth once daily for 5 days resolved the infection with no recurrence after 30 months.[31] In-water dimetridazole at 400 mg/L for a minimum of 3 days was required to successfully treat experimental infection with T gallinae in C livia housed individually in laboratory conditions; lower concentrations and/or shorter time periods had reduced efficacy.[32]

Clinically healthy finches of mixed species naturally infected with Cochlosoma sp, housed separately in small cages, gave negative results on fecal examinations with in-water metronidazole (40–2000 mg/L) or ronidazole (60 mg/mL) within 24 to 48 hours.[33]

Krautwald-Junghanns and colleagues[34] recommended toltrazuril in drinking water to aid in the control of coccidia in C livia, dosing at 20 mg/kg body weight of toltrazuril, added to the predetermined daily water intake volume for the loft, each day for 2 days; 20 mg/L toltrazuril in drinking water for 3 days was reported to be ineffective.

Sandhill cranes showed no significant adverse effects when fed pellets medicated with clazuril (up to 5.5 mg/kg) or monensin (up to 495 mg/kg) based on recommended dosage regimens in pigeons and poultry.[35] Carpenter and colleagues[36] evaluated the anticoccidial efficacy of amprolium-, clazuril-, and monensin-medicated crumble fed to juvenile sandhill cranes in the face of experimental infection with Eimeria spp

---

Box 1

Relative advantages/disadvantages of herd/flock treatment by individual dosing versus group treatment in food or water

Individual Dosing	Group Treatment (in Food/Water)
Advantages	
Accurate dosing for each individual.	More efficient treatment delivery.
Better oversight of dose delivery success to each individual.	Generally minimal stress associated with drug delivery.
Disadvantages	
More labor intensive in preparation and delivery.	Increased uncertainty of dose delivery success to each individual.
Potential for adverse impacts (eg, stress, trauma) if restraint or separation from the group is required.	Potential for inconsistent dosing between individuals, with the level of variability generally unknown.

Box 2

Considerations for determining the appropriate mode of drug delivery

The following factors should be considered in the determination of the most appropriate mode of drug delivery (group treatment in food or water vs individual animal dosing) on a case-by-case basis.

1. What is the indication for treatment (eg, infectious/parasitic disease, vaccination, nutritional imbalance)?
2. What is the goal of treatment (eg, treatment vs prophylaxis, eradication vs suppression)?
   a Do all individuals require treatment, or only some proportion of the group?
3. What is the evidence base for the safe and effective treatment of the problem?
   a What is the therapeutic index of the medication to be used?
   b How similar is the scenario at hand to the conditions examined in the literature (species, age, flock/herd size and structure, health status, disease severity, climatic conditions, enclosure design, provision of food and water sources, reproductive activity, comorbidities, etc.)
4. What is the likelihood that all individuals will receive the required dose, and what are the implications if a proportion of the group receives an inappropriate dose or no dose (eg, treatment failure, drug overdose, antimicrobial resistance)?
   a Do individuals requiring treatment have reduced appetite/thirst and/or have reduced activity impacting their ability to access medicated food/water?
   b Are there animals of different sizes in the group, and can proportional dosing be facilitated?
   c What is the social structure within the group? How will dominance hierarchies, presence of parent-fed hatchlings, and so forth influence the delivery of safe and effective treatment?
   d Are there multiple species in the enclosure, and do all require treatment to satisfy treatment goals?
      i Are there dietary or other ecological factors that require differing approaches?
      ii Are there differing drug sensitivities between species requiring different dosing strategies or drug selection?
5. What is the likelihood that the client/keeper will administer the treatment and manage the herd/flock in such a way that treatment safety and effectiveness will be optimized?
6. Are there other disease management considerations, such as environmental treatments for some infectious/parasitic diseases? How successfully can these be applied, and what are the implications if they are not?

associated with disseminated visceral coccidiosis; only monensin at 99 mg/kg feed provided protection from disease and was subsequently used successfully as a preventative measure.

Rodents

Despite widespread use of in-water medication in laboratory mice, relatively few studies have formally evaluated efficacy. Marx and colleagues[37] investigated stability in water, consumption of medicated water, and PK of multiple antibiotics commonly used in water for laboratory mice. Enrofloxacin and doxycycline remained stable in water for 1 week, amoxicillin was stable in reverse osmosis but not acidic water, and trimethoprim-sulfamethoxazole had variable stability.[37] Mice consumed similar volumes of medicated and unmedicated water.[37] Plasma concentrations over 7 days in pair-housed mice provided with in-water enrofloxacin (250 mg/L), doxycycline (50 mg/L),

---

Box 3
Considerations for flock/herd drug delivery in food

The following factors should be considered to optimize the safety and effectiveness of flock/herd treatment when delivery in food is considered appropriate (**Box 2**).

Note the potential for in-feed medication strategies to result in lower plasma concentrations that may be subtherapeutic, or to risk toxicity if administered inappropriately.

1. What is the evidence base for safety and effectiveness of the medication when delivered in feed, and how applicable is that evidence base to the situation at hand?
2. What type of food will be used to deliver the medication?
   a Will the animals eat all parts of the food being offered (eg, granivorous parrots that husk seed may incompletely ingest drug distributed over unhusked seed)?
3. How much food will the medication be mixed into?
   a Aim is to use the amount of food that enables each animal to receive the required dose in the amount of food they will eat at that meal.
   b If too much, there is the potential for underdosing, food spoilage, and drug degradation.
   c If too little, there is the potential for overdosing in some individuals and underdosing or missed dosing in others.
4. What available formulation of medication is best suited?
   a Are premixed formulations (eg, medicated pellets, gels) available?
   b Is a liquid (solution, suspension, etc.) or solid (powder, granules, etc.) preferable?
   c What amount of the formulation is required relative to the amount of food to be used?
   d What is the palatability, environmental stability, solubility, and so forth of the medication?
5. How can the medication be most evenly distributed through the food?
   a Is it necessary to extend the dose of drug in some matrix (eg, propylene glycol, vegetable oil), and how will that be added to and mixed with the feed, to facilitate even distribution?
6. How will the medicated feed be presented?
   a How many feed stations are necessary to best ensure that all individuals will have ready access to medicated feed?
   b Are there any factors that could reduce drug availability (eg, ambient temperature, sunlight, wind, or rain; the composition of the food bowl/tray; contamination with organic/inorganic material in the enclosure)
7. How will the medicated feed be provided relative to any other components of the diet?
8. Is there a time of day that best suits consistent intake of the medicated feed?
9. Is there a risk that nontarget animals (eg, pest species) will access and ingest medicated feed, reducing access of the target group?
10. Can drug intake be objectively assessed (eg, observation, weighing food in and out)?

amoxicillin (250 mg/L), or trimethoprim-sulfamethoxazole (800 mg/L) were all well below therapeutic levels questioning the validity of such treatment approaches.[37]

In-water tetracycline (4500 mg/L) and trimethoprim-sulfamethoxazole (130–660 mg/L) for 4 to 6 weeks was unsuccessful in eliminating *Bordetella pseudohinzii* from laboratory mice; in contrast, a cross-foster rederivation technique successfully established a *B pseudohinzii*-free population.[38]

Laboratory mice housed individually were successfully cleared of experimental *Tritrichomonas* sp. and *Tetratrichomonas* sp. with 5 days of in-water metronidazole (2500 mg/L) or tinidazole (2500 mg/L); lower concentrations of both drugs, and dimetridazole (1200–10,000 mg/L), failed to eliminate infections.[39]

Ivermectin 48 mg/L in-water administered to laboratory rats (housed in groups of 5) for 72 hours suppressed fecal shedding of *Syphacia* spp, *Giardia* spp, and *Hymenolepis nana*; based on total water intake it was estimated that rats received approximately 5 mg/kg ivermectin over the 3 days.[40]

GENERAL PRINCIPLES AND CONSIDERATIONS FOR THE USE OF THERAPEUTIC AGENTS IN HERDS AND FLOCKS

- **Box 1** outlines the pros and cons of individual dosing and group treatment.
- **Box 2** outlines considerations for determining the most appropriate treatment approach for a herd/flock.
- **Boxes 3** and **4** outline factors to consider for the optimization of treatment safety and effectiveness in situations in which in-feed or in-water medication, respectively, is determined to be the appropriate treatment option.

Box 4
Considerations for flock/herd drug delivery in water

The following factors should be considered to optimize the safety and effectiveness of flock/herd treatment when delivery in water is considered appropriate (see **Box 2**).

Note the potential for in-water medication strategies to result in low plasma concentrations that may be subtherapeutic.

1. What is the evidence base for safety and effectiveness of the medication when delivered in water, and how applicable is that evidence base to the situation at hand?
2. What volume of water will each individual consume in the relevant time period (eg, over 24 hours)?
   a Will this be influenced by species' ecology, climate, water content of food provided, palatability of medicated water, etc.
3. Is the drug sufficiently soluble in water to ensure even distribution to the required concentration?
4. What is the minimum drug concentration required to ensure adequate dosing?
   a Is the medicated water palatable at the required drug concentration?
5. How will the medicated water be presented?
   a How many watering stations, and what type of delivery system (bowl, dripper, etc.), will be used?
   i Are there any factors that could reduce drug availability (eg, ambient temperature, sunlight, wind or rain, the composition of the water delivery system, contamination with organic/inorganic material)?
6. How much evaporation of medicated water is expected under the prevailing conditions, and to what extent will this affect the concentration of medication?
7. Are there other potential sources of water that animals might preferentially drink from (eg, rainfall, water features)?
8. Can water and drug intake be objectively assessed (eg, volume of water in and out, accounting for evaporation)?

The evidence base for the safety and efficacy of reported treatments, including the validity of that evidence to the clinical scenario at hand, should be considered when deciding on an appropriate treatment strategy. Across veterinary medicine, there is an extensive range of peer-reviewed and non-peer-reviewed sources with evidence of variable quality.[41] Veterinarians should familiarize themselves with study design and research methods to enable critical evaluation of the available literature.[42] Where the evidence base for the treatment of exotic pets and zoo animals is deficient, veterinarians should still adopt a science-based approach, drawing on clinical experience and expert opinion, to make informed decisions for their patients.

ANTIMICROBIAL STEWARDSHIP AND REGULATORY CONSIDERATIONS

Administering antimicrobials as a herd/flock treatment exposes a large number of animals to antimicrobials. In-feed and in-water administration of antimicrobials frequently results in lower plasma concentrations than individual dosing, which may be subtherapeutic.[1] Increased use and inappropriate use of antimicrobials both promote the development of antimicrobial resistance[43] and should be considered in any decision to deliver antimicrobials as a group treatment. Spillage of medicated feed/water, inappropriate disposal of unconsumed medicated feed/water, and consumption of medicated feed/water by nontarget animals including wildlife can also contribute to the development and dispersal of antimicrobial resistance in the environment and should be managed appropriately.[44]

Veterinarians prescribing herd/flock treatments such as in-feed or in-water medication should adhere to relevant legislation and regulations in the jurisdiction in which they are practicing. Many jurisdictions regulate the use of medications in food-producing animals, which may include certain pet and zoo species, to prevent drug

---

Box 5
Flock treatment of airsac mites in Gouldian finches (*Chloebia gouldiae*)

Airsac mite (*S tracheacolum*) was identified clinically and on postmortem examination in a flock of approximately 100 Gouldian finches in a large naturalistic mixed-species aviary. Owing to the challenges of capturing birds in the aviary, in-seed treatment was initiated. Ivermectin 0.8 mg/mL oral liquid was mixed with propylene glycol (total volume 10 mL) and whisked thoroughly into 1 kg seed (the amount fed out each morning) and divided across 5 feed stations. The dose of ivermectin was titrated up from 0.8 to 3.2 mg/kg seed over 4 doses every 10 days to evaluate safety and then continued at 3.2 mg/kg every 7 days for a further 4 doses, with intent to provide a dose of 1 mg/kg per bird. No signs of toxicity were identified. Mortalities associated with airsac mite reduced, although clinical signs persisted.

All Gouldian finches were then captured and moved to holding aviaries for individual dosing with ivermectin 1 mg/kg by mouth every 7 days for 4 doses. Subsequently, airsac mites were not identified clinically or at postmortem for 12 months, but then recurred.

In-seed ivermectin was reinstituted at 1.2 mg/kg seed every 7 days for 4 months with intent to suppress parasitic load and prevent mortality while breeding in the flock was completed. Mortality was controlled, although clinical signs such as beak wiping continued to be observed throughout this period of in-seed treatment. When nest boxes were removed, all birds in the aviary, including Gouldian finches, elegant parrots (*N elegans*), white-winged trillers (*L sueurii*), rufous whistlers (*P rufiventris*), diamond doves (*G cuneata*), and spinifex pigeons (*P plumifera*), were removed from the exhibit to holding aviaries for individual dosing with moxidectin 1 mg/kg by mouth every 7 days for 4 doses. Removing all birds from the aviary for this time also effected the elimination of environmental stages of mites. Two years later, there remained no evidence of airsac mite in the aviary.

residues entering food supply chains. There may be restrictions on how antimicrobials of importance to human and animal health are used in animals, and specific additional conditions for extra-label drug use.[13,44,45] In the United States, the Food and Drug Administration (FDA) strictly regulates the use of in-feed medications, including the Veterinary Feed Directive, which restricts the use of in-feed antimicrobials (https://www.fda.gov/animal-veterinary/resources-you/fda-regulation-medicated-feed). An FDA Policy Guide for the "Extra-label Use of Medicated Feeds for Minor Species" outlines provisions for exotic pet and zoo veterinarians to prescribe such treatments where indicated (https://www.fda.gov/media/71960/download).

CASE STUDY

Box 5 presents a case study that illustrates potential limitations of flock treatments in large complex aviaries.

REFERENCES

1. Flammer K. Antimicrobial drug use in companion birds. In: Giguère S, Prescott JF, Dowling PM, editors. Antimicrobial therapy in veterinary medicine. 5th edition. Ames: John Wiley & Sons; 2013. p. 589–600.
2. Flammer K, Whitt-Smith D. Plasma concentrations of enrofloxacin in psittacine birds offered water medicated with 200 mg/L of the injectable formulation of enrofloxacin. J Avian Med Surg 2002;16:286–90.
3. Bowman MR, Waldoch JA, Pittman JM, et al. Enrofloxacin and ciprofloxacin plasma concentrations in sandhill cranes (*Grus canadensis*) after enrofloxacin administration in drinking water. J Avian Med Surg 2004;18:144–50.
4. Flammer K, Aucoin DP, Whitt DA, et al. Plasma concentrations of enrofloxacin in African grey parrots treated with medicated water. Avian Dis 1990;34:1017–22.
5. Flammer K, Whitt-Smith D, Papich M. Plasma concentrations of doxycycline in selected psittacine birds when administered in water for potential treatment of *Chlamydophila psittaci* infection. J Avian Med Surg 2001;15:276–82.
6. Bailey TA, Apo MM. Pharmaceutical products commonly used in avian medicine. In: Samour J, editor. Avian medicine. St Louis: Elsevier; 2016. p. 637–78.
7. Carpenter JW, Hawkins MG, Barron H. Table of common drugs and approximate doses. In: Speer BL, editor. Current therapy in avian medicine and surgery. St. Louis: Elsevier; 2016. p. 795–824.
8. Carpenter JW, Marion CJ, editors. Exotic animal formulary. 5th edition. St Louis: Elsevier; 2018.
9. Doneley B. Appendix 1: formulary. In: Avian medicine and surgery in practice: companion and aviary birds. 2nd edition. Boca Raton: CRC Press; 2016. p. 425–46.
10. Lewbart GA, editor. Invertebrate medicine. 2nd edition. Ames: John Wiley & Sons; 2012.
11. Noga EJ. Pharmacopoeia. In: Fish disease: diagnosis and treatment. 2nd edition. Ames: John Wiley & Son; 2010. p. 375–420.
12. Weibe VJ, Forsythe LE. Pharmacotherapeutics for non-traditional pets. In: Mealey K, editor. Pharmacotherapeutics for veterinary dispensing. Ames: John Wiley & Sons; 2019. p. 519–42.
13. Karreman GA, Gaunt PS, Endris RG, et al. Therapeutants for fish. In: Smith S, editor. Fish diseases and medicine. Boca Raton: CRC Press; 2019. p. 321–48.
14. Noga EJ. General concepts in therapy. In: Fish disease: diagnosis and treatment. 2nd edition. Ames: John Wiley & Son; 2010. p. 347–74.

15. Evans EE, Wade LL, Flammer K. Administration of doxycycline in drinking water for treatment of spiral bacterial infection in cockatiels. J Am Vet Med Assoc 2008; 232:389–93.
16. Flammer K, Massey JG, Roudybush T, et al. Assessment of plasma concentrations and potential adverse effects of doxycycline in cockatiels (*Nymphicus hollandicus*) fed a medicated pelleted diet. J Avian Med Surg 2013;27:187–93.
17. Flammer K, Trogdon MM, Papich M. Assessment of plasma concentrations of doxycycline in budgerigars fed medicated seed or water. J Am Vet Med Assoc 2003;223:993–8.
18. Padilla LR, Flammer K, Miller RE. Doxycycline-medicated drinking water for treatment of *Chlamydophila psittaci* in exotic doves. J Avian Med Surg 2005;19: 88–91.
19. Powers LV, Flammer K, Papich M. Preliminary investigation of doxycycline plasma concentrations in cockatiels (*Nymphicus hollandicus*) after administration by injection or in water or feed. J Avian Med Surg 2000;14:23–30.
20. Santos MD, Vermeersch H, Remon JP, et al. Administration of doxycycline hydrochloride via drinking water to turkeys under laboratory and field conditions. Poult Sci 1997;76:1342–8.
21. Knoll U, Glünder G, Kietzmann M. Comparative study of the plasma pharmacokinetics and tissue concentrations of danofloxacin and enrofloxacin in broiler chickens. J Vet Pharmacol Ther 1999;22:239–46.
22. De Herdt P, Devriese LA, de Groote B, et al. Antibiotic treatment of *Streptococcus bovis* infections in pigeons. Avian Pathol 1993;22:605–15.
23. Vanhaecke E, De Backer P, Remon JP, et al. Pharmacokinetics and bioavailability of erythromycin in pigeons (*Columba livia*). J Vet Pharmacol Ther 1990;13: 356–60.
24. Soenens J, Vermeersch H, Baert K, et al. Pharmacokinetics and efficacy of amoxycillin in the treatment of an experimental *Streptococcus bovis* infection in racing pigeons (*Columba livia*). Vet J 1998;156:59–65.
25. Baron HR, Stevenson BC, Phalen DN. Inconsistent efficacy of water-soluble amphotericln B for the treatment of *Macrorhabdus ornithogaster* in a budgerigar (*Melopsittacus undulatus*) aviary. Aust Vet J 2020;98:333–7.
26. Poleschinski JM, Straub JU, Schmidt V. Comparison of two treatment modalities and PCR to assess treatment effectiveness in macrorhabdosis. J Avian Med Surg 2019;33:245–50.
27. Kheirandish R, Salehi M. Megabacteriosis in budgerigars: diagnosis and treatment. Comp Clin Pathol 2011;20:501–5.
28. Phalen D. Macrorhabdosis. In: Speer BL, editor. Current therapy in avian medicine and surgery. St. Louis: Elsevier; 2016. p. 78–82.
29. Ratzlaff K, Papich MG, Flammer K. Plasma concentrations of fluconazole after a single oral dose and administration in drinking water in cockatiels (*Nymphicus hollandicus*). J Avian Med Surg 2011;25:23–31.
30. Reiss AE, Badcock NR. Itraconazole levels in serum, skin and feathers of Gouldian finches (*Chloebia gouldiae*) following in-seed medication. In: Proc Am Assoc Zoo Vet. Omaha, NE: American Association of Zoo Veterinarians; 1998. p. 142–3.
31. Zadravec M, Slavec B, Krapež U, et al. Trichomonosis outbreak in a flock of canaries (*Serinus canaria* f. domestica) caused by a finch epidemic strain of *Trichomonas gallinae*. Vet Parasitol 2017;239:90–3.
32. Inghelbrecht S, Vermeersch H, Ronsmans S, et al. Pharmacokinetics and antitrichomonal efficacy of a dimetridazole tablet and water-soluble powder in homing pigeons (*Columba livia*). J Vet Pharmacol Ther 1996;19:62–7.

33. Filippich LJ, O'Donoghue PJ. Cochlosoma infections in finches. Aust Vet J 1997; 75:561–3.
34. Krautwald-Junghanns ME, Zebisch R, Schmidt V. Relevance and treatment of coccidiosis in domestic pigeons (*Columba livia* forma domestica) with particular emphasis on toltrazuril. J Avian Med Surg 2009;23:1–5.
35. Carpenter JW, Novilla MN, Hatfield JS. The safety and physiologic effects of the anticoccidial drugs monensin and clazuril in sandhill cranes (*Grus canadensis*). J Zoo Wildl Med 1992;23:214–21.
36. Carpenter JW, Novilla MN, Hatfield JS. Efficacy of selected coccidiostats in sandhill cranes (*Grus canadensis*) following challenge. J Zoo Wildl Med 2005;36: 391–400.
37. Marx JO, Vudathala D, Murphy L, et al. Antibiotic administration in the drinking water of mice. J Am Assoc Lab Anim Sci 2014;53:301–6.
38. Clark SE, Purcell JE, Bi X, et al. Cross-foster rederivation compared with antibiotic administration in the drinking water to eradicate *Bordetella pseudohinzii*. J Am Assoc Lab Anim Sci 2017;56:47–51.
39. Roach PD, Wallis PM, Olson ME. The use of metronidazole, tinidazole and dimetridazole in eliminating trichomonads from laboratory mice. Lab Anim 1988;22: 361–4.
40. Foletto VR, Vanz F, Gazarini L, et al. Efficacy and security of ivermectin given orally to rats naturally infected with *Syphacia* spp., *Giardia* spp. and *Hymenolepis nana*. Lab Anim 2015;49:196–200.
41. Huntley SJ, Dean RS, Massey A, et al. International evidence-based medicine survey of the veterinary profession: information sources used by veterinarians. PLoS One 2016;11:e0159732.
42. Davidson G. Introduction to veterinary pharmacology. In: Mealey K, editor. Pharmacotherapeutics for veterinary dispensing. Ames: John Wiley & Sons; 2019. p. 1–24.
43. Weese JS, Page SW, Prescott JF. Antimicrobial stewardship in animals. In: Giguère S, Prescott JF, Dowling PM, editors. Antimicrobial therapy in veterinary medicine. 5th edition. Ames: John Wiley & Sons; 2013. p. 117–32.
44. Törneke K, Boland C. Regulation of antimicrobial use in animals. In: Giguère S, Prescott JF, Dowling PM, editors. Antimicrobial therapy in veterinary medicine. 5th edition. Ames: John Wiley & Sons; 2013. p. 443–53.
45. Bermingham E. Regulation of veterinary pharmaceuticals. In: Mealey K, editor. Pharmacotherapeutics for veterinary dispensing. Ames: John Wiley & Sons; 2019. p. 25–42.

Managing the Health of Captive Flocks of Birds

Ellen K. Rasidi, BBiomedSc, BSc (Vet) (Hons), BVSc[a],*, Juan Cornejo, BSc(Bio), PhD[b]

KEYWORDS

- Aviary • Aviculture • Compatibility • Diet • Environment • Husbandry • Hygiene
- Preventive health

KEY POINTS

- The natural history of the species kept in aviaries should be considered to fulfill their environmental, social, nutritional, and behavioral requirements, and to prevent individual or taxonomic incompatibilities.
- Proper avicultural practices, as well as comprehensive hygiene and preventive health programs, are key to manage the health of bird flocks in aviaries.

INTRODUCTION

Sound avicultural knowledge and practices are required to maintain the health of birds in captivity.[1,2] The dietary and husbandry requirements of the flock must be understood and met for captive birds to thrive. In this article we primarily consider single- and mixed-species aviaries whose primary purpose is exhibition and/or education. Usually the intention of these exhibits is to display the collection of species in an environment where they can demonstrate natural behaviors such as social grouping and interaction with their surroundings.[3]

Managing the health of flocks in such aviaries is a multifactorial exercise, with considerable intersection of species compatibility, diet, environment, hygiene, and preventive health programs. Maintenance of a healthy flock is reliant on attention to all 5 areas.[4]

INDIVIDUAL AND SPECIES COMPATIBILITY

When selecting a species for an already established aviary, or designing an exhibit for a particular species, the natural history of the species and its suitability for the space and conditions must be considered.

[a] Veterinarian, Conservation, Research and Veterinary Services, Jurong Bird Park, Wildlife Reserves Singapore, 80 Mandai Lake Road, Singapore 729826, Singapore; [b] Attractions Development, Mandai Park Development Pte. Ltd, 80 Mandai Lake Road, Singapore 729826, Singapore
* Corresponding author.
E-mail address: ellen.rasidi@wrs.com.sg

Vet Clin Exot Anim 24 (2021) 521–530
https://doi.org/10.1016/j.cvex.2021.05.004
1094-9194/21/© 2021 Elsevier Inc. All rights reserved.

vetexotic.theclinics.com

In a single-species aviary, the number and proportion of birds of different sex could be a source of aggression and stress. Noncolonial birds show different levels of territoriality toward their own species, and especially the males during the breeding season may not accept the presence of other males nearby. In most territorial species, groups of a single sex show tolerance with each other as long as there are no members of the opposite sex in the surroundings. This has proved to be a valuable strategy to display flocks of Cracidae males, *Cacatua* sp females, or single-sex Musophagidae. In Psittaciformes and other cavity nesters, the absence of nesting opportunity is usually enough to suppress the breeding activity allowing the coexistence of multiple pairs without aggression. In some colonial species, such as in some Anatidae, a specific ratio of adult sexes is critical to maintain the social dynamics and an imbalance could incite aggression and nest disturbance.

In single-species aviaries, the tolerance of other birds will vary depending on the species as well as the environment in the aviary. The space available, the presence of visual barriers, the perching space, and access to nests and nesting materials are all factors to be considered in the collection plan.

A mixed-species exhibit not only allows birds with preference for different physical niches to cohabit[5,6] but also requires different levels of intraspecific compatibility. If a mixed-species aviary is to be established, or if troubleshooting is required in an established aviary, then the following considerations should be made.

Habitat Compatibility

Species that are from similar climatic and vegetation zones are more likely to thrive when grouped together in mixed-species aviaries.[6] Where the prevailing climate favors one species over another, the favored one is likely to thrive, perhaps at the detriment of the other. For example, in a tropical climate, a mixed aviary of a tropical species and a temperate species may provide an advantage to the former, whereas the climatic constraints (too humid, too hot) may limit the performance of the temperate species, limiting its competence for space, breeding sites, or access to food.[4] The temperate species may, over time, be relatively less robust and more susceptible to disease. A temperate species housed in a tropical climate may also be more naturally susceptible to parasitism by endemic organisms, where a tropical bird species may be more resistant.[7]

Species from particular habitats are best housed together so the right environmental conditions are more easily provided.[5,6] Birds from arid regions may require loose dry substrate in which to dust bathe and tend to not use water bodies if provided. In fact, the provision of water bodies in aviaries housing arid region species may increase the incidence of infection with organisms such as *Mycobacterium* spp., *Pseudomonas*, and *Giardia*, as birds from arid regions may have little natural exposure to these organisms.[4] Conversely, avian species that normally inhabit the ecological niches around water bodies may not be so susceptible to infection with these types of organisms and are likely to require the presence of water bodies to maintain optimal health of plumage and integument.[5] For example, waders and waterbirds often develop plantar pododermatitis lesions if appropriate water bodies and associated substrate are not provided.[8] Species that naturally cohabit may often exhibit complementary social, feeding, and breeding behaviors.[5] The behavior of one species may encourage the behavior of another. For example, psittacines may eat only a scant percentage of the fruit that they drop, providing a varied diet for foraging species below. Buntings, tits, and other passerines found in the same habitat may well have evolved to understand the calls and song of other local species and avoid conflict over food and nesting resources.[9–11]

Resource Compatibility

Species that may compete directly for similar ecological resources may be better housed separately and not together in mixed-species aviaries, unless sufficient resources can be ensured.[12] For example, some passerines such as Sturnidae, and small psittacines such as *Aratinga* sp and *Pyrrhura* sp, may compete directly for nesting sites in small hollows, encouraging interspecific aggression and trauma morbidity and mortality.[13] Special attention should be paid when holding predatory species such as raptors and corvids as the lack of space or insufficient provision of feeding stations may turn them to predate other species or their own.

Seasonal Compatibility

Species that share an ecological and geographic niche are likely to show similar seasonality in breeding and social behaviors; this may mean that territorial aggression and competition for key resources are heightened at similar times of the year, which may reduce compatibility in the aviary. In these cases, close attention must be made to the provision of adequate resources, including nesting materials, shelter from competitors, and access to key feeding items. Temperate species from different hemispheres, with opposed breeding seasons in the wild, may maintain their different seasonality and may be more compatible as breeding may not occur simultaneously.

Behavioral Compatibility

Behavioral characteristics and personality of a species in captivity can be a significant source of distress if overlooked,[14] particularly in aviaries containing more intelligent species such as corvids or psittacines.[9,15] These birds can cause havoc in a mixed-species aviary due to their need for cognitive stimulation and capacity for problem solving.[16] Some individuals may be particularly prone to bullying behavior or interference in food provisions or nesting sites of other birds or have a predilection for destruction of the aviary habitat or structure. The latter behavior may put the individual at risk of ingested foreign bodies or toxicosis, whereas the former behavior may increase aggressive interactions and traumatic injuries in both bully and victim.

Certain species may outcompete others due to a generally more boisterous/bolder nature. In mixed psittacine aviaries this may often be noted. Walkthrough aviaries of mixed lory and lorikeet species are very popular throughout the world, as these birds readily adapt to hand feeding and visitor interaction. However, some of the larger *Chalcopsitta* and *Lorius* species may dominate the available resources and outcompete the smaller, less-robust species.[15]

Nutritional Compatibility

As diet and nutrition play such a significant role in avian individual and flock health, diet compatibility is an important consideration in mixed-species aviaries.[6] Nutritional management can be more closely controlled when species have similar dietary requirements that can be fed similar rations. A common mistake occurs when mixing fruit-eating birds susceptible to hemochromatosis together with insect-eating or carnivore species, providing them access to a diet high in iron.[17]

DIET AND NUTRITION

Nutrition is a vital component in avian health, and therefore close attention must be paid to the diet formulation and composition. In a captive flock environment, it is often challenging to control the type and the amount of the different food items ingested by a given species. It is common that preferred items are monopolized by a particular species or individual or that the diet targeted for one species is ingested by a different one. In both cases the result is the consumption of an unbalanced diet, which may lead to different health concerns and disease states.[18] Different food provision strategies and restricted feeding access need to be considered to avoid this in a mixed-species aviary.

ENVIRONMENT

It is intuitive to assume that maintaining birds in an environment that mimics the native environment as much as possible will be the most beneficial for maintaining health and preventing disease. Temperate species maintained in warm climates or tropical species kept in temperate zones will expend a considerable amount of energy in thermo-regulation and therefore not thrive as well as they might. Hence, not only is species selection important but also temperature modulation may be required depending on the enclosure design.[7]

Photoperiod, Temperature, and Humidity

As there are seasonal variations in nutrition, there are also seasonal cycles of photo-period and ambient temperature, which may contribute to the overall health of the flock.[7,19] An extreme example is the maintenance of Antarctic species of penguins in zoologic collections. The seasonal cycle of these species is governed by the most extreme change in photoperiod, as well as extremely cold temperatures, from 10°C during the endless daylight in summer to −20°C in the endless night of winter. Many penguin species undergo a catastrophic molt during the summer months and undertake all reproductive activities (courtship, egg laying and incubation, and chick feeding) during the same season. Energy demands peak during the summer months, and birds may increase their body mass significantly in the weeks or months leading up to this. Captive king penguins, for example, may increase their bodyweight by 50% in the weeks preceding the molt and become inappetant, staying out of the water and relatively immobile during the process.[20,21] Without the strong environmental anteced-ents of increasing photoperiod and rising temperatures, this seasonal event may become disrupted; weight gain may be insufficient to provide the energy for a full molt, causing the molt to be incomplete. Incomplete molt creates uneven plumage and may reduce the thickness of the subcutaneous fat layer if energy stores are depleted. Downstream effects include reduced thermoregulatory ability and immune function, leaving the bird vulnerable to opportunistic infection. In the authors' institu-tion, it is noted that persistent temperatures greater than the natural environmental range for some species may prevent molt entirely.

A lack of strong seasonal environmental antecedents may have particular impact on colonial breeding species such as flamingos. If molt and reproductive cycles are delayed or interrupted at the individual level, then the colony falls out of sync and the critical mass effect is lost. Overall fertility of the group is reduced and disrupted reproductive cycles may result in a higher incidence of reproductive disease, egg abandonment, and intraspecific conflict. All these associated stressors are likely to in-crease the incidence of disease or contribute to ill thrift.[18,21]

Polar species are of course an extreme example, but all avian species rely on envi-ronmental cues for seasonal events. Tropical species may tend to rely on humidity and precipitation, rather than ambient temperature or photoperiod, to trigger normal sea-sonal behaviors.

In addition to providing cues to normal seasonal behavior, temperature and humid-ity are also known to directly influence health and plumage quality, either in structural or surface integrity in pet birds[22] or in respect to ectoparasitic tolerance. The ecogeographical Gloger rule, in an extremely simplified form, describes the observation that birds in warmer, more humid geographic regions tend to have darker plumage and be exposed to more virulent feather-degrading keratinolytic bacteria than conspecifics inhabiting colder, more arid regions. Birds in colder, drier regions tend to have lighter plumage due to the lower prevalence of such bacteria.[23] Although not every species conforms to this rule, it is worth considering in captive collections that birds from arid climactic regions may show a higher susceptibility to ectoparasites and environmental pathogens, including *Aspergillus*, when maintained in enclosures with higher humidity.[24,25] Conversely, species with native ranges encompassing geographic areas of high humidity, such as most tropical and subtropical psittacine species, may show higher incidence of respiratory disease if the captive environment is too dry. Desiccation of the respiratory epithelium may predispose to sinusitis, airsacculitis, and entry of opportunistic pathogens.[26,27]

Landscaping and Furnishing

Enclosure design and furnishing is one of the most important aspects of the captive management, particularly for collections on exhibition. For the latter, the enclosure needs to fulfill certain esthetic requirements and allow the viewing of the species on display. However, in regard to the health of the captive flock, the esthetic design need not conflict with the needs of the avian species housed within.

Fabregas and colleagues[6] (2012) describe 7 aspects to be evaluated when assessing enclosure suitability for a particular species. The first 2 aspects concern temperature and humidity, as we have previously discussed: that the enclosure conditions allow the occupants to keep their body temperature within the species' specific range and that the occupants have an appropriate supply of water and humidity.[6] When thermal homeostasis and hydration can be maintained with ease, physiologic stressors are reduced and birds are more likely to thrive.

Two aspects of enclosure design are directly related to size, structure, and furnishing of the environment: that there is appropriate space and structural elements to perform each of the species' specific locomotion patterns and that there is appropriate space and furnishings for the occupants to remain in resting position. These environmental aspects directly affect energy expenditure, mobility, and social interactions.[6] The Aves taxonomic class shows a huge variation in species size and natural behavior, and so the space requirements of these species will vary considerably as well.[18] Most flying species will require a significant consideration to 3-dimensional space, depending on the style of flight. Passerines and small psittacines may be able to use an enclosure with greater height than width; larger, heavier birds such as vultures or Anseriformes require significant horizontal space for flight. Flightless land birds may not need much vertical space; highly aquatic Sphenisciformes require large volumes of water in which to swim and feed.[7]

If there is insufficient space for free movement of all birds, energy expenditure of the enclosure occupants is forcibly restricted. The frustration this causes can lead to the development of stereotypic behaviors such as circling or route tracing[28] (whether flying, walking, or swimming), feather destruction of the self or of others, and other repetitive motor or oral behaviors, in an attempt to expend energy in a minimal space.[6,18,29] Stereotypic behavior may not only cause the bird direct physical harm, as in feather or soft tissue mutilation, but allow ingress of opportunistic pathogens. Stereotypic behavior is also associated with elevated levels of stress hormones and increased oxidative damage, reducing the function of the immune system and increasing susceptibility to disease.[29,30] Chronic motor and oral stereotypies may lead to secondary physical abnormalities such as asymmetric muscle development, beak and talon wear, or pododermatitis.[28]

Insufficient or inappropriate space for the particular species or number of birds (overstocking) will also negatively impact social interactions within the group.[6] Without room to avoid each other or to be able to move freely around or away from each other, intraspecific or interspecific conflicts will increase.[31] The result of continued conflict may be the exclusion of some birds from resources such as food and water, leading to increased susceptibility of these birds to disease, or an escalation of aggressive behavior and traumatic injury among the flock.[12,31,32]

The enclosure and furnishings should provide not only shelter but also a sense of security to the occupants.[6] In this sense, the character or personality of the different species should be taken into account, as well as the social structure and natural habitat. Gregarious species adapted to socializing in large flocks in open spaces, like psittacines of the *Cacatua* genus, are unlikely to become stressed or agitated by human observers or the visual stimulus provided by human activity or other zoologic displays.[9,33] Such species are unlikely to suffer the effects of chronic stress from these particular conditions. However, smaller species, those that are nocturnal or those that prefer the shelter of undergrowth, are more likely to exhibit signs of stress if nearby human activity is evident, if aviary mates are boisterous, or if there are insufficient visual barriers in which to shelter.[33,34] Species selection is an important element here, as is the provision of shelter and visual barriers both within the aviary or between the aviary and the human observers or visitors.[5,18]

Both the vegetation and the built environment within the aviary play a role in providing multiple microhabitats within the one enclosure[6]. Provision of multiple microhabitats is particularly important in mixed-species aviaries, where different species use different levels of the 3-dimensional space, where Galliformes may inhabit the undergrowth and brushy areas[5] and passerines may dominate the more elevated areas.[7] It also may have significant impact on breeding success, in the provision of adequate nesting sites, whether these might be individual sites or territories, with visual barriers and measured distance between them, or in a colony arrangement or structure.[16]

Careful consideration of the environment also supports the last aspect of enclosure design and furnishing, which is to house the birds in a suitable social environment. Some species are solitary (most raptor species), but many are social to some degree.[6] Social hierarchies are often visible when birds are at rest or roosting, as in many species those individuals occupying the higher perches may be assumed to hold higher social status, although this is often highly dynamic. The aviary furnishing must provide ample space and perching opportunities for social interactions, conflicts, and resolutions to occur[5] and ensure a variety and range of perching heights to allow for fluidity in social standing; this is also true of the provision of nesting sites—they should be of sufficient number and variety to allow choice and change in the social dynamic, if that is typical of the species.[13] There should be adequate locations throughout the enclosure for birds to congregate in smaller groups or in pairs, for courtship and for bathing and feather care to occur.[7,31]

HYGIENE

It should go without saying that adoption and adherence to the principles of the closed aviary concept, including monitoring and regulation of traffic flow, quarantine of incoming birds, and scrupulous hygiene practices, are an essential part of maintaining a captive flock in good health. In the closed aviary, disease is relatively controlled by limiting the flow of birds, humans, and other materials through designated areas and paths. In this way, disease pathogens are not spread from untested incoming birds to established birds and not spread by humans from one part of a facility to another. A complete closed aviary management system would neither be feasible in an open-to-air-type aviary because the birds inside will be in contact with the wild ones to a lesser or larger extent nor will it be possible to implement in walkthrough aviaries, where visitors pass through and may have direct contact with the birds. High standards of record keeping, operating protocols, and monitoring should be maintained, so that diagnostic testing and intervention can be easily performed if necessary.[1,2,7,25]

Cleanliness of the environment and all equipment used in the maintenance of the flock should be kept to a high standard.[25] Cleaning regimens will vary depending on the size and furnishing of the enclosure and the types and number of species and individuals maintained. However, in all aviaries, leftover food should be disposed of at least daily and food and water bowls cleaned. Fecal material should be removed as much as possible and food and water provided in such a way as to avoid fecal fouling and contamination.[7]

Substrate and enclosure design often determine the extent to which an aviary can be cleaned. An enclosure representing an arid region environment, with sand or gravel substrate, and housing arid region species is likely to harbor less environmental pathogens than a densely planted aviary with deep soil and leaf litter substrate, misting sprays, and housing nectivorous or frugivorous species. However, the principles of the closed aviary and the points on husbandry discussed earlier will still apply in both situations. Areas of the built environment that can be cleaned should be, and temporary or removable items such as nest boxes, feeding platforms, or enrichment items should be regularly removed and disinfected thoroughly before reuse.[7]

As determined by the closed aviary operating protocols, any incoming materials, including food, should be checked for quality, contamination, and spoilage before proper storage and use. Good food hygiene practices should be in place around preparation of food and food storage, to avoid cross-contamination.[1,2,25]

As mentioned previously, disease may find its way into the aviary not via the regulated routes but using pests as vectors. Bird-safe methods of pest control and prevention are an important consideration in any enclosure. Barriers to entry are best, but often pest control needs to extend to the surrounding environment to reduce or eliminate the local population and potential reservoirs of disease. Mosquito control often requires the identification and elimination of potential breeding grounds (stagnant water),[35] and humane traps, nest identification, and elimination can be used to reduce the rodent population. The use of poisons or baits is not recommended in or around aviaries due to the risk of toxin ingestion in nontarget species, both inside and outside the aviary.

PREVENTIVE HEALTH

Good nutrition, husbandry, and management are key to maintaining the health of any captive flock, and it is generally desired to use as little pharmaceutical therapy as possible in usual practice. However, a preventive health program should be in place to monitor disease and to identify potential concerns before they impact the overall health of the flock.[1,2,25,36] Disease screening should be part of the quarantine procedures, particularly if there are specific diseases from which the flock is to be kept free. Testing for certain viral diseases, such as beak and feather disease virus, or Pacheco disease virus, is advised for psittacine flocks. Parasite screening, and treatment if necessary, should be included in quarantine protocols for all incoming birds.[7,36,37]

For ongoing flock monitoring, a pooled fecal sample can be screened at regular intervals for the presence of endoparasitic organisms.[36–38] Low levels of some organisms may be tolerated, and may be beneficial within a flock, whereas others may be less so, depending on the host-pathogen interaction.[16] Flock treatment may be necessary in these instances and the route of entry identified and addressed.[38,39] Regular observation of the individual bird's behavior and feeding habits will provide early warning signs of disease development and of individuals under environmental or behavioral stress. Leg bands for individual bird identification, especially those colors coded to allow identification from a distance, are an invaluable tool for the management of aviary flocks. In large aviaries, trapping cages are a necessary feature to allow the removal of individuals when required for health or management reasons.

Other preventive health or monitoring programs may be more complicated, depending on the aviary size, species kept, specific disease concerns, and risk factors involved.[7]

SUMMARY

When managing the health of flocks in aviaries, extensive knowledge of the natural history of the species kept is key to fulfilling the environmental, social, nutritional and behavioral requirements of the birds, whether in a mixed- or sole-species aviary. Species compatibility with environment, climate, and other co-occupants plays a role as well, as does hygiene, good avicultural management, and veterinary involvement and consultation. In understanding and meeting these requirements, optimal health can be maintained through the reduction or elimination of stressors and the maintenance of normal physiologic function.

CLINICS CARE POINTS

- The avian veterinary clinician is already well-versed in the application of nutrition, hygiene, and preventive health concepts as they pertain to captive companion birds. These principles remain the same in the application to captive collections, although in most cases they will be extended to the flock rather than the individual.
- Individual and species compatibility, as well as the captive environmental conditions, need to be considered in the holistic approach to the health management of captive flocks. The clinician should be prepared to work closely with avicultural colleagues to ensure that all aspects of a species' natural history are considered

DISCLOSURE

The authors have nothing to disclose.

REFERENCES

1. Speer BL. A current view of veterinary flock health management: Developing "growing paiv". Semin Avian Exot Pet Med 2001;10:105–11.
2. Speer BL. Avicultural medical management - an introduction to basic principles of flock medicine and the closed aviary concept. Vet Clin North Am Small Anim Pract 1991;21:1393–404.
3. Hosey G, Melfi V, Pankhurst S. Zoo animals: behaviour, management, and welfare. 2 ed. Oxford, UK: Oxford University Press; 2013.
4. Magno MN. 1 - Housing, environment, and public awareness. In: Samour J, editor. Avian medicine. 3rd edition. Maryland Heights, MO: Mosby; 2016. p. 1–7.

5. Jeggo D, Young HG, Darwent M. The design and construction of the Madagascar teal aviary at Jersey Zoo. Dodo 2001;37:50–9.
6. Fabregas MC, Guillen-Salazar F, Garces-Narro C. Do naturalistic enclosures provide suitable environments for zoo animals? Zoo Biol 2012;31:362–73.
7. Crosta L, Timossi L, Burkle M. Management of zoo and park birds. In: Harrison GJ, Lightfoot TL, editors. Clinical avian Medicine. Palm Beach, FL, USA: Spix Publishing, Inc.; 2011. p. 991–1004.
8. Nielsen AMW, Nielsen SS, King CE, et al. Risk factors for development of foot lesions in captive flamingos (Phoenicopteridae). J Zoo Wildl Med 2012;43:744–9.
9. Sol D, Duncan RP, Blackburn TM, et al. Big brains, enhanced cognition, and response of birds to novel environments. Proc Natl Acad Sci U S A 2005;102: 5460–5.
10. Hansen B, Johannessen L, Slagsvold T. Interspecific cross-fostering of great tits (*Parus major*) by blue tits (*Cyanistes caeruleus*) affects inter- and intraspecific communication. Behaviour 2010;147:413–24.
11. Payne RB. Ecological consequences of song matching: breeding success and intraspecific song mimicry in indigo buntings. Ecology 1982;63:401–11.
12. Valuska AJ, Leighty KA, Ferrie GM, et al. Attempted integration of multiple species of turaco into a mixed-species aviary. Zoo Biol 2013;32:216–21.
13. Brazill-Boast J, Pryke SR, Griffith SC. Nest-site utilisation and niche overlap in two sympatric, cavity-nesting finches. Emu 2010;110:170–7.
14. McDougall PT, Reale D, Sol D, et al. Wildlife conservation and animal temperament: Causes and consequences of evolutionary change for captive, reintroduced, and wild populations. Anim Conserv 2006;9:39–48.
15. Diamond J, Bond AB. A comparative analysis of social play in birds. Behaviour 2003;140:1091–115.
16. Burgess MD, Woolcock D, Hales RB, et al. Captive husbandry and socialization of the red-billed chough (*Pyrrhocorax pyrrhocorax*). Zoo Biol 2012;31:725–35.
17. Sheppard C, Dierenfeld E. Iron storage disease in birds: speculation on etiology and implications for captive husbandry. J Avian Med Surg 2002;16:192–7.
18. Mason GJ. Species differences in responses to captivity: stress, welfare and the comparative method. Trends Ecol Evol 2010;25:713–21.
19. Beebe K, Bentley GE, Hau M. A seasonally breeding tropical bird lacks absolute photorefractoriness in the wild, despite high photoperiodic sensitivity. Funct Ecol 2005;19:505–12.
20. Olsson O. Seasonal effects of timing and reproduction in the King Penguin: a unique breeding cycle. J Avian Biol 1996;27:7–14.
21. Groscolas R, Robin JP. Long-term fasting and re-feeding in penguins. Comp Biochem Physiol A Mol Integr Physiol 2001;128:645–55.
22. Koski MA. Dermatologic diseases in psittacine birds: an investigational approach. Semin Avian Exot Pet Med 2002;11:105–24.
23. Delhey K. A review of Gloger's rule, an ecogeographical rule of colour: definitions, interpretations and evidence. Biol Rev 2019;94:1294–316.
24. Moyer BR, Drown DM, Clayton DH. Low humidity reduces ectoparasite pressure: implications for host life history evolution. Oikos 2002;97:223–8.
25. Black D. Ostrich flock health. Semin Avian Exot Pet Med 2001;10:117–30.
26. Morrisey JK. Diseases of the upper respiratory tract of companion birds. Semin Avian Exot Pet Med 1997;6:195–200.
27. Hillyer EV. Clinical manifestations of respiratory disorders. In: Altman RB, Clubb SL, Dorrenstein GM, et al, editors. Avian medicine and surgery. Philadelphia: Saunders; 1996. p. 394–411.

28. Phillips CJC, Farrugia C, Lin CH, et al. The effect providing space in excess of standards on the behaviour of budgerigars in aviaries. Appl Anim Behav Sci 2018;199:89–93.
29. van Zeeland YRA, Spruit BM, Rodenburg TB, et al. Feather damaging behaviour in parrots: a review with consideration of comparative aspects. Appl Anim Behav Sci 2009;121:75–95.
30. Larcombe SD, Tregaskes CA, Coffey J, et al. Oxidative stress, activity behaviour and body mass in captive parrots. Conservation Physiol 2015;3.
31. Poot H, ter Maat A, Trost L, et al. Behavioural and physiological effects of population density on domesticated Zebra Finches (*Taeniopygia guttata*) held in aviaries. Physiol Behav 2012;105:821–8.
32. Hanselmann R, Hallager S, Murray S, et al. Causes of morbidity and mortality in captive kori bustards (*Ardeotis kori*) in the United States. J Zoo Wildl Med 2013; 44:348–63.
33. Blumstein DT. Developing an evolutionary ecology of fear: how life history and natural history traits affect disturbance tolerance in birds. Anim Behav 2006;71: 389–99.
34. Ellenberg U, Mattern T, Seddon PJ, et al. Physiological and reproductive consequences of human disturbance in Humboldt penguins: The need for species-specific visitor management. Biol Conservation 2006;133:95–106.
35. Le Net R, Provost C, Lalonde C, et al. Whole genome sequencing of an avipox-virus associated with infections in a group of aviary-housed snow buntings (*Plectrophenax nivalis*). J Zoo Wildl Med 2020;50:803–12.
36. Clubb SL. Avicultural Considerations. Semin Avian Exot Pet Med 2000;9:217–20.
37. Papini R, Girivetto M, Marangi M, et al. Endoparasite infections in pet and zoo birds in Italy. ScientificWorldJournal 2012;9.
38. Clyde VL, Patton S. Diagnosis, treatment, and control of common parasites in companion and aviary birds. Semin Avian Exot Pet Med 1996;5:75–84.
39. Delaski KM, Nelson S, Dronen NO, et al. Detection and management of air sac trematodes (*Szidatitrema* species) in captive multispecies avian exhibits. J Avian Med Surg 2015;29:345–53.

Managing Disease Outbreaks in Captive Flocks of Birds

Ellen K. Rasidi, BBiomedSc, BSc(Vet) (Hons), BVSc*,
Shangzhe Xie, BSc/BVMS, MVS (Conservation Medicine), PhD, Dipl ABVP (Avian)

KEYWORDS

- Flock management • Avian diseases • *Escherichia coli* • *Salmonella* typhimurium
- *Plasmodium relictum* • *Erisypelothrix rhusopathiae* • *Chlamydia psittaci*

KEY POINTS

- As the level of veterinary medicine and standard of care for avian patients increases, ante-mortem diagnoses and individualized medication/treatment regimens allow for earlier diagnoses of disease in a flock, as well as better treatment outcomes.
- Isolation of the infected focus from the population at risk is imperative and requires consideration of the disease presentation.
- Once the infected focus is removed, disease containment should be performed within the aviary. This may involve disinfection, removal of substrate or fomites, removal or modification of water bodies, pest control, or repairs to prevent ingress of wildlife. This may also involve restricting movement of birds, humans, and equipment into and out of the aviary.
- Once the isolated and affected birds have been treated and cleared of disease, they can be reintroduced to the main population. Before this occurs, a suitable amount of time should have passed to ensure there are no new cases.

INTRODUCTION

Flock management of diseases traditionally involves using postmortem diagnoses and in-water/in-food medications. However, as the level of veterinary medicine and standard of care for avian patients increase, ante-mortem diagnoses and individualized medication/treatment regimens allow for earlier diagnoses of disease in a flock, as well as better treatment outcomes. These advances will be demonstrated by using examples of disease outbreaks, for example, pathogenic *Escherichia coli* in a large flock of mixed lorikeet species, *Salmonella* Typhimurium in a flock of oriental white-eyes, *Chlamydia psittaci* in Columbiformes birds within a mixed species aviary and

Conservation, Research and Veterinary Services, Jurong Bird Park, Wildlife Reserves Singapore, 80 Mandai Lake Road, Singapore 729826
* Corresponding author.
E-mail address: ellen.rasidi@wrs.com.sg

Vet Clin Exot Anim 24 (2021) 531–545
https://doi.org/10.1016/j.cvex.2021.05.001
1094-9194/21/© 2021 Elsevier Inc. All rights reserved.

Erysipelothrix rhusiopathiae in a mixed colony of penguins. There will also be discussion of epidemiologic principles that can be used to analyze these outbreaks after the events have concluded.

The Closed Aviary Concept and Principles of Avicultural Medicine as they Pertain to Exhibition Collections

A series of publications from 1991 to 2001 laid down basic principles for avian flock medicine and health management targeted at aviculturists and the veterinarians with whom they might consult.[1-5] These publications outlined the concept of the "closed aviary", whereby infectious disease is avoided through a system of strict traffic control in regard to the movement of birds, humans, materials, and equipment. While these publications focused the application of these principles on avicultural facilities (those focused on breeding avian species), the modern avian veterinarian may be called upon to manage avian flock disease outbreaks where some of these principles may not be applicable. With the popularity of large backyard pet bird aviaries, and the consultation of avian veterinarians by the operators of both small and larger collections, it may be more useful to draw experience from the management of flock disease outbreaks in zoologic exhibits.

Table 1 lists some of the original principles discussed by Speer (1991) and modifications to the applicability to pet and exhibit bird flocks.

Principles of Disease Outbreak Investigation

The Office International des Epizooties (OIE) guidelines for the management and investigation of outbreaks of animal disease can be simplified into the following steps,[6] as shown in **Fig. 1**.

As the level of veterinary medicine and standard of care for avian patients increases, antemortem diagnoses and individualized medication/treatment regimens allow for earlier diagnoses of disease in a flock, as well as better treatment outcomes. Routine health checks of a flock based on epidemiologic principles, combined with improved antemortem diagnoses and individualized medication/treatment regimens, will allow for earlier diagnoses of disease in a flock, as well as better treatment outcomes.

Surveillance of pet, exhibition, or collection birds may be part of an established preventive health program and be conducted on a regular or ad hoc/opportunistic basis. The extent and frequency of screening after the initial quarantine period will vary between flocks and aviaries, as outlined in the principles listed in **Table 1**. Diagnostic testing for surveillance purposes should be guided by historical veterinary records and evaluation of the aviary/facility records to identify potential diseases or pathogens of concern. If closed aviary procedures are adhered to, testing for particular conditions will have been performed during the initial quarantine period and the aviary can therefore be considered to be free of these conditions.

In a small number of private aviaries, the number of occupants is small enough that each bird can be given an annual wellness examination, similar to that usually recommended for pet birds.[7] In these cases, and testing may be comprehensive enough to assure complete absence of any diseases of pathogens of concern. However, most collection aviaries will not fall into this subset, and the veterinarian must turn to epidemiologic principles to evaluate the health of the flock as a whole.

Epidemiology is the study of the distribution and determinants of health-related states or events in specified populations, and the application of this study to the control of health problems.[8] In regard to disease surveillance and preventive health management of a captive flock, epidemiologic principles are used to answer the following questions:

Table 1
Speer's original principles of avicultural medical management[2] (left) and the applicability to veterinary management of pet bird and collection/exhibition aviaries

Original Principles	Modified Principles
1. Aviculture is essentially a bird farm; therefore, productivity is the most important measure of the aviculturist's success.	• Very few pet bird flocks exist for the purpose of increasing population numbers for monetary profit, so productivity is not an important reason for owners of these flocks to maintain the birds in the aviaries. • In zoologic institutions, productivity is measured by number of visitors to the institution, which may not have direct correlation with the numbers and species of birds in the exhibit, but rather the overall presentation of the institution.
2. Veterinary service to aviculturists should be tailored to their individual needs and goals.	• This is still applicable, regardless of the type of client. The owner of each flock may have different needs and goals, for example, preferences of certain species within the aviary.
3. The time and cost of any veterinary recommendations must always be justified against the productivity of the aviculturist.	• This is less applicable for pet bird aviaries. The compliance to veterinary recommendations is more associated with the capabilities and willingness of each pet bird aviary owner to follow them.
4. The health of the flock always has priority over the health of an individual bird.	• This is still an important consideration, but some pet bird aviary owners may have preferences for certain individuals and/or species of birds, and may be more willing to go the extra mile for them over other birds in the flock.
5. Culling/euthanasia and replacement of birds are fundamental for improvement of the flock productivity.	• As productivity is not an important factor for pet bird aviaries, improvement of flock productivity is not a priority. However, euthanasia and replacement of birds may still be applicable when some birds in the flock become geriatric or incompatible with others.
6. Stock management protocols are dictated by measurements of productivity.	• Less applicable for pet bird aviaries, but husbandry and management protocols should still be focused on minimizing the chances of introducing pathogens and diseases into the flock.
7. Productivity success is best achieved by focusing on a few taxonomic orders of birds.	• This depends on the preference of each pet bird aviary owner. Some take pride in the number of species within an aviary, and may focus on increasing, rather than decreasing, the number of taxonomic orders.
8. The closed aviary concept provides the best chance for success.	• This is still important and should form the basis of any discussion on disease prevention. However, in zoologic institutions with open walk-through aviaries, there will always be human traffic and potential wild bird interaction.

(continued on next page)

Table 1
(continued)

Original Principles	Modified Principles
9. Prevention is better than cure. 10. Most flock diseases symptoms of management and husbandry issues rather than the primary diagnosis itself. 11. Consultation with specialist and utilization of technology each specialist field has to offer is important. 12. Fulfilment of short-term goals will result in achievement of long-term goals. 13. Avicultural medical management requires a combination of pet bird medicine and avicultural experience.	• These are still applicable.
14. Medications cannot replace good husbandry and management practices.	• This is still applicable, but medications may be required depending on the type of disease involved.
15. Strict client confidentiality is important.	• This is important, but the legal reporting requirements to the authorities for notifiable diseases needs to be adhered to.

- For a particular disease, what is the current prevalence within the population? (and as a follow-up question, is this an acceptable prevalence?)
- How many individuals out of this population need to be sampled (randomly) to rule this disease out in this population?

To assist in these calculations, there are numerous online tools available. The authors prefer FreeCalc, found on the Epitools site managed by Ausvet, and available at https://epitools.ausvet.com.au/freecalctwo. Only a few numbers are required, which can be found either in the scientific literature or in the records maintained by the owner of the aviary or the avian veterinarian.

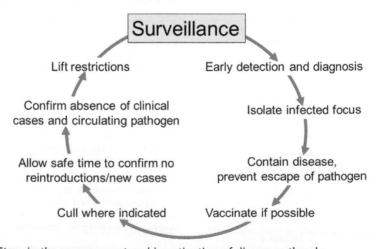

Fig. 1. Steps in the management and investigation of disease outbreaks.

The number of diagnosed cases
- prevalence of the disease 5 the population size
- sensitivity and specificity of the diagnostic test used to confirm the disease (from the literature)

Fig. 2 is an example using a hypothetical scenario.

The use of these methods permits the *early detection and diagnosis of disease* in the flock, particularly in conditions such as mycobacteriosis where incubation periods may be extended.[9,10]

In the event that the prevalence of a particular disease is noted to increase, either through routine surveillance or increased morbidity or mortality, then the clinician proceeds with the investigation of the outbreak. A disease outbreak may also occur of a novel or unknown disease, in which case it is identified by the OIE definition of an outbreak; the occurrence of one or more cases in an epidemiologic unit (such as an aviary or contained flock), or an increase in the number of disease cases over and mora than an "expected" number per given place or time period.[11]

Disease outbreaks may present in the following ways:

- Unknown pathogen affecting a defined population:
  - A common point source exposure may be discovered
- Defined pathogen affecting an unknown population:
  - The best clues for exposure may be the demographic distribution of cases

A group of Nicobar pigeons is kept in a planted aviary on exhibition in a zoological setting. *Mycobacterium avium* ssp. avium was determined as the causative agent in 3 mortalities over the last 12 mon.

•prevalence of the disease $= \dfrac{3}{25} = 0.12$
•sensitivity and specificity of the PCR assay $= 1.0:1.0$
(This test detects mycobacterial DNA with primers specific for the 65-kD heat shock protein gene, using tissue samples, from Tell et al. (2003)[9])

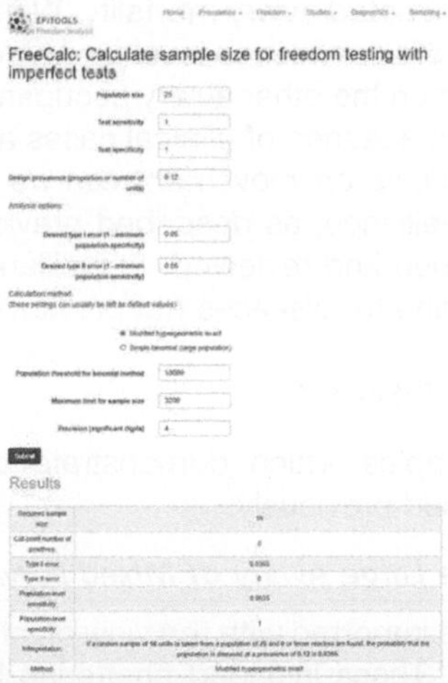

Interpretation: If a random sample of 16 units is taken from a population of 25 and 0 or fewer reactors are found, the probability that the population is diseased at a prevalence of 0.12 is 0.0365.

Therefore, 16 birds will need to be randomly tested to ensure that the prevalence of this disease has not increased.

Fig. 2. The use of a simple online epidemiologic calculator (FreeCalc) in aviary disease surveillance.

- Defined pathogen affecting a known population:
  - Look for the source and subsequent exposures
- Unknown pathogen affecting an unknown population:
  - a cluster of syndromic cases within the same aviary (or throughout multiple aviaries in the same facility), which may or may not be related.[11]

Isolation of the infected focus from the population at risk is imperative and requires consideration of the disease presentation. Isolation of potentially infected birds is considerably easier when the population at risk is known, and particularly when the pathogen is also known. However, in real-world situations, where diagnostic test results may take several days to return, isolation may be required before the pathogen is defined, to prevent further mortality. In most situations, isolation requires the removal of potentially infected birds from the aviary to a separate location (perhaps a separate on-site holding or hospital area), and potentially treatment.

Once the infected focus is removed, *disease containment* should be performed within the aviary. This may involve disinfection, removal of substrate or fomites, removal or modification of water bodies, pest control, or repairs to prevent ingress of wildlife. This may also involve restricting movement of birds, humans, and equipment into and out of the aviary.

Vaccination is rarely used in most avian disease outbreak events in exhibition aviaries,[12,13] although in many cases treatment of affected birds is possible, to avoid culling/euthanasia and enable them to return to the aviary once cleared of the pathogen. However, there are several diseases in which euthanasia is considered necessary, both for the welfare of the individual and the health of the flock; mycobacteriosis[9,14–16] and beak and feather disease virus are examples.[17]

Once the isolated and affected birds have been treated and cleared of disease, they can be reintroduced to the main population. Before this occurs, *a suitable amount of time should have passed to ensure there are no new cases.* The minimum length of time is at least one incubation period from the time of isolation of the last known infected bird, or from the last noted aviary mortality. Waiting for multiples of the incubation period may increase the confidence level for nonrecurrence. Screening or surveillance may be conducted on the other aviary occupants before the affected group being reintroduced. Once an absence of clinical cases and circulating pathogen has been confirmed, the *restrictions on movement can be lifted* and the treated birds returned to the aviary. Surveillance, as described previously, and preventive health programs should be continued and reviewed. Surveillance may be conducted more frequently or include screening for diseases not previously tested.

MANAGEMENT OF SPECIFIC DISEASES

The following are all examples which demonstrate the avicultural and disease response principles discussed previously.

Case 1: E. coli Outbreak in a Large Aviary of Mixed Lory/Lorikeet Species

A mixed group of lories were imported with the view of introduction to a large aviary of mixed lory/lorikeet species. These included chattering lories (*Lorius garrulous*), red lories (*Eos bornea*), rainbow/coconut lorikeets (*Trichoglossus haematodus*), dusky lories (*Pseudeos fuscata*), ornate lorikeets (*Trichoglossus ornatus*), and brown lories (*Chalcopsitta duivenbodei*). After a quarantine period of approximately 60 days, the newly imported lorikeets were introduced into the existing large aviary. They were negative for the standard quarantine tests of *C. psittaci*, *Salmonella*, beak and feather disease virus, avian bornavirus, avian polyomavirus, and Pacheco's disease virus.

Shortly after their introduction, mortalities began to occur in the newly introduced birds. In total, 34 birds died in a 24-day period after introduction.

Detection and diagnosis
The only consistent finding was enteritis of varying severities. *E. coli* was cultured from swabs of intestinal contents postmortem and submitted for further testing of virulence genes, including increased serum survivability (iss), ferric aerobactin receptor (iutA), and novel catecholate siderophore receptor (iroN).[18,19] A few *E. coli* colonies were positive for some of these virulence genes.

Isolation of infected focus
The newly introduced birds were removed from the large aviary, separate according to their species and isolated in a separate aviary building.

Disease containment/treatment
Cloacal swabs were collected from the isolated birds for bacterial culture and sensitivity testing. Treatment was initially attempted using in-water enrofloxacin but was stopped when repeated culture results suggested the pathogen was rapidly developing antibiotic resistance.

Euthanasia where indicated
A large number of the birds were euthanized as they consistently returned cloacal cultures with *E. coli*. This decision was made because of the high risk of mass mortality recurring if these birds were to be reintroduced into the large aviary.

Allow safe time to confirm no new cases
No further morbidities or mortalities were recorded in the aviary after the newly introduced birds were removed.

Confirm absence of clinical cases and circulating pathogen
A small number of the imported birds that returned *E. coli*–negative cloacal cultures were retained for breeding purposes but were housed in a separate aviary and not reintroduced to the existing population. The majority of the imported birds were euthanized to safeguard the existing flock.

Lift restrictions
No birds from the imported group were reintroduced to the aviary.

Clinical notes
- Despite being an important component of the closed aviary concept, quarantine periods and preintroduction testing are not infallible. It is impractical and impossible to test for every possible pathogen of concern, especially to the level of virulence factors in the case of *E. coli*.
- Therefore, risk exists every time new birds are introduced into an aviary. *The more stringent the quarantine requirements, the lower the risk becomes.*
- The health of the existing flock should have priority over the incoming flock. This is because the health status of the existing flock is better known than the incoming flock, and the existing flock has proven to be adapted to the local environment and has a stable host/pathogen relationship.

Case 2: Salmonella Typhimurium Outbreak in a Medium-Sized Aviary of Oriental White Eyes (Zosterops palpebrosus)

Over a period of 30 days, seven oriental white-eye and one red-faced parrotfinch carcass were presented to the authors' clinic from the same aviary. On day 7, an oriental white-eye was presented with nonspecific signs of weakness and lethargy but died 2 days later despite treatment with oral trimethoprim-sulfa, meloxicam and subcutaneous fluids. Pooled fecal samples from the aviary were positive for coccidian oocysts, and the aviary was treated with in-water toltrazuril for two consecutive days.

The first carcass was too autolyzed for postmortem examination, but 6 of the 7 oriental white-eyes showed hepatomegaly and splenomegaly on gross postmortem examination, and the remaining oriental white-eyes showed bacterial hepatitis. *Salmonella* Typhimurium was cultured from organ swabs of 6 of the 7 white-eyes and also from a choanal lesion on the red-faced parrotfinch.

Over the 30-day period of mortalities, several attempts at antibiotic treatment of the aviary were made, using in-water and in-food administration routes. Enrofloxacin (in water), doxycycline (in food), and trimethoprim-sulfamethoxazole (TMS) (in food) were all administered at different times based on the most recent sensitivity results. No mortalities were recorded during the 10-day course of TMS but recurred after the course was completed.

Detection and diagnosis

Salmonella Typhimurium infection was diagnosed on bacteria culture of postmortem intracelomic swabs collected from all oriental white-eye and finch carcasses. However, cloacal swabs from birds that were still alive returned negative *Salmonella* cultures and polymerase chain reactions (PCRs).

Isolation of infected focus

All birds (remaining oriental white-eyes and various finch species) in the affected aviary were removed and housed in the authors' clinic, divided into 3 groups based on visual assessment of hepatomegaly. This was performed by wetting and parting the feathers over the keel. Group 1 contained birds with no signs of hepatomegaly, group 2 birds with mild hepatomegaly, and group 3 consisted of birds with signs of moderate hepatomegaly.

Disease containment/treatment

Groups 1 and 2 were treated with enrofloxacin 20 mg/kg by mouth q24 h for 14 days, based on previous culture and sensitivity results. Visual assessment of hepatomegaly was repeated after the course of treatment and was found to be resolved in all birds in these groups. Group 3 experienced a further mortality 9 days after the commencement of enrofloxacin treatment. Postmortem examination confirmed hepatomegaly, but no *Salmonella* was cultured from the coelomic organ swab. Group 3 was treated with enrofloxacin 20 mg/kg by mouth q24 h for 28 days. Birds with resolved hepatomegaly after 28 days had treatment discontinued, while the remaining two birds continued treatment with enrofloxacin for a further 28 days. Hepatomegaly did not resolve, and treatment was changed to amoxicillin-clavulanate 125 mg/kg by mouth q12 h for 14 days. Personal protective equipment (PPE) was worn by staff to handle the birds during the period of hospitalization because of the zoonotic potential of *Salmonella* Typhimurium.[20,21]

The structure of the aviary was thoroughly disinfected with F10 quaternary ammonium veterinary disinfectant, and the perches, plants, nest boxes, and top layer of soil were removed and replaced anew.

Euthanasia where indicated

Hepatomegaly (as determined by visual assessment) persisted in the remaining two birds despite the change in antibiotics, and they were euthanized because of nonresponse to treatment. Postmortem examination and histopathology revealed underlying iron storage disease in both birds.

Allow safe time to confirm no new cases

Groups 1 and 2 were held in hospital for 15 days (many multiples of the incubation period for salmonellosis) after conclusion of treatment prior to discharge to the aviary.[21] Group 3 birds continued treatment but were discharged at the same time as group 1 and 2. Birds were returned to the aviary 21 days after the last mortality event (death of group 3 bird in hospital).

Confirm absence of clinical cases and circulating pathogen

Posttreatment culture swabs were not performed, as Salmonella was unable to be cultured from live birds before treatment.

Lift restrictions

Birds were discharged to the aviary on completion of treatment and resolution of hepatomegaly. The surviving birds continue to thrive and reproduce in the aviary with no further mortalities from *Salmonella*.

Clinical notes

- Ten birds died during outbreak. Eight out of 24 birds died in the aviary, before hospitalization, and 1 out of 18 birds treated in hospital died, with a further 2 euthanized.
- The odds ratio for surviving in hospital compared with surviving in the aviary during this outbreak of *Salmonella* Typhimurium was 2, that is, a bird was twice as likely to survive this outbreak of *Salmonella* Typhimurium in hospital than in the aviary.
- Therefore, in similar situations, in-hospital treatment should be preferred as the outcome of treatment is more likely to be successful because of the possibility of individualized medication regimens compared with a shotgun approach using in-water or in-food medications.
- Despite the availability of diagnostic tests, for example, bacteria culture and PCR, the most useful assessment tool in this case was a good physical examination, including direct visual examination of the celom for hepatomegaly.

Case 3: C. psittaci Outbreak Affecting Columbiformes Birds in a Large Aviary of Mixed Species

Over a period of 51 days, multiple Columbiformes birds from a large mixed species aviary presented to the authors' clinic, either sudden deaths, or obtunded and dying shortly after presentation.

Patient #1: Male tambourine dove (*Turtur tympanistria*) carcass. Postmortem showed emaciation, coelomic hematomas, hepatomegaly, necrotizing hepatitis, and bacterial interstitial nephritis.

Patient #2: Tambourine dove presented with generalized nonspecific signs and died overnight despite treatment with amoxicillin-clavulanate, meloxicam, and subcutaneous fluids. Postmortem showed hepatomegaly and coelomic hematoma.

Patient #3: Blue-spotted wood dove (*Turtur afer*) presented with weakness and lethargy and died despite treatment with ceftiofur and subcutaneous fluids. Postmortem showed hepatomegaly, cranial hematoma, and endoparasitism. Histopathology showed renal trematodes, hepatitis, and ventriculitis.

Patient #4: Blue-spotted wood dove presented with weakness and lethargy and died despite supportive care with subcutaneous fluids. Postmortem showed emaciation and mild thickening of the right air sac. Histopathology showed bacterial infection of the heart, lungs, kidneys, and the liver. On the same day, a crestless fireback pheasant (*Lophura erythrophthalma*) carcass from the same aviary was presented. Postmortem showed severe lymphoplasmacytic enteritis.

Patient #5: Female blue-spotted wood dove carcass was presented. Postmortem showed salpingitis, chlolangiohepatitis, and renal trematodes.

Patient #6: Malagasy turtle dove (*Nesoenas picturatus*) chick carcass was presented. Postmortem showed lung congestion, but no evidence of *Chlamydia sp.* noted.

Patient #7: Tambourine dove carcass was presented. Postmortem showed splenomegaly with organisms suspicious of *C sp.* observed on histopathology.

Patient #8: Blue-spotted wood dove presented with weakness and lethargy, and died despite treatment. No macroscopic lesions were noted postmortem.

Patient #9: Blue-spotted wood dove carcass was presented.

Detection and diagnosis

Samples from patient #7 were tested and positive for *C. psittaci* on PCR which led to the retesting of patients #1 to 6, which were all found to be positive for *C. psittaci* on PCR. Patient #8 and #9 were tested at the time of PM and were PCR positive. *C. psittaci* PCR was performed on pooled coelomic organs of affected birds,[22,23] and only the Columbiformes birds in the aviary returned positive results. Multisite (conjunctiva, choana, cloaca) swabs from unaffected birds were also collected for the PCR, and only a few Columbiformes birds returned positive tests. Representative Galliformes, Anseriformes, Psittaciformes, and Passeriformes birds all tested negative.

Isolation of infected focus

Owing to the size of the aviary population, and the significant proportion of Columbiformes birds, the at-risk population was determined to be the majority of the aviary. The aviary was therefore isolated as a single unit and traffic restrictions used to maintain isolation.

Disease containment/treatment

The entire aviary was treated with in-water doxycycline by adding the medication to all available water sources in the aviary for 56 days. This required the pond in the aviary to be drained, as the volume of water in the pond was too large to be medicated. Relevant government bodies were notified of the disease because of the zoonotic potential,[24,25] and PPE measures were put in place for staff.

Euthanasia where indicated

No euthanasia was performed or deemed necessary in this case.

Allow safe time to confirm no new cases

There were no further morbidities or mortalities after doxycycline treatment was started.

Confirm absence of clinical cases and circulating pathogen

Ten days after the conclusion of doxycycline treatment, a representative sample of the population (20% of all birds, representing all taxonomic orders within the population) were tested (multisite swabs for PCR). No birds returned positive tests after 8 weeks of in-water doxycycline treatment.

Restrictions

Traffic restrictions were lifted from the aviary after posttreatment test results were returned.

Clinical notes

- The genotype of the *C. psittaci* involved in this outbreak was not determined, but as only Columbiformes birds were affected, it is more likely genotype B.[22,23,26] The zoonotic potential was recognized, but as human infections are usually associated with genotype A,[24,27] a decision was made to not close the aviary down completely. Additional biosecurity measures, such as increased reminders for visitors to use the provided hand sanitizer and hand washing stations after visiting the aviary, were introduced. There was no reported zoonotic spread of the disease throughout the outbreak.

- The source of the pathogen was never identified, but there were no birds added to the aviary in at least 12 months preceding the outbreak. The keepers taking care of the birds in this aviary were also dedicated to this aviary and did not work in other parts of the park. However, as it was an open aviary covered by mesh all around, it was possible that droppings from wild birds could enter the aviary. This was considered a more likely source than human or fomites transferring the pathogen into the aviary.

- The pathogen took 33 days to be diagnosed. This was longer than for the *Salmonella* Typhimurium outbreak described in case 2 because this aviary was much larger than that of the oriental white-eyes, with a larger number of species and taxonomic orders within it. This meant that the baseline mortality rate was higher than the aviary in case 2, and the initial mortality rate of 1 every 7 to 10 days did not raise immediate alarm bells. *C. psittaci* was also not a pathogen that could be diagnosed on a routine bacteria culture, and the additional test was not considered until classical histopathological lesions were seen at postmortem examination of patient #7. Further testing should be considered early on during increases in mortality rates, even if noninfectious causes of death are considered more likely initially.

Case 4: *Erysipelas rhusiopathiae* Outbreak in an Exhibit of Mixed Penguin Species

A mixed colony of 25 Humboldt penguins (*Spheniscus humboldti*), 18 king penguins (*Aptenodytes patagonicus*), 2 Macaroni penguins (*Eudyptes chrysolophus*), and 1 rockhopper penguin (*Eudyptes chrysocome*) were moved out of their exhibit into temporary holding facilities for a period of 5 weeks, while the exhibit underwent renovations. Terbinafine 15 mg/kg by mouth q24 h was administered for prophylactic treatment against aspergillosis throughout this period of stress, but the holding period was otherwise uneventful. The birds were moved back to their exhibit once renovations were complete, but 1 week later, 5 Humboldt penguins (patients #1 - #5) started displaying nonspecific signs of illness, including lethargy, inappetence, and regurgitation. Treatment with enrofloxacin 10 mg/kg by mouth q24 h day was commenced, but there was no clinical improvement after 5 days.

Patient #1 died on day 5, and gross postmortem examination revealed multifocal white nodules throughout the liver, purulent material surrounding the left lung and a grossly enlarged right testicle, later confirmed to be a seminoma. Liver swab was taken for culture.

Patient #2 died on day 11, and postmortem examination also showed similar multifocal white nodules throughout the liver. Liver swab was taken for culture.

Patient #6, a previously healthy Humboldt penguin died suddenly without showing any clinical signs, and similar multifocal white nodules throughout the liver were noted on postmortem examination. Liver swab was taken for culture.[28]

Detection and diagnosis

A full physical examination, hematology, and serum biochemistry tests were performed initially on the clinically sick Humboldt penguins (patients #1-#5), and repeated 3 days later when no clinical improvement was observed. Swabs from the livers of all three deceased patients grew *E rhusiopathiae*.

Water samples were collected from the pools within the exhibit and swabs were collected from selected areas inside the exhibit. Cloacal swabs were collected from 5 Atlantic puffins (*Fratercula arctica*) and 1 silver gull (*Chroicocephalus novaehollandiae*) that were in the adjacent exhibit sharing the same water system. Swabs of the slime on the fish that were fed to the penguins were collected. Only the water samples collected grew *E. rhusiopathiae*.

Isolation of infected focus. As *E. rhusiopathiae* is a known environmental pathogen and water contaminant, on day 13, all penguins were moved out of the exhibit back into temporary holding facilities while disease investigation continued.

Disease containment/treatment. Starting on day 5, patients #2-#5 were treated with amoxicillin/clavulanic acid 125 mg/kg by mouth q12 h, enrofloxacin 10 mg/kg by mouth q24 h, itraconazole 8.5 mg/kg by mouth q12 h, and silymarin 10 mg/kg by mouth q24 h for 10 days. The addition of amoxicillin/clavulanic acid was based on culture and sensitivity results. Despite the new treatment regime, patient #2 died on day 11.

The clinical signs in patients #3-#5 resolved by the end of the 10-day course of medications. During this time, it was discovered that the temperature of the water in the pool had increased to 29 °C because of a fault in the water circulating system. This fault was rectified on day 46, which brought the water temperature down to 13°C before the penguins were reintroduced to the exhibit.[28]

Euthanasia where indicated. No euthanasia was performed or deemed necessary in this case.

Allow safe time to confirm no new cases. The significance of the fault in the water circulating system was unknown, but there were no further Humboldt penguin deaths due to *E. rhusiopathiae* after it was corrected. The water temperature continued decreasing, before reaching the lowest point of 9 °C. Further water samples collected after the temperature was decreased did not culture *E. rhusiopathiae*.

Confirm absence of clinical cases and circulating pathogen. Water samples collected after the temperature was decreased did not culture *E. rhusiopathiae*.

Lift restrictions. Penguins were reintroduced to the exhibit on day 53. However, on day 58, patient #7, a previously healthy Humboldt penguin had a seizure and passed away despite treatment. Necropsy of this Humboldt penguin revealed renal adenocarcinoma and a single focal white nodule on the liver. A swab from the liver grew *E. rhusiopathiae*.[28]

Clinical notes

- Four Humboldt penguins died, while two Humboldt penguins displaying clinical signs of illness recovered with treatment. The remaining colony did not display

---

Box 1
Actions taken in managing disease outbreak in an aviary.

Dealing with Aviary Disease Outbreak

- *Detection and diagnosis:* An outbreak is noted. A diagnosis may or may not be known.

- *Isolate infected focus:* Remove the species, demographics, or other groups that appear to be at risk and isolate or hospitalize. Sort these birds into subgroups to allow targeted testing and treatment.

- *Contain the disease and treat:* Prescribe appropriate treatment for each group, based on diagnostic testing. Some groups may require different drugs, routes of administration, or supportive care based on severity of disease or clinical signs, species physiology, or susceptibility or age.

- *Euthanasia:* Birds that do not show clinical improvement, deteriorate despite treatment, or return repeated positive tests for the pathogen (and may be carriers or potential reservoirs for future outbreaks) may be euthanized to protect the rest of the flock.

- *Allow a safe amount of time to pass, confirm absence of further cases or pathogen:* Once affected birds have been treated and resolved cases are confirmed through posttreatment testing, wait several incubation periods to ensure there are no further new cases.

- *Lift restrictions:* traffic restrictions on the aviary can be lifted and the birds returned. Surveillance should continue as part of the preventive health program.

---

any signs of illness throughout the outbreak. During the time of elevated water temperatures, the Humboldt penguins were the only species that continued to swim in the pool, which is most likely why they were the only species affected.

- The primary source of *E. rhusiopathiae* was not determined. It was hypothesized that the conspecific species or the fish could have been the source of the pathogen, but swabs collected from them were negative on *E. rhusiopathiae* culture. Nevertheless, the cause of the outbreak was most likely due to the elevated water temperatures that created ideal conditions for the proliferation of *E. rhusiopathiae*, and decreasing the water temperature was the key to curbing the outbreak. The penguin exhibit water parameters and temperature are now closely monitored, with water samples tested for *E. rhusiopathiae* once a month.[28]

- Environmental surveillance, as well as disease surveillance within the birds themselves, may be necessary for early detection and diagnosis of disease in an aviary or exhibition flock.

SUMMARY

Each response to avian disease outbreak will be different because of factors including the characteristics of the aviary, the species and the number of birds at risk, the type of pathogen, and its zoonotic potential. However, overall morbidities and mortalities may be reduced by implementation of a surveillance or preventive health program based on epidemiologic principles, and ongoing avicultural management of the aviary following the closed aviary concept. Response to outbreaks is steered by simplified international guidelines, which can be modified or adapted to the situation but outline the way in which the disease investigation will be conducted. **Box 1** describes in practical terms, what this may look like for the avian practitioner.

From the examples discussed, in the authors' experience it appears that the key to minimizing the impact of any disease outbreak is early diagnosis, assisted by regular disease surveillance, and early formulation of an action plan. This requires the close cooperation and coordination of a team of experts including avian veterinarians, pathologists, aviculturists, and caregivers.

CLINICS CARE POINTS

- Most collection aviary populations are too large to allow for examination of each individual bird, and the veterinarian must turn to epidemiologic principles to evaluate the health of the flock as a whole.

- If closed aviary procedures are adhered to, testing for particular conditions will have been performed during the initial quarantine period, and the aviary can therefore be considered to be free of these conditions.

- Despite being an important component of the closed aviary concept, quarantine periods and preintroduction testing are not infallible. It is impractical and impossible to test for every possible pathogen of concern.

- Despite the availability of diagnostic tests, for example, bacteria culture and PCR, the most useful assessment tool in some cases can be a good, thorough physical examination.

- Environmental surveillance, as well as disease surveillance within the birds themselves, may be necessary for early detection and diagnosis of disease in an aviary or exhibition flock.

DISCLOSURE

The authors have nothing to disclose.

REFERENCES

1. Echols MS, Speer BL. Management of avian flock emergencies. Veterinary Clin North Am Exot Anim Pract 1998;1:59–75.
2. Speer BL. Avicultural medical management - an introduction to basic principles of flock medicine and the closed aviary concept. Vet Clin North Am Small Anim Pract 1991;21:1393–404.
3. Speer BL. A current view of veterinary flock health management: Developing "growing pains. Semin Avian Exot Pet Med 2001;10:105–11.
4. Clubb SL. Avicultural Considerations. Semin Avian Exot Pet Med 2000;9:217–20.
5. Black D. Ostrich Flock Health. Semin Avian Exot Pet Med 2001;10:117–30.
6. Brückner GK. Managing outbreaks, . OIE Global Conference on Wildlife: animal health and Biodiversity - Preparing for the future. Paris: France; 2011. p. 30.
7. Welle KR. Maximizing Avian Wellness Examinations. J Exot Pet Med 2011;20: 86–97.
8. Porta M, Greenland S, Last JM. A dictionary of epidemiology. 4 ed. New York, NY, USA: Oxford University Press; 2008.
9. Tell LA, Woods L, Cromie RL. Mycobacteriosis in birds. Rev Sci Tech Off Int Epizoot 2001;20:180–203.
10. Witte CL, Hungerford LL, Papendick R, et al. Investigation of characteristics and factors associated with avian mycobacteriosis in zoo birds. J Vet Diagn Invest 2008;20:186–96.
11. Abila RC, Cocks PC, Stevenson M, et al. A Field Manual for Animal Disease Outbreak Investigation and Management In: Asia OS-RRfS-E, ed. Paris, France: world Organisation for animal health, 2018.
12. Jazayeri SD, Poh CL. Recent advances in delivery of veterinary DNA vaccines against avian pathogens. Vet Res 2019;50:13.

13. Meunier M, Chemaly M, Dory D. DNA vaccination of poultry: The current status in 2015. Vaccine 2016;34:202–11.
14. Tell LA, Foley J, Needham ML, et al. Diagnosis of avian mycobacteriosis: Comparison of culture, acid-fast stains, and polymerase chain reaction for the identification of Mycobacterium avium in experimentally inoculated Japanese quail (Coturnix coturnix japonica). Avian Dis 2003;47:444–52.
15. Kul O, Tunca R, Haziroglu R, et al. An outbreak of avian tuberculosis in peafowl (Pavo cristatus) and pheasants (Phasianus colchicus) in a zoological aviary in Turkey. Vet Med 2005;50:446–50.
16. Andre JP. Cage and aviary birds tuberculosis. Revue De Medecine Veterinaire 1996;147:907–12.
17. Raidal SR, Sarker S, Peters A. Review of psittacine beak and feather disease and its effect on Australian endangered species. Aust Vet J 2015;93:466–70.
18. Sen K, Shepherd V, Berglund T, et al. American Crows as Carriers of Extra Intestinal Pathogenic E. coli and Avian Pathogenic-Like E. coli and Their Potential Impact on a Constructed Wetland. Microorganisms 2020;8:17.
19. Ikuta N, Sobral FDS, Lehmann FKM, et al. Taqman Real-Time PCR Assays for Rapid Detection of Avian Pathogenic Escherichia coli Isolates. Avian Dis 2014; 58:628–31.
20. Dar MA, Ahmad SM, Bhat SA, et al. Salmonella typhimurium in poultry: a review. Worlds Poult Sci J 2017;73:345–54.
21. Jajere SM. A review of Salmonella enterica with particular focus on the pathogenicity and virulence factors, host specificity and antimicrobial resistance including multidrug resistance. Vet World 2019;12:504–21.
22. Geens T, Dewitte A, Boon N, et al. Development of a Chlamydophila psittaci species-specific and genotype-specific real-time PCR. Vet Res 2005;36:787–97.
23. Sachse K, Vretou E, Livingstone M, et al. Recent developments in the laboratory diagnosis of chlamydial infections. Vet Microbiol 2009;135:2–21.
24. Gaede W, Reckling KF, Dresenkamp B, et al. Chlamydophila psittaci infections in humans during an outbreak of psittacosis from poultry in Germany. Zoonoses and Public Health 2008;55:184–8.
25. Vanrompay D, Harkinezhad T, van de Walle M, et al. Chlamydophila psittaci transmission from pet birds to humans. Emerg Infect Dis 2007;13:1108–10.
26. Vanrompay D, Butaye P, Sayada C, et al. Characterization of avian Chlamydia psittaci strains using omp1 restriction mapping and serovar-specific monoclonal antibodies. Res Microbiol 1997;148:327–33.
27. Vanrompay D, Harkinezhad T, Van de Walle M, et al. Chlamydophila psittaci transmission from pet birds to humans. Emerg Infect Dis 2007;13:1108.
28. Xie S, Hsu CD, Tan BZY, et al. Erysipelothrix Septicaemia and Hepatitis in a Colony of Humboldt Penguins (Spheniscus humboldti). J Comp Pathol 2019; 172:5–10.

Managing the Health of Captive Herds of Exotic Companion Mammals

Kim Le, BSc, BVSc, MVS, DABVP (Exotic Companion Mammal)[a],*,
Joanne Sheen, BVMS, CertZooMed, DABVP (Exotic Companion Mammal)[b]

KEYWORDS

- Nutrition • Husbandry • Ethology • Rabbit • Ferret • Guinea pig • Rats
- Exotic companion mammals

KEY POINTS

- Knowledge of animal husbandry and appreciation of a species-specific requirements is key in optimizing the health and welfare of exotic companion species.
- Provision of diet and housing in a captive environment should resemble those of wild counterparts as closely as possible.
- Environmental enrichment should be incorporated in order to meet minimal welfare standards.
- Regional and local jurisdictions should be consulted in order to meet legal requirements for the context of care.

Exotic companion mammal species continue to become popular pets as the human-animal bond expands. Exotic veterinary care beyond treating the individual animal is changing: more owners are becoming educated in the benefits of social enrichment through additional conspecifics. Furthermore, there is increasing awareness of the need for herd care practices among zoologic collections, laboratories, welfare and disaster response, pet stores, hobbyists, and private and commercial breeding facilities. Veterinarians treating exotic companion mammals should be knowledgeable about species ethology and key concepts in husbandry, including appropriate diet, housing, environmental enrichment, socialization, and exercise. A single set of guidelines cannot completely describe appropriate care for all species in all situations. It should be kept in mind that this information is mostly gained by comparing various conditions that represent all deviations from what could be considered optimal.[1]

[a] Bulger Veterinary Hospital, 141 Winthrop Avenue, Lawrence, MA 01843, USA; [b] Sydney Exotics and Rabbit Vets, North Shore Veterinary Specialist Hospital, 63 Herbert Street, Artarmon, Sydney, New South Wales 2064, Australia
* Corresponding author.
E-mail address: kle@ethosvet.com

Vet Clin Exot Anim 24 (2021) 547–566
https://doi.org/10.1016/j.cvex.2021.05.006
1094-9194/21/© 2021 Elsevier Inc. All rights reserved.
vetexotic.theclinics.com

PROVISION OF CARE
Biosecurity, Cleaning, Disinfection, Sanitation, and Hygiene

Sound principles of epidemiology are required when developing protocols to maintain disease-free herds of animals. The foundation for disease prevention and control based on host-pathogen-environment interplay[2-5] involves incorporating appropriate husbandry protocols, fulfillment of animal welfare, and good management by animal caregivers.[6]

Readers are encouraged to seek additional resources in the literature pertaining to veterinary epidemiology,[3,5] biosecurity, and infection control.[7-9]

Personnel should be trained in the performance of their duties addressing animal, personal, and public safety. Formal documentation on standard operating procedures, animal medical records, disaster plans, cleaning schedules, and equipment maintenance should be accessible and the activities routinely performed.

The goal of cleaning and disinfection is to significantly decrease pathogen loads in order to minimize the risk of disease transmission.[9-12] Cleaning improves disinfection efficacy, and involves the removal of visible foreign material and organic matter. Disinfection decreases the bioburden of the environment and limits cross-transmission of pathogens. Techniques and agents should be chosen based on the nature and composition of surfaces to be disinfected, level of contamination, degree of microbial killing desired, and efficacy and safety of disinfectant.[12,13]

The decision and feasibility to provide certain housing and feedstuff should incorporate appropriate hygiene measures. Housing surfaces should be made of materials that allow for effective sanitation and are resistant to damage from normal use and manipulation. Frequent bedding changes, regular cage cleaning, low animal stocking densities, and the provision of optimal temperature and humidity, reduce bacterial loads from excrement accumulation.[1] All feed should be sourced from reputable sources. Appropriate storage is required to minimize nutrient degradation, limit vermin and pest contamination, and prevent spoilage. The manufacturer's recommendations for proper storage should be followed to preserve nutritional quality and prevent contamination.[14] Food containers must be sanitized frequently. Vitamins and minerals can quickly become oxidized in the presence of light, heat, or moisture.[15]

All waste must be removed regularly and in compliance with all federal, state, and local regulations.[14] Waste receptacles should be leak proof, have tight-fitting lids, and be stored in areas separated from animal housing and kept free of vermin.

Feeding

Exotic companion mammals should receive dietary provisions that are as close to their free-ranging counterparts as possible. This requirement can be significantly challenging for caregivers, because delivery may not be feasible, practical, or economical.[16,17]

Literature citing the nutritional requirements of exotic companion mammal species is focused on animals in intensive farming systems and those in laboratories. Intensively farmed animals require nutrition for rapid growth and short lifespans, whereas laboratory and companion animals require diets that maintain health and promote longevity.[18-24] Despite the availability of commercially prepared complete diets, the exact nutritional requirements of these animals are not fully determined.[18] There is additionally limited information on the nutritional requirements of growing, pregnant and lactating individuals. Furthermore, although the farming and laboratory environments do not necessarily reflect the practices or recommendations of animals that are kept for companionship, requirements established in these animals should be considered as minimum standards.[25,26]

In group-housed animals, water should be delivered in more than 1 manner.[27] Delivery through a nipple bottle as well as a bowl avoids reduced consumption caused by equipment failure or contamination by ingesta or excrement.[20,28–30] In intensive systems, automated water delivery systems are more common and often provide water for up to 15 animals in communal pens. It is recommended that animals are observed regularly and acclimatized appropriately to ensure regular usage. Appropriate and regular sanitation of all water delivery systems includes flushing or disinfection to prevent pathogen contamination.[24]

HUSBANDRY AND ENRICHMENT

An environment that takes into account the animal's behavior and emotional needs is imperative for animal welfare. Observing preferences expressed by animals given free choice allows caregivers to detect discomfort induced by husbandry conditions. Animals should be housed in solid-bottom rather than wire-bottom cages to prevent pododermatitis, with appropriate substrate as a form of enrichment. The decision for choosing one substrate rather than another should be based on species preferences, cost, and availability. Animals housed outdoors should have access to shelter from the elements.

By incorporating the knowledge of species ethology, veterinarians can devise a suitable plan to ensure that the psychological needs of the animals are being met. Enrichment interactions contribute to the welfare of animals and provide additional options for bonding between the caregivers and their animals. Broad overlapping categories include[6,31,32]:

- Social: temporary or permanent conspecific and contraspecific contact, gender
- Physical: caging alterations, accessories that may be permanent, such as furniture, hanging objects, rotation of toys, manipulation of puzzles/games
- Nutritional: feeding schedules, rotations of food presentation or processing time, foraging options
- Occupational: designated exercise areas or runs, tasks or puzzles, allowing environmental control or habitat enhancement
- Sensory: visual, auditory, taste, or other stimuli

Legislation, Regulations, and Restrictions

Navigating legislation, regulations, and codes surrounding exotic companion mammal species and their care can be challenging. Most countries around the world have legal minimal standards for the housing of laboratory animals, a considerable number have regulations for farm animals, very few for zoologic collections, and none for the housing of companion animals.[6] It is best to consult the appropriate local regulatory authorities in the relevant jurisdictions.

Ownership of certain exotic companion mammals as pets may be restricted, although their possession in biomedical research and as a farming commodity may be classified under other mandates. Ferrets are the most frequently encountered species with restrictions on ownership. In the United States, the states of California[33] and Hawaii[34] prohibit pet ferret ownership, citing public health concerns as rabies vectors.[35] Their ownership is also strictly controlled in various Asian and Oceania countries.[36] Other species limitations include the prohibition of hamster and gerbil ownership in Hawaii[34] and Australia,[37] and chinchillas as pets are forbidden in Australia.[37]

Requirements for laboratory animals in the United States is governed by the Animals Welfare Act (AWA) 1990, regulation PL 89-544 (US Department of Agriculture 1985), and the Public Health Service policy (2002). Similarly, the European Union has adopted Directive 86/609/EEC – for its member states to apply a minimal standard of laws, regulations, and administrative provisions regarding the protection of animals used for experimental and scientific purposes. Each country may also implement higher measures of protection.

The protection of fur animals is poorly described in US federal laws. Animals that are used or intended for use as food or fiber are exempt from both the Animal Welfare Act and the Humane Methods Slaughter Act.[38] Welfare standards in production rabbits currently lag behind other farmed species and, frequently, the current legislation does not meet the modern welfare needs of rabbits in farmed systems.[39]

Rabbits

Ethology

The European wild rabbit (Oryctolagus cuniculus) is the sole progenitor of the domestic rabbit.[40,41] Although wild European rabbits exist only in their native habitat of the Iberian Peninsula, the ubiquity of the species is primarily caused by the unintended consequence of human introduction into non-native habitats.[41] Domestication reportedly occurred during the fifth and sixth century, when monks cultivated them as a sustainable food source during Lent.[40,42,43] There are more than 100 breeds and more than 500 varieties of domestic rabbits identified by the American Rabbit Breeders Association and the British Rabbit Council.

The relationship of the rabbit to humans is unique compared with other exotic companion mammal species: it is farmed for meat and fiber, used in laboratory research, and included as a household pet. The New Zealand white is the main breed of rabbit used in research laboratories and in industry. Numerous inbred and transgenic strains have been developed by medical researchers[44] and are used across multiple disciplines, including immunology, vaccine development, genetics, and infectious disease research.[41]

During the depression and the Second World War in Europe, the rabbit was the main source of animal protein for many people.[20,45] Eastern Europe currently produces 60% of the world's commercial production of rabbit meat,[46] with China second.[20] Compared with other livestock species, approximately 30% of rabbit meat consumed in the European Union is sourced from backyard farms compared with conventional intensive farming.[47] Breed selection depends on feed conversion efficiency with noncompetitive feeds, high reproductive potential, rapid growth rates, and carcass quality.[46,48] Commonly selected breeds include Flemish giant, French lop, Belgian hare, Champagne d'Argent, Thuringer, Chinchilla, and British.[46]

The Angora breed is the most recognized in the textile industry, with 90% of the world's production located in China.[49,50]

Husbandry

Wild rabbits are social animals that live in stable groups of up to 14 individuals, with clearly defined hierarchies.[51] They spend most of their resting time in close contact in underground burrows, leaving during dusk and dawn to feed, patrol, and mark their territories.[52] Individual rabbits have high dispersal rates of up to 20 km, with the average home range being up to 2000 m^2.[26,45]

The recommended ambient temperature for keeping rabbits is 16°C to 21°C with lower and upper critical temperatures being 15°C and 30°C respectively.[23,24,53,54] In the wild, rabbits remain well sheltered in underground runs during temperature extremes. They are more comfortable when kept at the lower end of the range, provided there are no draughts or moisture, sufficient bedding is provided, and have conspecifics to share body heat.[26] A relative humidity of 30% to 70% for rabbits is rec-ommended.[24,55] Heat prostration occurs at temperatures greater than 35°C because the sweat glands are confined to the lips, and obligate nasal respiration limits their ability to pant effectively.[23,43]

Laboratory rabbits are often housed individually in stainless steel cages in a rack-style system or group housed in floor pens.[55,56] Individual housing may be required for health or experimental reasons. In such cases, pens should be modified by dividing into smaller areas, with direct visual and olfactory access to conspecifics. When given an opportunity to use larger spaces, rabbits increase their activity levels.[26,57,58] Higher levels of inactivity and restricted behavior patterns are observed in smaller enclo-sures.[57,58] Singly housed animals show a higher incidence of stereotypical behavior patterns[23,58–60] and higher levels of corticosterone in their feces.[61] Pen arrangements should include substrate such as straw, shavings, or paper. It is recommended to pro-vide 6000 to 8000 cm^2 per rabbit for groups of up to 6 individuals.[56]

Environmental enrichment in rabbits is considered an important aspect of appropriate housing. Group housing is recommended to allow species-specific expression of normal behavior.[59] Rabbits housed individually with no social interactions with conspe-cifics show stereotypical behaviors such as biting and/or licking of bars, food hoppers, walls, and floor, and are more likely to be timid.[58,62,63] Interactions with enrichment de-vices such as toys decrease over time, indicating the need for frequent rotation of different devices and that novelty is an important aspect of environmental enrichment.[64]

On rabbit farms, breeding males and breeding females are individually caged due to fighting and competition for nest boxes. Fattening rabbits are kept in collective cages, in which group sizes depend on cage dimensions. The European Food Safety Author-ity survey[65] into the housing systems of production rabbits revealed that 20% were kept in conventional cages, followed by 18% in elevated pens, 12% floor pens, 16% indoor/outdoor systems, and 14% organic systems.

High variations in pet rabbit housing, combined with a lack of research concerning the behavioral needs of companion rabbits, make recommendations to veterinarians ambiguous. A survey performed in the United Kingdom with pet rabbits found that a good proportion of rabbits are housed in hutches that are smaller than the required regulations in laboratory rabbits.[66] The People's Dispensary for Sick Animals in the United Kingdom reports that half of all pet rabbits are housed singly despite recom-mendations for paired housing.[67]

Diet

The best diet for rabbits is one that mimics as closely as possible the grass-based diet that wild rabbits have evolved to eat.[15,25] Wild rabbits are crepuscular feeders that pri-marily consume grass as the major component of their diet. Forbs, herbs, leaves, tree shoots, branches, and bark are variably consumed as grass availability changes.[43,68,69] They spend 30% to 70% of the day foraging and eating during the early morning and late afternoon.[59] Daylight hours are spent underground in warrens.

The hindgut fermentative digestive strategy of the rabbit allows efficient conversion of a high-fiber, low-energy diet. Cecotrophy acts as a valuable source of microorgan-isms, amino acids, volatile fatty acids, and vitamins. During periods of food scarcity, all cecotropes are consumed.

Carbohydrates, including starch and simple sugars, are digested and absorbed in the upper gastrointestinal tract as the major source of energy. Excess levels of carbo-hydrates entering the caecum may cause alterations in cecal microflora, resulting in dysbiosis and enteritis.[23,70,71] The digestibility of cereals (grains and seeds) is higher than that of roots and tubers, and increases with heating during manufacturing.[15]

Optimum levels of protein for growth and lactation are 16% and 19% respectively though these levels are likely to be excessive in pet and laboratory rabbits because these animals are prone to obesity.[15,55] Recommended levels in this group are 12% to 17%. The essential fatty acid requirements of rabbits are met by plant materials.

The justification for feeding forage to rabbits is plentiful. Feeding low-fiber diets is implicated in dental disease,[72–74] gastrointestinal disease,[70,75,76] increases in stereo-typical behavior,[77–79] obesity,[17,22,55] reduction in water intake predisposing the animal to urolithiasis,[80–84] and myiasis.[85] Analysis of the natural diet of rabbits indicates levels of crude fiber of 25% to 30%.[86] When given the opportunity, rabbits selectively feed on food that is high in energy, protein, sugar and concentrates in preference to forage.[15,17,19,55] Coarse concentrate mixes that contain cereals, legumes, extruded biscuits, and pellets are commonly fed, and can lead to an unbalanced diet because of selective eating.[22,80,87] Extruded and pelleted foods can overcome the issue of selective feeding and ensure a consistent level of nutrition is delivered. Current recommended fiber levels in commercial pellets are 20% to 25% for pet or maintenance rabbits, and 18% to 20% for those in production.[23,25,87] Current dietary guidelines for rabbits recommend that a mixture of hays, fresh grass, herbs, and green leafy vegetables make up 95% of the diet, and should be available ad libitum.[15,17]

Rabbits in laboratory settings are fed a limited ration of 90 to 120 g of high-quality commercially produced, laboratory-grade pellets, once or twice a day.[55] These pellets tend to be high in carbohydrates with the fiber content close to 25%.[88] The provision of hay and vegetables for enrichment is restricted.[88]

The feeding practices in commercial meat rabbits emphasize growth and reproduction.[21] Feed restrictions occur in bucks, whereas young and growing animals, late-gestation and lactating does, and finisher rabbits are fed ad libitum.[20,65] Animals are almost exclusively fed extruded pellets according to their life stage. The pellets are low in fiber and high in carbohydrates, to encourage rapid growth before slaughter.[20,88] Forage supplementation to concentrate diets only occurs in intensive systems that are classified as indoor/outdoor or organic farms. The cost per unit of nutrients is often too high for commercial producers and high water content renders them too bulky and low in energy for feed conversion efficiency.

Angora breed rabbits used for fur or wool production are housed individually in open-wire cages. Feeding of hay can be associated with fleece contamination, which drastically reduces its commercial value. Thus, commercial Angora rabbits are fed pelleted concentrates.[23] Current practices recommend fasting once a week with access to straw or bulky forage to avoid the formation of stomach hair balls, which may cause fatal obstruction.[23] Nutritional requirements of Angora rabbits for optimal production have not been well studied, but dietary levels of sulfur-containing amino acids such as methionine and cysteine can act as limiting factors for wool production in this breed.[48,89]

Water requirements in rabbits are higher than those of other species. Consumption is approximately 120 mL/kg/d and it should be available ad libitum. Rabbits prefer to drink from open bowls than from nipple drippers,[80] which is likely a reflection of their preference to forage in a natural grazing posture.[90]

Guinea Pigs

Ethology

The domestic guinea pig (*Cavia porcellus*) is a hystricomorph rodent originating from the grasslands and Andes mountains of South America.[91,92] Domestication of guinea pigs was recorded in 5000 BC in South America, primarily raised for food and for use in religious ceremonies.[93,94] They remain an economically significant commodity for the Andean culture as a vital high-protein and low-fat source of food.[93,95] Their high proliferation rates, rapid growth, and dietary requirements that do not compete directly with human food resources such as corn and wheat, have made them popular as a livestock animal.[96–98]

C porcellus is a resultant species of domestication, and wild caviomorph species such as the *Cavia aperea*, *Cavia fulgida*, and *Cavia tschudii* still exist in open grasslands and marshy areas of South America.[91,94] The domestic guinea pig was introduced to Europe between the sixteenth and seventeenth centuries. Their ease of maintenance and docile temperament saw them raised as a companion animals and then, later, as laboratory research animals.[94] As research animals, they are used in toxicology research, product development, and medical quality control.[28]

There are currently approximately 16 recognized breeds of domestic guinea pigs.[94] These range from the short-haired coat of the American (or English) breed to the Abyssinian, with unique hair growth patterns, and the long-haired Peruvian breed.[91] The Dunkin-Hartley, an out-bred strain of short-haired pink-eyed white guinea pig, is the most commonly used strain in research. Some hairless strains have been developed for research.[91,94]

Husbandry
Guinea pigs are social animals, and housing in small groups of either single or mixed genders provides important social enrichment opportunities. Single housing should be avoided.[28,92] Social hierarchies are usually male dominated.[92] Studies of group-housed guinea pigs have identified variations in social structure depending on population density. Male guinea pigs at lower population densities typically organize into linear or occasionally despotic dominance hierarchies, and females form loose, flexible dominance hierarchies. Males can become territorial at higher population densities.[99,100] Fighting is usually limited to intense vocalizations, nipping, and prevention of subordinate animals from accessing resources. Dominant guinea pigs may barber subordinates, but this behavior can also be seen with overcrowding or in stressful situations.[101]

Guinea pigs require simple housing with good, draught-free ventilation.[28,102] Enclosures should provide sufficient space for exercise and grazing.[28] Guidelines for laboratory animals recommend a minimum enclosure size of 0.25 m^2 and a floor area of 0.09 m^2 per adult animal weighing greater than 0.7 kg.[103] Guinea pigs are tolerant of colder temperatures, with the optimal environmental temperature considered to be between 18°C and 24°C, and a relative humidity between 30% and 70%.[28,92,104]

As with other rodents, guinea pigs are thigmotactic and choose to avoid open spaces, preferring to huddle with conspecifics next to a wall or in a tunnel or shelter. They show preference for moving along the periphery of the enclosure rather than crossing into the middle.[92,105,106] At minimum, an enclosed solid-sided nesting area or shelter should be provided for housing and for security.[92]

Enclosures should be constructed from secure materials because there is a risk of chewing and thus escape with wooden and some plastic enclosures. Outdoor enclosures should be secure to prevent attacks from predators and access by wild rodents and birds.[92] Smooth, solid flooring should be provided to reduce the risk of pododermatitis and leg injuries. Shredded or pelleted recycled paper and hay are suitable substrates that also serve as environmental enrichment, offering burrowing and hiding opportunities.[28,92,102] Large-diameter plastic drainpipes and fabric bedding sacs can additionally be used. Wood chips or shavings have been associated with respiratory disease and should be avoided.[102]

In the homes of rural smallholders in the South American Andes, guinea pigs have free range of the kitchen area, or are confined to a corner near the stove or fire.[96] Commercial meat production in South America involves having 10 to 15 growers in a 1-m^2 solid-floor pen with a wall height of 0.6 m.[96] Grain straw or rice hulls are used as bedding substrate, laid with a thickness of approximately 70 mm.[96] Water is provided via fresh forage, and supplemental grains are fed using a simple trough.

Nutrition

Guinea pigs are strict herbivores, and are hindgut fermenters showing coprophagy.[30] A crude protein level of 18% to 20% is considered sufficient for growth and lactation, and a minimum crude fiber level of 10% is recommended.[28,102] Food should be available ad libitum.[28,29]

Guinea pigs require a dietary source of vitamin C (ascorbic acid), because they lack L-gulonolactone oxidase, an enzyme in the synthesis pathway of ascorbic acid from glucose. Adult guinea pigs require 10 to 25 mg/kg of vitamin C daily for maintenance.[102] Fresh vegetables can contribute to their daily requirement, and commercial guinea pig pellets supplemented with vitamin C should be used.[92] Vitamin C oxidizes rapidly on exposure to heat, light, and air; commercial pellets now typically contain the stabilized form of vitamin C, but storage in a cool, dark, dry area remains important to maintain a shelf-life of around 6 months.[29,102]

Unlimited clean, fresh drinking water should be available at all times. Guinea pigs consume approximately 100 mL/kg/d of water, depending on diet and the environment.[29,30,102] Supplementation of vitamin C into the drinking water has been a common recommendation,[28,92] but it is currently thought to potentially reduce water consumption by altering palatability, and thus is no longer recommended.[102] Guinea pigs do not show a drinking preference for nipple drinkers or open bowls.[27]

Ferrets

Ethology

The domestic ferret (*Mustela putorius furo*) is an obligate carnivore belonging to the Mustelidae family and related to polecats, weasels, minks, otters, and martens. There are currently 3 species of wild ferrets naturally found through Europe, Asia, and North America: the European polecat (*Mustela putorius*), the steppe or Siberian polecat (*Mustela eversmanni*), and the black-footed ferret (*Mustela nigripes*).[107]

The ferret has been domesticated for more than 2000 years and is most likely a descendant of the European polecat, although its exact origins remains unclear.[108] Around 63 BC to 24 AD, Greek and Roman writers described ferretlike, rabbit-catching animals during periods of rabbit plagues,[108] which is considered to have been the start of its domestication.

Ferreting currently remains popular in parts of Europe as a means of rabbit hunting and pest control.[109,110] A British survey in 2009 indicated that nearly 20% of owned ferrets were considered working ferrets.[111] This practice in the United States is, at present, banned to protect native rabbit species in certain states.[107,112]

In a laboratory setting, the ferret is the animal model used for biomedical research into viral diseases, especially for influenza, the severe acute respiratory syndrome (SARS)–associated virus, and, more recently, the severe acute respiratory syndrome coronavirus 2.[113,114] They have also played a secondary role in neuroscientific, oncological, cardiovascular physiology, and emesis research.[115–117]

Ferrets as companion pets are popular because of their small size, playful nature, and engaging personality.

Husbandry

Domestic ferrets can be housed either indoors or outdoors, although indoor housing is more common in pet and laboratory ferret populations.[112,115] Ferrets do not tolerate high ambient temperatures of greater than 30°C because their sweat glands are poorly developed. The recommended temperature range in laboratory settings is between 15°C and 24°C, with a relative humidity between 40% and 60%.[117]

Working ferrets in northeastern Spain are usually housed in pairs in wire cages, or in outdoor enclosures in groups of 4 to 8 animals.[109] Although there are minimum size recommendations for housing in laboratory ferrets,[117] it has been considered that this is less important in pet ferrets as long as the ferret receives sufficient supervised play time outside its enclosure.[112] The enclosure should be sufficiently high to enable the ferret to stand on its hindlimbs, and large enough to provide a dark, enclosed sleeping/nesting area, a litter box, a feeding area, and some room to play. Outdoor housing should provide sufficient protection against the elements.[112,117] Ferrets are extremely social animals, and take readily to group housing.[118] Ferrets of either gender or age may accept conspecifics,[112] although it has been suggested that there is reduced aggression among ferrets that have been housed together from a young age.[119] Aggression can be noted between entire males during breeding season.[119]

A consideration in designing ferret housing should be to ensure that escape is impossible.[112] In free-range situations, ferrets dig and spend much of their time in underground tunnels. Environmental enrichment in pet and laboratory ferrets can be provided in the form of pipes or similar tunnel-like structures to encourage crawling and hiding, and soft bedding to allow burrowing behaviors.[117,119] Rough-and-tumble social play between conspecifics has also been shown to be important for their well-being.[120] Many pet ferrets choose to sleep in hammocks when offered. Group-housed ferrets often sleep together, thus it is important to provide a sufficiently large sleeping area and also multiple sleeping sites for individual solitude.[112,119]

Nutrition
Ferrets are obligate carnivores with a short intestinal tract, rapid gut transit time, and unsophisticated intestinal flora.[107,117,121] As such, ferrets require highly digestible diets that are high in protein and fat, and low in carbohydrates and fiber.[18,112,115,117] Diets containing protein content of 30% to 40% and fat content of 9% to 28% have been recommended, although the exact nutritional requirements are yet to be fully established via feeding trials.[112,115,117,121] Protein sources in ferret diets should be primarily of animal origin.[121] Avoidance of raw fish protein sources has also been recommended because of excessive levels of thiaminase.[117] High dietary levels of plant protein can be associated with urolithiasis in ferrets.[122]

Specific ferret extruded diets are available commercially, but premium-quality high-protein feline diets can also be used when not available. The feeding of extruded diets in ferrets is thought to have negative effects on their dental hygiene, because ferrets are adapted for a whole-prey diet.[121,123] Feeding clean sources of whole-prey animals, such as chicks, rats, and mice, may be considered on occasion and can serve as a valuable source of environmental enrichment.[112,121] This practice is commonly performed in working ferrets used for hunting.[18,109] Certain pet ferret owner perceptions and the nutritional uniformity required for laboratory ferrets may limit this practice.[18]

The water intake required in adult ferrets is estimated at 75 to 100 mL/animal/d[117,124] and they prefer to drink from a dish rather than a dropper bottle.[121] Clean sources of water should always be available, and this is particularly important in ferrets fed an extruded diet.[112,115,121] Mixing pelleted food with water improves palatability, increases water intake, and is an excellent form of enrichment.[118]

Mice, Rats, Hamsters, Gerbils

Ethology
Mice. Most pet and laboratory mice are domesticated from the wild house mouse (*Mus musculus*). Their ancestral range was likely in present-day India.[125,126] House mice live in close proximity to humans and their prevalence stems from their adaptability to new

environments, prolific breeding rates, and omnivory.[127] They exist in feral populations, are commonly found in residential, agricultural, and commercial structures, and provide a vital role as food sources for predatory reptiles, birds, and mammals.

The laboratory mouse was used in comparative anatomic studies as early as the seventeenth century, but interest in biology accelerated during the nineteenth century. Research requirements for a small, economical mammal that was easily housed and bred were instrumental in the development of the modern-day laboratory mouse.[125,128] They are the most commonly used mammals in biomedical and behavioral research.[128,129]

Rats. Also belonging to the family Muridae, the rat is likely a domesticated form of the Norway rat (*Rattus norvegicus*) and likely originated in Asia.[130,131] Domestication and the development of albino rats likely began in the 1800s as high-volume prey available for sport baiting, with albinos selected out as a hobby breed.[126,131] Albino rats were standardized by researchers at the Wistar Institute by means of mass breeding.[130,131] The rat is the second most frequently used mammal in biomedical research after the mouse.[129,131] The American Fancy Rat and Mouse Association recognizes more than 65 different varieties of each species.

Hamsters. Hamsters belong to the suborder Myomorpha and are in the family Cricetidae.

The native habitats of the various hamsters range from the Middle East to areas of Europe as well as Asia. Different species are frequently encountered as pets, although the Syrian hamster (*Mesocricetus auratus*) is the dominant species for laboratory studies.

The natural habitat of Syrian hamsters is northwest Syria in the area of Aleppo. It seems that most of the Syrian hamsters used as laboratory animals or pets are decedents of the original 3 or 4 surviving littermates captured in 1930.[132] Other species of hamster in the pet industry include the dwarf Djungarian (*Phodopus sungorus*), Campbell's (*Phodopus campbelli*), Roborovskii (*Phodopus roborovskii*), and Chinese hamsters (*Cricetulus griseus*).

Gerbils. The Mongolian gerbil (*Meriones unguiculatus*) belongs to the Muridae family. It is the most common gerbil species in biomedical research and as a companion pet. In the wild, they are diurnal with crepuscular tendencies. They are widely distributed and originate in the dry and desert grasslands of northern Africa, regions of eastern Europe, India, Russia, Mongolia, and northern China.[133] In recent wild survey studies, colonies have been prevalent near agricultural areas, especially those of old cultivated fields.[134]

Domestication occurred relatively recently when wild-caught stock were sent to Japan, and the animals that are available today originated from 20 pairs captured in 1935.[135] In 1954, 11 pairs were imported from Japan and distributed to the United States to establish a foundation farming colony in New York.[135]

Housing

As a general rule, different species of rodents should be housed separately to prevent interspecies disease transmission. In addition, housing males and females together results in mating and subsequent litters.

The Guide for the Care and Use of Laboratory Animals recommends mice, rats, hamsters, and gerbils be kept at room temperatures of 18°C to 26°C and a controlled relative humidity of 30% to 70%.[24] Hamsters hibernate if environmental temperatures decrease to less than 10°C.

Mouse cages should provide at least 0.033 m^2 of floor space per animal,[136] whereas rat cages should provide at least 0.08 m^2 of floor space per animal.[137] Hamsters require 0.0064 to 0.0122 m² each, and gerbils are recommended to have 0.0116 m². Multilevel cages with solid sloping ramps, hides, and hammocks are well used by mice and rats.

The opportunity to retreat into burrows, provided in the form of shelters, are as important as the provision of bedding in cages with solid floors. Suitable bedding material also acts as a form of enrichment, and hamsters show preference for bedding material suited to nest construction (pine or aspen shavings) rather than granular material (corn cob or wood pellets).[138] Reduced stereotypical behaviors are seen in hamsters provided with deep bedding of 0.4 to 0.8 m to allow burrowing,[139] and a running wheel.[140]

Mice. House mice in the wild have variable social structures, ranging from discrete demes with a single male incorporating several adult females and juveniles, to high-density aggregations with adults that are socially gregarious and have largely overlapping ranges.[125] Home ranges of 600 to 1200 m² have been reported.[141] Demes of mice in local areas are likely to be related, because females tend to live in extended family groups and can nest and nurse offspring communally.[142] For mouse colonies kept as companions or in laboratories, female mice do well housed together, but adult intact males should be kept separately.[126]

Rats. The rat is found in urban areas globally and is ubiquitous in urbanized areas.[143–145] For a species that exists in social colonies in underground burrow systems, wild rats show a surprising lack of cooperative behavior, tending to ignore other members of their own colony except during times of mating or communal sleeping in nests.[144,146,147] Hostility is observed toward strange individuals, and heavier individuals tend to dominate smaller ones in a social heirachy.[147] Male rats have larger home ranges than females.[148] Female rats establish burrow systems underneath the ground that increase in size as litters and family groups grow.[149] Domesticated rats as pets and in laboratory settings are more communal and do well housed in mixed groups of several males and females.[126]

Hamsters. The natural habitats of hamsters are dry, rocky steppes or brush slopes,[132] but recent data reveal increasing population densities in agricultural land cultivating grain.[150] Hamsters spend a considerable amount of time underground in burrows.[150,151] Nesting material in these burrows included textile remnants, bird feathers, and shredded plastic sack pieces in colonies that were housed adjacent to agricultural fields.[150] In the wild, hamsters are solitary, living either singly or as nursing females with pups in burrow systems.[151] In captive settings, it is recommended to house female Syrian hamsters separately, because they tend to be aggressive. Other hamster species may be kept in groups, but fighting may occur.[152]

Gerbils. Gerbils live in extended family groups of up to 30 individuals, consisting of 1 adult male, 1 to 3 adult females, and their offspring.[133,134,153] Complex burrows systems are excavated in dry and sandy soil.[134,154,155] Family groups are territorial, which must be considered when introducing or reintroducing animals into groups.[152,156] Behavioral observations suggest that Mongolian gerbils are socially monogamous until one of the dominant adults dies or disperses.[155] Familial control of reproductive activity in young females in a family unit is complex and hierarchies of alloparental care exist.[154,156–158]

Diet
Rats and mice. Rats and mice are omnivorous, opportunistic, and adapt to a variety of foods, including grasses, seeds, grains, and insects.[1,126,144] Commercial laboratory rodent pellets are easily accessible and are typically high in fat and low in fiber.

They should contain greater than 14% protein for mice and 20% to 27% protein for rats.[159] Ad libitum feeding, as used in laboratory animals,[131] can lead to obesity. It is recommended in companion rats and mice that the number of pellets should be limited, with supplement and food variety provided by vegetables and small amounts of fruit.[1] Selective feeding is seen when seed-based diets are offered and are discouraged because of their high fat content and poor nutritional maintainence.[159] Mice consume about 3 to 5 g of feed per day, whereas rats consume about 15 g of feed per day.[160]

Hamsters and gerbils. Hamsters are primarily granivorous but also forage for green plant parts, shoots, roots, insects, and fruits.[132] Similar to hamsters, gerbils feed mainly on plant seeds, especially during winter as they consume their hoards. In summer, green stems, leaves, underground parts of plants, and insects are consumed.[161] Gerbils require very little water and they obtain most or all of their water requirements from metabolic processes and any available fruit or vegetable matter[152]; however, this does not preclude their access to water in captivity.

Hamsters and gerbils have similar dietary requirements. In order to prevent selective feeding, a balanced commercial diet specific to the species is recommended rather than seed-based diets.[151,159] Recommended minimal protein levels are 16% for hamsters and 20% for gerbils, with a 4% to 5% fat level.[159] Specific pelleted diets for each species are recommended in companion pets,[152] although diets formulated for other rodent species, such as rats and mice, are more commonly fed to laboratory animals.[151]

Water should be provided through a bottle with a conventional nipple to prevent contamination in rodents, as seen with bowls. Bottles should be changed daily and inspected for debris or malfunction. Water intake for laboratory rats and mice has been reported to be 10 mL per 100 g of body weight.[131] This amount has been similarly reported in hamsters as well.[151,159] Because of gerbils' arid origins, their total daily water intake is notably less and has been estimated as 8% to 13% of body weight[160] or approximately 4 mL of water per day.[159]

CLINICS CARE POINTS

- Consult local jurisdictions on species-specific practices and welfare legislation.
- Species-specific knowledge on husbandry and diet is vital for veterinarians to educated caretakers on animal health and welfare.
- Understanding species ethology provides insight for domestication and the human-animal bond.

DISCLOSURE

The authors have nothing to disclose.

REFERENCES

1. Brown CJ, Donnelly TM. Rodent husbandry and care. Veterinary Clin North Am Exot Anim Pract 2004;7(2):201–25.
2. Engering A, Hogerwerf L, Slingenbergh J. Pathogen-host-environment interplay and disease emergence. Emerg Microbes Infect 2013;2(1):1–7.

3. Thrusfield M, Christley R. Veterinary epidemiology. 4th edition. Cornwall, Great Britain: Blackwell Publishing; 2018.
4. Dunowska M. "Links in the chain" of disease transmission. In: Caveney L, Jones B, Ellis K, editors. Veterinary infection prevention and control. UK: John Wiley & Sons; 2012. p. 99–148.
5. Robertson ID. Disease control, prevention and on-farm biosecurity: The role of veterinary epidemiology. Engineering 2020;6(1):20–5.
6. Young R. Environmental enrichment for captive animals. Great Britain: Blackwell Publishing; 2003.
7. Stull JW, Bjorvik E, Bub J, et al. 2018 AAHA Infection control, prevention, and biosecurity guidelines. J Am Anim Hosp Assoc 2018;54(6):297–326.
8. Caveney L, Jones B, Ellis K. Veterinary infection prevention and control. West Sussex, UK: Wiley Blackwell; 2012.
9. Byers CG. Biosecurity measures in clinical practice. Vet Clin North Am - Small Anim Pract 2020;50(6):1277–87.
10. Weese JS. Cleaning and disinfection of patient care items, in relation to small animals. Vet Clin North Am - Small Anim Pract 2015;45(2):331–42.
11. Traverse M, Aceto H. Environmental cleaning and disinfection. Vet Clin North Am - Small Anim Pract 2015;45(2):299–330.
12. Caveny L. Guidelines for effective cleaning and disinfection. In: Caveney L, Jones B, Ellis K, editors. Veterinary infection prevention and control. UK: John Wiley & Sons; 2012. p. 246–86.
13. Rutala WA, Weber DJ. Selection of the ideal disinfectant. Infect Control Hosp Epidemiol 2014;35(7):855–65.
14. Association AV. Companion animal care guidelines. Available at: https://www.avma.org/resources-tools/avma-policies/companion-animal-care-guidelines.
15. Prebble J. Nutrition and feeding. In: Meredith A, Lord B, editors. BSAVA manual of rabbit medicine. 2018. p. 27–35.
16. Böhmer C, Böhmer E. Shape variation in the craniomandibular system and prevalence of dental problems in domestic rabbits: A case study in evolutionary veterinary science. Vet Sci 2017;4(4):5.
17. Clauss M. Clinical technique: Feeding hay to rabbits and rodents. J Exot Pet Med 2012;21(1):80–6.
18. Fox JG, Schultz CS, Vester Boler BM. Nutrition of the ferret. In: Fox JG, Marini RP, editors. Biology and diseases of the ferret. 3rd edition. Somerset, United States: John Wiley & Sons, Incorporated. 2014. p. 123–46.
19. NRC. Nutrient requirements of rabbits 1977.
20. Lebas F, Coudert P, Rochambeau H de, et al. The rabbit: husbandry, health and production. Rome, Italy: FAO - Food and agriculture organization of the United Nations; 1997.
21. Smith S. Gastrointestinal physiology and nutrition of rabbits. In: Quesenberry K, Orcutt C, Mans C, et al, editors. Ferrets, Rabbits and rodents: Clinical Medicine and Surgery. 4th ed. Canada: Elsevier; 2021. p. 162–73.
22. Prebble JL, Meredith AL. Food and water intake and selective feeding in rabbits on four feeding regimes. J Anim Physiol Anim Nutr (Berl) 2014;98(5):991–1000.
23. de Blas C, Wiseman J. Nutrition of the rabbit. 2nd ed. United Kingdom: CAB International; 2010.
24. NRC. Guide for the care and Use of laboratory animals. 8th edition. Washington DC: National Academies Press; 2011.
25. Clauss M, Hatt JM. Evidence-based rabbit housing and nutrition. Vet Clin North Am - Exot Anim Pract 2017;20(3):871–84.

26. Saunders R. Husbandry. In: Meredith A, Lord B, editors. BSAVA manual of rabbit medicine. Gloucester, UK: BSAVA; 2018. p. 13–26.

27. Hagen K, Clauss M, Hatt JM. Drinking preferences in chinchillas (Chinchilla laniger), degus (Octodon degu) and guinea pigs (Cavia porcellus). J Anim Physiol Anim Nutr (Berl) 2014;98(5):942–7.

28. Kaiser S, Kruger C, Sachser N. The guinea pig. In: Hubrecht R, Kirkwood J, editors. The UFAW Handbook on the care and management of laboratory and other research animals. 8th edition. Herts (United Kingdom): Universities Federation for Animal Welfare. 2010. p. 380–98.

29. Gresham VC, Haines VL. Management, husbandry, and colony health. In: Suckow MA, Stevens KA, Wilson RP, editors. The laboratory rabbit, Guinea pig, hamster, and other rodents. San Diego (CA): Elsevier Science & Technology. 2011. p. 603–20.

30. Kohles M. Gastrointestinal anatomy and physiology of select exotic companion mammals. Veterinary Clin North Am Exot Anim Pract 2014;17(2):165–78.

31. Bloomsmith MA, Schapiro SJ. Guidelines for developing and managing an environmental enrichment program for nonhuman primates. Lab Anim Sci 1991; 41(4):372–7.

32. Wells DL. Sensory stimulation as environmental enrichment for captive animals: A review. Appl Anim Behav Sci 2009;118(1–2):1–11.

33. California S of. Fish and Game code of California. United States of America. Available at: https://leginfo.legislature.ca.gov/faces/codesTOCSelected.xhtml?tocCode=FGC.

34. State of Hawaii D of A. List of prohibited animals. USA. Available at: https://hdoa.hawaii.gov/wp-content/uploads/2019/08/List-of-Prohibited-Animals.pdf. Accessed January 3, 2021.

35. Hitchcock JC. The European ferret, Mustela putorius, (family Mustelidae) its public health, wildlife and agricultural significance, . Proceedings of the Sixteenth Vertebrate pest Conference. p. 207–12.

36. Department HKAF and C. Personal Communication.

37. Australian Government Department of Agriculture W and the E. Unique or Exotic Pets. Available at: https://www.agriculture.gov.au/travelling/bringing-mailing-goods/unique-exotic-pets. Accessed January 3, 2021.

38. Peterson LA. Detailed discussion of fur animals and fur production. Animal Legal & Historical Center - Michigan State University College of Law.

39. Dorning J, Harris S. The welfare of farmed rabbits in commercial production systems 2017.

40. Alves JM, Carneiro M, Afonso S, et al. Levels and patterns of genetic diversity and population structure in domestic rabbits. In: Paiva SR, editor. PLoS One 2015;10(12):e0144687.

41. Naff K, Craig S. The domestic rabbit, Oryctolagus cuniculus: origins and history. In: Suckow M, Stevens K, Wilson R, editors. The laboratory rabbit, Guinea pig, hamster, and other rodents. 1st edition. London: Academic Press, Inc.; 2012. p. 157–63.

42. Carneiro M, Afonso S, Geraldes A, et al. The genetic structure of domestic rabbits. Mol Biol Evol 2011;28(6):1801–16.

43. Donnelly TM, Vella D. Basic anatomy, physiology and husbandry of rabbits. In: Quesenberry K, Orcutt C, Mans C, et al, editors. Ferrets, rabbits and rodents: Clinical medicine and Surgery. 4th Edition; 2021. p. 131–49.

44. Christensen ND, Peng X. Rabbit genetics. In: Suckow M, Stevens K, Wilson R, editors. The laboratory rabbit, Guinea pig, hamster, and other rodents. USA: Academic Press, Inc.; 2012. p. 165–93.
45. Williams K, Parer I, Coman B, et al. Managing Vertebrate pests: rabbits 1995.
46. Bolet G, Monnerot M, Arnal C, et al. A programme for the inventory, characterisation, evaluation, conservation and utilisation of European rabbit (Oryctolagus cuniculus) genetic resources. Anim Genet 1999;59.
47. European Commission Directorate-General For Health And Food Safety DG (SANTE). Overview report commercial rabbit farming in the European union 2017.
48. Cheeke P. Rabbit feeding and nutrition. USA: Academic Press, Inc.; 1987.
49. Gerken M, Renieri C, Allain D, et al. Advances in fibre production science in South American Camelids and other fibre animals 2012.
50. Rochambeau H de, Thebault RG. Genetics of the rabbit for wool production. Anim Breed Abstr 1990;51(1):1–15.
51. Szendro Z, McNitt JI. Housing of rabbit does: Group and individual systems: A review. Livest Sci 2012;150(1–3):1–10.
52. Dixon LM, Hardiman JR, Cooper JJ. The effects of spatial restriction on the behavior of rabbits (Oryctolagus cuniculus). J Vet Behav Clin Appl Res 2010; 5(6):302–8.
53. Sohn J, Cuoto M. Anatomy, physiology and behavior. In: Suckow M, Stevens K, Wilson R, editors. The laboratory rabbit, Guinea pig, hamster, and other rodents. USA: Academic Press, Inc.; 2012. p. 195–216.
54. McEwen GN, Heath JE. Resting metabolism and thermoregulation in the unrestrained rabbit. J Appl Phys 1973;35(6):884–6.
55. Quinn RH. Rabbit colony management and related health concerns. In: Suckow M, Stevens K, Wilson R, editors. The laboratory rabbit, Guinea pig, hamster, and other rodents. London: Academic Press, Inc; 2012. p. 217–41.
56. Morton D, Jennings M, Batchelor G, et al. Refinements in rabbit husbandry. Laboratory Animals 1993;27:301-329.
57. Dixon LM, Hardiman JR, Cooper JJ. The effects of varying floor area on the behaviour of pet rabbits (Oryctolagus cuniculus). In: 7th International veterinary Behavior meeting. Edinburgh. 2009. p. 115–8.
58. Hansen LT, Berthelsen H. The effect of environmental enrichment on the behaviour of caged rabbits (Oryctolagus cuniculus). Appl Anim Behav Sci 2000;68(2): 163–78.
59. Trocino A, Xiccato G. Animal welfare in reared rabbits: a review with emphasis on housing systems. World Rabbit Sci 2010;14(2):77–93.
60. McBride EA. Normal behaviour and behavioural problems. In: Meredith A, Lord B, editors. BSAVA manual of rabbit medicine. Gloucester, UK: BSAVA; 2018. p. 45–58.
61. Lisiewicz N, Waters M, Jackson B. Social stress in rabbits. In: Proceedings of the 7th International behaviour meeting. Belgium. 2009. p. 29–42.
62. Poggiagliolmi S, Crowell-Davis SL, Alworth LC, et al. Environmental enrichment of New Zealand White rabbits living in laboratory cages. J Vet Behav Clin Appl Res 2011;6(6):343–50.
63. Bozicovich TFM, Moura ASAMT, Fernandes S, et al. Effect of environmental enrichment and composition of the social group on the behavior, welfare, and relative brain weight of growing rabbits. Applied Animal Behaviour Science 2016;182:72-79.

64. Johnson CA, Pallozzi WA, Geiger L, et al. The effect of an environmental enrichment device on individually caged rabbits in a safety assessment facility. Contemp Top Lab Anim Sci 2003;42(5):27–30.
65. Saxmose Nielsen S, Alvarez J, Bicout DJ, et al. Health and welfare of rabbits farmed in different production systems. Eur Food Saf Auth J 2020;18(1).
66. Rioja-Lang F, Bacon H, Connor M, et al. Rabbit welfare: Determining priority welfare issues for pet rabbits using a modified Delphi method. Vet Rec Open 2019; 6(1):363.
67. PDSA animal Wellbeing report.
68. Katona K, Bíró Z, Hahn I, et al. Competition between European Hare and European Rabbit in a Lowland Area, Hungary: A long-Term Ecological Study in the period of rabbit Extinction. Folia Zoologica 2004;53(3):255-268.
69. Marques C, Mathias ML. The diet of the European wild rabbit, Oryctolagus cuniculus (L.), on different coastal habitats of Central Portugal. Mammalia 2001; 65(4):437–49.
70. Gidenne T, Jehl N, Lapanouse A, et al. Inter-relationship of microbial activity, digestion and gut health in the rabbit: effect of substituting fibre by starch in diets having a high proportion of rapidly fermentable polysaccharides. Br J Nutr 2004;92(1):95–104.
71. Gidenne T. Dietary fibres in the nutrition of the growing rabbit and recommendations to preserve digestive health: A review. Animal 2014;39(11).
72. Meredith AL, Prebble JL, Shaw DJ. Impact of diet on incisor growth and attrition and the development of dental disease in pet rabbits. J Small Anim Pract 2015; 56(6):377–82.
73. Crossley DA. Oral biology and disorders of lagomorphs. Vet Clin North Am - Exot Anim Pract 2003;6(3):629–59.
74. Harcourt-Brown FM. The progressive syndrome of acquired dental disease in rabbits. J Exot Pet Med 2007;16(3):146–57.
75. Meredith AL, Prebble JL. Impact of diet on faecal output and caecotroph consumption in rabbits. J Small Anim Pract 2017;58(3):139–45.
76. Oglesbee BL, Lord B. Gastrointestinal diseases of rabbits. In: Quesenberry K, Orcutt C, Mans C, et al, editors. Ferrets, rabbits and rodents: Clinical medicine and Surgery. 4th ed. Canada: Elsevier; 2021. p. 174–87.
77. Berthelsen H, Hansen LT. The effect of hay on the behaviour of caged rabbits (Oryctolagus cuniculus). Anim Welf 1999;8(2):149–57.
78. Harris LD, Custer LB, Soranaka ET, et al. Evaluation of objects and food for environmental enrichment of NZW rabbits. Contemp Top Lab Anim Sci 2001;40(1): 27–30.
79. Lidfors L. Behavioural effects of environmental enrichment for individually caged rabbits. Appl Anim Behav Sci 1997;52(1–2):157–69.
80. Tschudin A, Clauss M, Codron D, et al. Water intake in domestic rabbits (Oryctolagus cuniculus) from open dishes and nipple drinkers under different water and feeding regimes. J Anim Physiol Anim Nutr (Berl) 2011;95(4):499–511.
81. Clauss M, Burger B, Liesegang A, et al. Influence of diet on calcium metabolism, tissue calcification and urinary sludge in rabbits (Oryctolagus cuniculus). J Anim Physiol Anim Nutr (Berl) 2012;96(5):798–807.
82. White RN. Management of calcium ureterolithiasis in a French lop rabbit. J Small Anim Pract 2001;42(12):595–8.
83. Kamphues J. Calcium metabolism of rabbits as an etiological factor for urolithiasis. J Nutr 1991;121(11 Suppl):S95–6.

84. Harcourt-Brown FM. Diagnosis of renal disease in rabbits. Veterinary Clin North Am Exot Anim Pract 2013;16(1):145–74.
85. Cousquer G. Veterinary care of rabbits with myiasis. Pract 2006;28(6):342–9.
86. Wallage-Drees JM, Deinum B. Quality of the diet selected by wild rabbits (Oryctolagus cuniculus) in autumn and winter. Neth J Zool 1986;36(4):438–48.
87. Irlbeck NA. How to feed the rabbit (Oryctolagus cuniculus) gastrointestinal tract. J Anim Sci 2001;79(E-Suppl):E343.
88. Kylie J, Weese JS, Turner PV. Comparison of the fecal microbiota of domestic commercial meat, laboratory, companion, and shelter rabbits (Oryctolagus cuniculi). BMC Vet Res 2018;14(1):1–15.
89. Lebas F, Thebault RG, Allain D. Nutritional recommendations and feeding management of Angora rabbits. In: de Blas C, Wisewan J, eds. Nutrition of the rabbit. 2nd edition, Oxfordshire, UK: CABI Publishing; :308-316.
90. Prebble JL, Langford FM, Shaw DJ, et al. The effect of four different feeding regimes on rabbit behaviour. Appl Anim Behav Sci 2015;169:86–92.
91. Pritt S. Taxonomy and history. In: Suckow MA, Stevens KA, Wilson RP, editors. The laboratory rabbit, Guinea pig, hamster, and other rodents. United States of America: Elsevier Science & Technology. 2011. p. 56375.
92. Johnson-Delaney CA. Guinea pigs, chinchillas, degus and duprasi. In: Meredith A, Johnson-Delaney C, editors. BSAVA manual of exotic pets. Gloucester, UK: BSAVA; 2018. p. 28–62.
93. Morales E. The Guinea pig: Healing, food, and Ritual in the Andes. Tucson, Arizona: University of Arizona Press; 1995.
94. Barthold SW, Griffey SM, Percy DH. Guinea pig. In: Barthold SW, Griffey SM, Percy DH, editors. Pathology of laboratory rodents and rabbits. 4th ed. United States of America: John Wiley & Sons, Incorporated; 2016. p. 213–52.
95. Morales E. The guinea pig in the Andean economy: from household animal to market commodity. Lat Am Res Rev 1994;29(3):129–42.
96. Lammers PJ, Carlson SL, Zdorkowski GA, et al. Reducing food insecurity in developing countries through meat production: The potential of the guinea pig (Cavia porcellus). Renew Agric Food Syst 2009;24(2):155–62.
97. Barba L, Sánchez-Macías D, Barba I, et al. The potential of non-invasive pre- and post-mortem carcass measurements to predict the contribution of carcass components to slaughter yield of guinea pigs. Meat Sci 2018;140:59–65.
98. Sánchez-Macías D, Castro N, Rivero MA, et al. Proposal for standard methods and procedure for guinea pig carcass evaluation, jointing and tissue separation. J Appl Anim Res 2015;44(1):65–70.
99. Sachser N. Different Forms of Social Organization At High and Low Population Densities in Guinea Pigs. Behaviour 1986;97(3–4):253–72.
100. Fuchs S. Spacing patterns in a colony of guinea pigs: Predictability from environmental and social factors. Behav Ecol Sociobiol 1980;6(4):265–76.
101. Harper LV. Behavior. In: Wagner JE, Breazile JE, Manning PJ, editors. The biology of the Guinea pig. New York: Academic Press; 1976. p. 31–48.
102. Pignon C, Mayer J. Guinea pigs. In: Quesenberry K, Mans C, Orcutt C, et al, editors. Ferrets, rabbits and rodents: clinical medicine and surgery. St Louis, Missouri: Elsevier - Health Sciences Division; 2021. p. 270–97.
103. Union OJ of the E. Directive 2010/63/EU of the European parliament and of the council of 22 September 2010 on the protection of animals used for scientific purposes 2010. p. 2020.
104. National Research Council (NRC). Guide for the care and use of laboratory animals. Washington DC: National Academies Press; 2011.

105. White WJ, Balk MW, Lang CM. Use of cage space by guineapigs. Lab Anim 1989;23(3):208–14.
106. Hargaden M, Singer L. Anatomy, physiology, and behavior. In: Suckow MA, Stevens KA, Wilson RP, editors. The laboratory rabbit, Guinea pig, hamster, and other rodents. San Diego, United States: Elsevier Science & Technology. 2011. p. 576–602.
107. Powers LV, Brown SA. Ferrets: Basic anatomy, physiology and husbandry. In: Quesenberry KA, Carpenter JW, editors. Ferrets, rabbits and rodents: Clinical medicine and Surgery. 3rd Edition. Philadelphia, PA: Saunders; 2012. p. 1–12.
108. Thomson APD. A History of the Ferret. J Hist Med Allied Sci 1951;VI(Autumn): 471–80.
109. Martorell J, Cabezon O, Castella J, et al. Health status of working ferrets in Northeastern Spain. In: ExoticsCon. Portland: Oregon; 2016. p. 445–6.
110. Bessant D. Hunting with ferrets. Malaysia: The Crowood Press; 2008.
111. Cooper JE. Ferrets: Working ferrets: Forgotten and neglected? Vet Rec 2011; 168(19):518–9.
112. Schoemaker NJ. Ferrets, skunks and otters. In: Meredith AL, Johnson-Delaney CA, editors. BSAVA manual of exotic pets. 5th ed. Gloucester, UK: British Small Animal Veterinary Association; 2018. p. 127–38.
113. Ryan KA, Bewley KR, Fotheringham SA, et al. Dose-dependent response to infection with SARS-CoV-2 in the ferret model and evidence of protective immunity. Nat Commun 2021;12(1):1–13.
114. Ball RS. Issues to consider for preparing ferrets as research subjects in the laboratory. ILAR J 2006;47(4):348–57.
115. Mayer J, Marini RP, Fox JG. Biology and diseases of ferrets. In: Anderson LC, Otto G, Pritchett-Corning KR, et al, editors. Laboratory animal medicine. United States of America: Elsevier Science & Technology; 2015. p. 577–622.
116. Fox JG, Marini RP. Biology and diseases of the ferret. United States of America: John Wiley & Sons, Incorporated; 2014.
117. Plant M, Lloyd M. The ferret. In: Hubrecht R, Kirkwood J, editors. The UFAW Handbook on the care and management of laboratory and other research animals. 8th edition. Herts (United Kingdom): Universities Federation for Animal Welfare. 2010. p. 418–31.
118. Fox JG, Broome R. Housing and management. In: Fox JG, Marini RP, editors. Biology and diseases of the ferret. 3rd ed. United States of America: John Wiley & Sons, Incorporated; 2014. p. 145–56.
119. Bulloch MJ, Tynes VV. Ferrets. In: Tynes VV, editor. Behavior of exotic pets. United Kingdom: Wiley-Blackwell. 2010. p. 69–77.
120. Chivers SM, Einon DF. Effects of early social experience on activity and object investigation in the ferret. Dev Psychobiol 1982;15(1):75–80.
121. Johnson-Delaney CA. Ferret nutrition. Veterinary Clin North Am Exot Anim Pract 2014;17(3):449–70.
122. Orcutt CJ. Ferret urogenital diseases. Veterinary Clin North Am Exot Anim Pract 2003;6(1):113–38.
123. Church RR. The impact of diet on the dentition of the domesticated ferret. Exot DVM 2007;9(2):30–9.
124. Moody KD, Bowman TA, Lang CM. Laboratory management of the ferret for biomedical research. Lab Anim Sci 1985;35(3):272–9.
125. Phifer-Rixey M, Nachman MW. Insights into mammalian biology from the wild house mouse Mus musculus. eLife 2015;2015(4):1–13.

126. Frohlich J. Rats and mice. In: Quesenberry K, Orcutt C, Mans C, et al, editors. Ferrets, Rabbits and rodents: Clinical Medicine and Surgery. 4th edition. St Louis, Missouri: Elsevier; 2021. p. 345–67.
127. Latham N, Mason G. From house mouse to mouse house: The behavioural biology of free-living Mus musculus and its implications in the laboratory. In: Applied animal behaviour science, vol. 86. Elsevier; 2004. p. 261–89.
128. Jacoby RO, Fox JG, Davisson M. Biology and diseases of mice. In: Fox J, Anderson L, Loew F, et al, editors. Laboratory animal medicine. 2nd ed. London: Elsevier; 2002. p. 34–119.
129. Council on Animal Care C. Canadian council on animal care guidelines: animal data report 2019. 2019. Available at: www.ccac.ca. Accessed January 3, 2021.
130. Modlinska K, Pisula W. The natural history of model organisms: The Norway rat, from an obnoxious pest to a laboratory pet. eLife 2020;9.
131. Kohn DF, Clifford CB. Biology and diseases of rats. In: Fox J, Anderson L, Loew F, et al, editors. Laboratory animal medicine. 2nd ed. Elsevier; 2002. p. 121–66.
132. Smith G. Hamsters: Taxonomy and history. In: Suckow M, Stevens K, Wilson R, editors. The laboratory rabbit, Guinea pig, hamster, and other rodents. United States of America: Academic Press, Inc; 2012. p. 747–51.
133. Wang Y, Liu W, Wang G, et al. Home-range sizes of social groups of Mongolian gerbils Meriones unguiculatus. J Arid Environ 2011;75(2):132–7.
134. Gromov VS, Severtsov AN. Rodents and space: What behavior do we study under semi-natural and laboratory conditions?, . Rodents: habitat Pathology and environmental Impact. p: 43–59.
135. Batchelder M, Keller LS, Sauer MB, et al. Gerbils. In: Suckow M, Stevens K, Wilson R, editors. The laboratory rabbit, Guinea pig, hamster, and other rodents. London: Academic Press, Inc; 2012. p. 1132–49.
136. Council on Animal Care C. Canadian Council on Animal Care Guidelines: Mice. 2019. Available at: http://www.ccac.caacknowledgements. Accessed December 1, 2020.
137. Council on Animal Care C. Canadian Council on Animal Care Guidelines: Rats. 2019. Available at: http://www.ccac.caacknowledgements. Accessed December 1, 2020.
138. Lanteigne M, Reebs SG. Preference for bedding material in Syrian hamsters. Lab Anim 2006;40(4):410–8.
139. Hauzenberger AR, Gebhardt-Henrich SG, Steiger A. The influence of bedding depth on behaviour in golden hamsters (Mesocricetus auratus). Appl Anim Behav Sci 2006;100(3–4):280–94.
140. Gebhardt-Henrich SG, Vonlanthen EM, Steiger A. How does the running wheel affect the behaviour and reproduction of golden hamsters kept as pets? Appl Anim Behav Sci 2005;95(3–4):199–203.
141. Fitzgerald BM, Karl BJ, Moller H. Spatial organization and ecology of a sparse population of house mice (Mus musculus) in a New Zealand forest. J Anim Ecol 1981;50(2):489.
142. Laurie CC, Nickerson DA, Anderson AD, et al. Linkage disequilibrium in wild mice. In: Barsh G, editor. PloS Genet 2007;3(8):1487–95.
143. Combs M, Puckett EE, Richardson J, et al. Spatial population genomics of the brown rat (Rattus norvegicus) in New York City. Mol Ecol 2018;27(1):83–98.
144. Feng AYT, Himsworth CG. The secret life of the city rat: A review of the ecology of urban Norway and black rats (Rattus norvegicus and Rattus rattus). Urban Ecosyst 2014;17(1):149–62.

145. Gardner-Santana LC, Norris DE, Fornadel CM, et al. Commensal ecology, urban landscapes, and their influence on the genetic characteristics of city-dwelling Norway rats (Rattus norvegicus). Mol Ecol 2009;18(13):2766–78.

146. Inglis IR, Shepherd DS, Smith P, et al. Foraging behaviour of wild rats (Rattus norvegicus) towards new foods and bait containers. Appl Anim Behav Sci 1996;47(3–4):175–90.

147. Barnett SA, Spencer MM. Feeding, social behaviour and interspecific competition in wild rats. Behaviour 1951;3(3):229–42.

148. Macdonald DW, Fenn MGP. Rat ranges in arable areas. J Zool 1995;236(2): 349–53.

149. Calhoun JB. The Ecology and Sociology of the Norway rat. No. 1008. Bethesda, Maryland: US Department of Health, Education, and Welfare, Public Health Service; 1936.

150. Gattermann R, Fritzsche P, Neumann K, et al. Notes on the current distribution and the ecology of wild golden hamsters (Mesocricetus auratus). J Zool 2001; 254(3).

151. Mulder GB. Hamsters: management, husbandry, and colony health. In: The laboratory rabbit, Guinea pig, hamster, and other rodents. Suckow (MA): 2012. p. 765–75.

152. Miwa Y, Mayer J. Hamsters and gerbils. In: Quesenberry K, Orcutt C, Mans C, et al, editors. Ferrets, rabbits and rodents: Clinical medicine and Surgery. 2021. p. 368–84.

153. Ågren G, Zhou Q, Zhong W. Ecology and social behaviour of Mongolian gerbils, Meriones unguiculatus, at Xilinhot, Inner Mongolia, China. Anim Behav 1989; 37(PART 1):28–32.

154. Swanson HH, Lockley MR. Population growth and social structure of confined colonies of mongolian gerbils: Scent gland size and marking behaviour as indices of social status. Aggress Behav 1978;4(1):57–89.

155. Scheibler E, Weinandy R, Gattermann R. Social categories in families of Mongolian gerbils. Physiol Behav 2004;81(3):455–64.

156. Roper TJ, Polioudakis E. The Behaviour of Mongolian Gerbils in a semi-natural environment, with special reference to ventral marking, dominance and sociability. Behaviour 2008;61(3–4):207–36.

157. Clark MM, Galef BG. Socially induced infertility: familial effects on reproductive development of female Mongolian gerbils. Anim Behav 2001;62:897–903.

158. Clark MM, Galef BG. Why some male Mongolian gerbils may help at the nest: testosterone, asexuality and alloparenting. Anim Behav 2000;59:801–6.

159. Sayers I, Smith S. Mice, rats, hamsters and gerbils. In: Meredith A, Lord B, editors. BSAVA manual of exotic pets. Gloucester, UK: BSAVA; 2018. p. 1–27.

160. Council NR. Nutrient requirements of laboratory animals 1995. United States of America.

161. Naumova EI, Zharova GK, Chistova TY. Isolating structures of gerbils' digestive tract (Gerbillidae, Rhombomys, Meriones) and their functional significance. Biol Bull 2011;38(4):379–85.

Managing Disease Outbreaks in Captive Herds of Exotic Companion Mammals

Amber Lee, BVSc, DABVP (Avian Practice)

KEYWORDS

- Herd health • Exotic companion mammals • Epizootic • Infectious diseases
- Outbreak

KEY POINTS

- Diseases that cause epizootics in small mammal herds occur subsequent to inadequate husbandry, inappropriate diet, and stress.
- Many diseases occur because of the stress of weaning so anticipating this and maximizing sanitation and ventilation, minimizing overcrowding and concurrent disease, and providing enough fiber for herbivores is prudent.
- When approaching the diagnosis of a disease in an outbreak, it is important to be knowledgeable in the common etiologic agents and their zoonotic potential.
- Knowledge of route of administration and the adverse effects of drugs used in these species is paramount from the standpoint of risk of enterotoxemia development postantibiotic use.
- Preventative medicine with vaccines, quarantine, and regular disease screening of herds allows for early disease detection and reduction in mortality in the face of an outbreak.

INTRODUCTION

The exotic animal veterinarian is likely comfortable with the medicine of individually owned animals, but may not be familiar with the treatment of exotic companion mammal herds. The diagnosis and treatment of epizootics in exotic companion mammal herds has foundations in laboratory and pet animal medicine; however, production aspects of husbandry and management must not be overlooked. Epizootics of multiple animals should use the same systematic approach as individual animal situations.[1]

Diseases that cause epizootics in small mammal herds occur subsequent to inadequate husbandry, inappropriate diet, and stress. Ventilation, sanitation, and observation are paramount in disease control. Air dilution through ventilation is an effective

The Unusual Pet Vets, 210 Karingal Drive, Frankston, VIC 3199, Australia
E-mail address: birdvetamber@gmail.com
Twitter: DrAmberLee (A.L.)

Vet Clin Exot Anim 24 (2021) 567–608
https://doi.org/10.1016/j.cvex.2021.04.003
1094-9194/21/© 2021 Elsevier Inc. All rights reserved.

method of reducing the numbers of some pathogens. Physical or chemical removal of organisms is also important. This includes removal of manure and hair, and disinfection of cages and the environment. Fluctuations in temperature, humidity, and dust have effects on host susceptibility, and environmental load and proliferation of pathogens. Likewise, the density of animals also affects sanitation levels and concentration of organisms. Control of insect vectors, wild rodents, and birds is also of importance in limiting spread of disease to naive populations. Prey species are capable of hiding signs of illness and careful observation for subtle changes in behavior, feed/water intake, stool production, and breathing patterns can lead to detection of disease if noticed early.

Organisms that cause disease affect a younger, immunologically incompetent population and are exacerbated by the stresses of weaning.[2] Additional stressors that affect these animals include transportation to veterinary facilities or from vendors, concurrent diseases, handling for physical examination and/diagnostic procedures, disruption of normal biorhythms, incorrect light intensity and cycles, overall room activity, overcrowding, and excessive noise.[1]

When approaching the diagnosis of a disease in an outbreak, it is important to be knowledgeable in the common etiologic agents and their zoonotic potential. The use of screening diagnostics (polymerase chain reaction [PCR], culture, serology) for certain pathogens is an important way of early disease detection in a herd. The use of necropsy in the face of an outbreak also becomes important in identifying characteristic organ lesions and submission of tissues for histopathologic and microbiologic confirmation of pathogens.

In the assessment of the prevalence of clinical disease, infection, or seropositive animals, samples are taken from individuals or may be obtained from groups, herds, or administrative regions.[3] The classification of herds as positive or negative for certain diseases is an important but crude measure for infection status. The prevalence of disease at the animal-level gives more accurate information.[4,5] Various mathematic models are used to estimate animal-level prevalence from pooled samples.[4,6] Samples from multiple animals or groups of animals may be pooled and tested to reduce costs.[7] The general pooled-sample testing approach for identifying individually infected animals is to initially test pools of samples, and then to retest individual samples from groups that were positive. This avoids testing most individual negative samples.[8] In herd testing typically 10 to 20 animals are tested, or even 5 to 60.[5] The main advantage of pooling is increased population-level coverage when disease prevalence is low (<10%) and most samples are expected to test negative.[7,8] Disadvantages of pooled-sample testing include false-negative results from sample dilution lower than the level detectable by the assay and false-positive results from cross-contamination of samples or pools and cross-reaction from other agents that may be detected by the assay.[8]

Treatment at the herd level is different from the individual. Often, for serious diseases depopulation and restocking with disease-free animals may be the best option, but may not be commercially viable. Therefore, focus may be on separation of affected individuals and limiting spread of disease through the herd. Knowledge of adverse effects of drugs used in these species is paramount from the standpoint of risk of enterotoxemia development postantibiotic use. Preventative medicine, with quarantine of new animals and vaccines where available, is also important to help reduce spread and minimize clinical signs associated with disease.

Route of administration of medications needs to be considered carefully, given the species involved (Appendix Table 1). For large groups in-water or in-feed treatment may be easy to administer but medications may not be as efficacious in those formulations. For skin diseases, such as dermatophytosis in rodents, bathing individuals may not be practical and probably causes excessive stress to the animal.[9] For many of the gastrointestinal pathogens of herbivores, reducing stress, providing a high-fiber diet, and optimal husbandry practices, such as appropriate disinfection and judicious use of antibiotics, helps control and prevent disease outbreaks.

RESPIRATORY PATHOGENS OF EXOTIC COMPANION MAMMALS
Bacterial and Viral Diseases of Rabbits and Rodents

Pasteurella multocida (zoonosis)
Pasteurella multocida is a gram-negative coccobacillus that is part of the microbiota of the respiratory tract of many domestic and wild animals (**Tables 1** and **2**).[10] Multiple zoonotic infections with P multocida have been reported, mostly through bites from dogs or cats but also nonbite transmissions have occurred from various species.[11] P multocida is one of the most common bacterial pathogens of rabbits and is spread rapidly by direct contact, fomites, and aerosolization within a room.[10,12] Infection occurs at a young age with transmission from dams to offspring during birth or lactation.[12] The disease begins in the nasal cavity resulting in rhinitis or asymptomatic chronic infection. Following this carrier state, the organism then spreads from the respiratory tract to the nasolacrimal ducts, eustachian tubes, trachea, hematogenously, or venereally.[10,12] Clinical manifestation of pasteurellosis in rabbits can include several syndromes (**Figs. 1** and **2, Table 3**).

Definitive diagnosis is made by culture of the organism.[12] Cultures of the nares are inexpensive and easy to perform; however, studies evaluating the reliability suggest about 30% of infected animals may not be detected on a single culture.[13,14] This may be caused by lower numbers of organisms in the nares or the infection is localized to other parts of the body.[12,15] The proportion of infected animals increases with age, with 60% to 90% of adult rabbits from endemically infected herds harboring the organism in the nasal passages.[12,15] In determining prevalence of infection within a herd, testing by age groups is recommended (preweanlings, 12 week old, 22 week old, and adults).[15] In laboratory settings, it seems prudent to perform three sequential cultures before an animal is considered Pasteurella-free.[12]

For screening colonies, enzyme-linked immunosorbent assay (ELISA) or PCR is helpful.[10,16] ELISA can detect antibody in up to 98% of nasal culture–positive animals.[12] Furthermore, ELISA was able to detect antibody about 10% of rabbits that were negative by nasal culture, suggesting false-negative culture results in those animals.[17] A P multocida–specific PCR assay has been described and shown to correlate well with conventional methods of identification.[18]

Treatment with antibiotics can reduce symptoms but does not eradicate disease.[16] Based on sensitivity results from Rougier and coworkers[19] and Quinton and coworkers,[20] fluoroquinolones, such as enrofloxacin and marbofloxacin, are likely to be effective against most bacterial strains with the exception of Bordetella bronchiseptica.[19] The clinical forms most likely to respond to therapy are rhinitis, conjunctivitis, and subcutaneous abscesses, because the other forms are diagnosed too late in the stages of disease.[21]

Control is focused on prevention with barrier housing, vaccination, and antimicrobial prophylaxis because therapy is only marginally effective.[21] Treatment of does with enrofloxacin (5 mg/kg intramuscularly or 200 mg/kg in water, treated from Day 14 of gestation to kindling) may be more effective than other antibiotics in producing Pasteurella-free offspring.[22] Control in rabbitries often entails testing and culling infected animals because antibiotics are not capable of eliminating disease.[12,16,22] Stress

Table 1
Bacterial respiratory pathogens of rabbits and rodents[1,23,26,28,32,35,39,40,47,57,59,62]

Species	Organisms	Comments
Rabbit (*Oryctolagus cuniculus*)	*Pasteurella multocida* *Bordetella bronchiseptica* *Pseudomonas* spp *Staphylococcus* spp	Most common bacteria isolated from respiratory tract of rabbits
Guinea pig (*Cavia porcellus*)	*B bronchiseptica** *Streptococcus pneumoniae** *Klebsiella pneumoniae* *P multocida* *Streptococcus equi* subsp. *zooepidemicus* *Citrobacter freundii* *Pseudomonas aeruginosa*	*Most common etiologic agents
Chinchilla (*Chinchilla lanigera*)	*Pasteurella* spp *Streptococcus* spp *B bronchiseptica* *Staphylococcus aureus* *P aeruginosa* *K pneumoniae* *Listeria monocytogenes*	Most common bacterial isolated from respiratory tract of chinchillas
Rat (*Rattus norvegicus*)	*Mycoplasma pulmonis** *S pneumoniae** *Corynebacterium kutscheri** Sendai virus[+] Pneumonia virus of mice[+] *Pneumocystis carinii* (a fungus)[+] CAR bacillus[+] *Haemophilus* sp[+]	*Major pathogens [+]Minor pathogens act synergistically with major pathogens as copathogens to produce 2 major clinical syndrome: chronic respiratory disease and bacterial pneumonia
Mice (*Mus musculus*)	*M pulmonis*	Primary bacterial pneumonia is uncommon unless immunosuppressed or stressed Concurrent infection with Sendai virus or CAR bacillus can lead to a fatal pneumonia
Hamsters (Family: Cricetidae)	*Streptococcus* spp *Pasteurella pneumotropica*	Uncommon
Gerbils (*Meriones unguiculatus*)	*P pneumotropica* *B bronchiseptica* CAR bacillus *M pulmonis* *S pneumoniae*	Disease caused by natural infection is rare

Abbreviation: CAR, cilia-associated respiratory.
* Designates "Most common etiologic agents" (in the Guinea pig row).
* Designates "Major pathogens" (in the rat row).
+ Designates "Minor pathogens that act synergistically with major pathogens as copathogens to produce 2 major clinical syndromes: chronic respiratory disease and bacterial pneumonia" (in the rat row).

Table 2
Viral respiratory pathogens of rodents[1,32,33,47,84,85]

Organism Features	Species and Age Susceptibility	Clinical Signs/Lesions	Diagnosis	Treatment/Comments
Sendai virus (Paramyxoviridae)	Mice, rats, hamsters, and guinea pigs Suckling and weanling mice most affected Usually self-limiting in rats	Weight loss, dyspnea, chattering sounds, eye crusting (mice) Reduction in litter sizes with occasional respiratory signs (rats)	Multiplex fluorescent immunoassay	Virus acts to suppress normal antibacterial activity of lungs, which predisposes mice to secondary bacterial infection (eg, *Mycoplasma pulmonis*) Antibiotics may be beneficial in prevention and treatment
Pneumonia virus of mice (Paramyxoviridae)	Mice, rats, hamsters, gerbils, guinea pigs, and rabbits	Multifocal, nonsuppurative vasculitis, and interstitial pneumonitis	Serology or PCR	Significant copathogen for *M pulmonis*
Rat respiratory virus (Bunyviridae) Zoonosis	Wild rodents (rats) are natural reservoirs	Chronic and subclinical		Serious zoonotic risk for humans from rats shedding Seoul Hantavirus causing hemorrhagic fever with renal syndrome
Sialodacryoadenitis virus (Coronavirus)	Young rats	Rhinitis, epithelial necrosis, and swelling of salivary and lacrimal glands and cervical lymph nodes Keratoconjunctivitis	Serology or PCR	Largely supportive with ophthalmic preparations Control wild rodent access Rats only shed virus for 1 wk, then they are immune and not latently infected

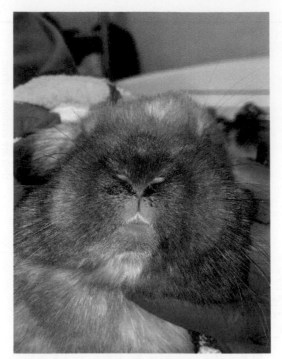

Fig. 1. Rabbit with nasal discharge typical of pasteurellosis.

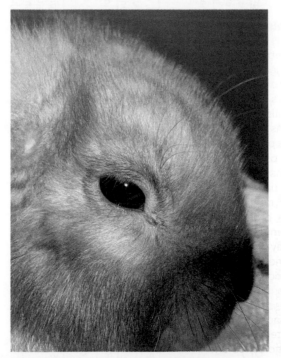

Fig. 2. Rabbit with conjunctivitis typical of pasteurellosis.

Table 3 Syndromes of pasteurellosis in rabbits[10,16,19,23,65]	
Rhinitis	Serous-mucopurulent nasal discharge (see **Fig. 1**) Exudate on the inside of forelimbs Turbinate atrophy with some strains
Conjunctivitis	Ocular discharge, chemosis, and conjunctival hyperemia (see **Fig. 2**) Epiphora as only sign, and infection limited to the nasolacrimal duct
Pneumonia	Acutely; variable consolidation of lungs with cyanosis Chronically; often asymptomatic, may have anorexia, depression, dyspnea, moist lung sounds, and sudden death Pulmonary abscesses, pleuritis, and pyothorax
Otitis	Vestibular signs; ataxia, head tilt, and torticollis Otitis media; signs can be absent Rule out infection with *Encephalitozoon cuniculi*
Genital	Pyometra, metritis, orchitis, or epididymitis Massive uterine dilation must be differentiated from uterine adenocarcinoma
Abscesses	Subcutaneous masses; thick, white-yellow caseous purulent debris Occur around the head, neck and shoulders or internal organs
Septicemia	Rapid death with or without other clinical forms of pasteurellosis
Miscellaneous	Any organ involved; osteomyelitis, iritis/uveitis and meningoencephalitis ± otitis media

reduction is another important part of prevention of disease through providing optimal husbandry, including diet, exercise, ventilation, and proper sanitation.[23]

Bordetella bronchiseptica (zoonosis)

B bronchiseptica is a gram-negative rod that is a common inhabitant of the upper respiratory tract of rabbits, dogs, cats, and guinea pigs.[10] High morbidity and mortality rates in guinea pigs have been seen.[24] Naturally infected rabbits generally remain free of respiratory disease unless concurrently infected with *P multocida* or other pathogens.[21] Hamsters and mice are not as susceptible as other rodents. The organism can cause zoonotic infections, although the risk in transmission from rodents and lagomorphs seems minimal compared with rates of infection from dogs.[25]

Younger guinea pigs and pregnant sows are particularly at risk and can have no clinical signs or may present with dyspnea, nasal discharge, sneezing, anorexia, ruffled fur, and weight loss (**Fig. 3**).[24,26] Otitis media with a head tilt may also be seen.[24] Transmission is primarily through aerosol, but also fomites and from other infected species, such as rabbits or dogs.[24,26,27] Of the several bacterial and viral agents that cause acute bronchopneumonia in guinea pigs, *Bordetella* sp infection has been the most common diagnosis because of its ease of culture. ELISA and immunofluorescence assay (IFA) serology are more sensitive than culture for organism detection; however, various antigenic variants should be used in serologic testing because of serotypic variation within guinea pigs.[26]

Treatment of bacterial pneumonia should be based on culture and sensitivity results but first-line options include: fluoroquinolones, trimethoprim-sulfa, and chloramphenicol.[27,28] The efficacy of canine, porcine, human, and autologous *Bordetella* vaccines have been evaluated and results suggest that although not completely protective they seem to reduce incidence and severity of disease in experimentally challenged animals.[24] Recovered guinea pigs may act as carriers for other in-contact guinea pigs,

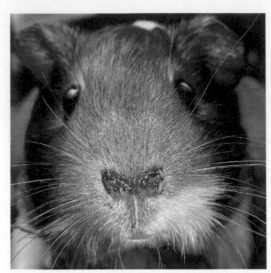

Fig. 3. Guinea pig with nasal discharge typical of infection with *Bordetella bronchiseptica*.

therefore restocking or testing and culling of a herd may be more beneficial than treatment.[24,29]

Streptococcus pneumoniae (zoonosis)

Streptococcus pneumoniae is gram-positive, α-hemolytic, and oval-lancet-shaped organism that has been isolated from several mammalian species. Rats and guinea pigs are most susceptible to this pathogen. Several different serotypes affect rats and guinea pigs and some of these serotypes can infect humans.[25] Transmission is through respiratory aerosol, direct contact with subclinical carriers (including humans), or vertically during birth.[24,26]

Clinical signs if present in guinea pigs include high mortality or depression, anorexia, oculonasal discharge, sneezing, coughing, dyspnea, torticollis, and stillbirths or abortion.[28] Diagnosis is based on gram-stained impression smears or culture. Antibiotic treatment usually leads to a subclinical carrier state so removal of affected animals is recommended. In the face of epizootic outbreak, chloramphenicol (30–50 mg/kg orally every 12 hours for 7–21 days[30]; or 1 mg/mL in water),[31] trimethoprim-sulfa (15–30 mg/kg orally every 12 hours),[29] and tetracyclines (10–20 mg/kg every 8–12 hours, with caution because toxicities reported)[28] are used.[24]

Bacterial pneumonia in rats is nearly always caused by *S pneumoniaiae*, usually in combination with *Mycoplasma pulmonis*, Sendai virus, or cilia-associated respiratory (CAR) bacillus.[32] The disease is usually subacute to acute in younger animals with sudden death usually the only clinical sign. Adults may have dyspnea, snuffling, and abdominal breathing with purulent nasal discharge. Treatment must be aggressive, and amoxicillin/clavulanic acid (20 mg/kg orally every 12 hours) is the antibiotic of choice.[32] Penicillin administered subcutaneously or oxytetracycline in drinking water are alternatives.[33]

Streptococcus zooepidemicus (zoonosis)

Streptococcus equi subsp. *zooepidemicus* is a gram-positive, β-hemolytic organism that guinea pigs can carry subclinically in the nasopharynx and conjunctiva.[26] This pyogenic bacterium is associated with suppuration and abscess formation in guinea

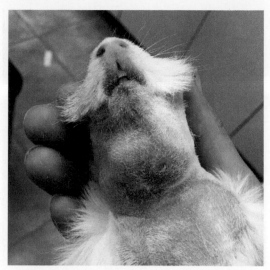

Fig. 4. Guinea pig cervical lymphadenitis caused by infection with *Streptococcus zooepidemicus*.

pigs, usually in the cervical lymph nodes (**Fig. 4**). *Streptobacillus moniliformis* (transmitted from wild rodents) and other *Streptococcus* spp are sometimes implicated.[26,29] Other signs may include torticollis, oculonasal discharge, dyspnea, cyanosis, hematuria and hemoglobinuria, cyanotic and engorged mammary glands, abortions and stillbirths, and sudden death.[24,28] Transmission is via aerosol onto respiratory, oropharyngeal, conjunctival, or female genital epithelium. Prevention in guinea pigs is aimed at feeding nonabrasive feed (crude fiber may abrade the pharyngeal mucosa), trimming overgrown or broken teeth, and using feeders that do not abrade the skin of the neck.[24,26] Control is best achieved by culling affected animals before the rupture of infectious abscess contents and appropriate environmental sanitation because animals treated with antibiotics may become carriers and remain infective.[28] Empirical antibiotic therapy includes enrofloxacin, gentamicin, trimethoprim-sulfa, or chloramphenicol.[24,26,28] There is the possibility for zoonotic transmission for humans working with guinea pigs.[29,34]

S *zooepidemicus* has been reported in chinchillas with increasing frequency over the past decade.[34–37] These reports include cases with conjunctivitis and subcutaneous abscesses, but pyometra and otitis have also been reported anecdotally.[37] For farmed chinchillas, sulfadimethoxine administered in water has been used in outbreaks.[37] It is currently unknown if chinchillas treated with antibiotics remain carriers and contagious to other individuals.[37]

Chlamydophilosis (zoonosis)

Chlamydophila caviae and *Chlamydophila psittaci* have been reported to cause conjunctivitis, rhinitis, bronchitis, and pneumonia in guinea pigs (**Fig. 5**).[27,29] *Chlamydophila* spp are gram-negative, obligate intracellular organisms. Diagnosis is with cytology or PCR or conjunctival scrapings and treatment with ophthalmic tetracyclines or fluoroquinolones with the addition or systemic antibiotics in severe cases.[27,29] C *caviae* should be considered a potential human pathogen because of a recent report describing respiratory failure in three people.[38]

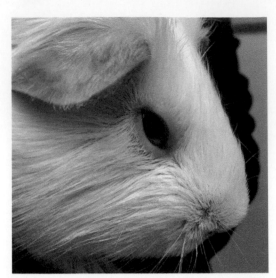

Fig. 5. Guinea pig with conjunctivitis typical of infection with *Chlamydophila caviae*.

Pseudomonas aeruginosa (zoonosis)

Pseudomonas aeruginosa is a gram-negative, aerobic, rod-shaped bacterium that causes infections and epizootics in chinchillas.[39] The organism is not a normal inhabitant of the enteric flora but is an opportunistic agent that occurs in moist environments or contaminated water supply.[37,40] The organism has been cultured from healthy pet and laboratory animals and infection occurs when host defenses are low or the animal has been exposed to high infective doses.[35,41,42] Clinical signs include conjunctivitis, otitis, dermal pustules, anorexia, weight loss, enteritis, mesenteric lymphadenopathy, pneumonia, sepsis, and death.[39,43]

Control focuses on water quality and reducing colonization of organisms through chlorination (10–13 ppm) or acidification (pH 2.5–3.0).[39] There are widespread multidrug-resistant strains whereby trimethoprim-sulfonamide combinations, chloramphenicol, and tetracyclines are ineffective; therefore, culture and sensitivity is recommended.[35,37] Typically, susceptible drugs include fluoroquinolones, third-generation cephalosporins, and aminoglycosides (amikacin). For ocular infections topical polymyxin B and gentamicin formulations are effective.[35] *P aeruginosa* can cause nosocomial infections in humans, so disinfection practices are important after handling animals or cleaning their cages.[41]

Mycoplasma pulmonis

M pulmonis is the major pathogen of chronic respiratory disease in rats, also known as murine respiratory mycoplasmosis. It can also be associated with genital tract infections. Other bacteria (eg, CAR bacillus, *S pneumoniae*, *B bronchiseptica*) and viruses (eg, Sendai, sialodacryoadenitis) are often isolated from the lungs of infected rats.[32,33] *M pulmonis* is transmitted by direct contact between an infected dam and her offspring, by intrauterine or venereal transfer, and by aerosol. The organism has a tropism for the epithelial cells of the respiratory tract, middle ear, and endometrium.[32] Clinical signs are variable; many cases are asymptomatic, although significant pulmonary lesions may exist. Generally clinical disease is slowly progressive with prevalence and severity of signs increased in older animals and with the presence of environmental stressors (eg, high ammonia), concurrent respiratory pathogens, genetic susceptibility of host, virulence of strain, and vitamin A or E deficiency.[33,44]

Serous nasal discharge, sneezing, nasal congestion, and chromodacryorrhea may be early clinical signs. Bronchitis presents with labored breathing, weight loss, lethargy, a hunched posture, and rough hair coat.[33,45] When the infection travels via the eustachian tube to the middle ear a head tilt can develop.[33] Clinical signs associated with genital mycoplasmosis include infertility and fetal and neonatal deaths.[45] Diagnosis is based on history, clinical signs, organism isolation, and gross and microscopic lesions. A serum ELISA is the most rapid tool for screening colonies.[33,45] Tetracycline antibiotics are efficacious in treating chronic respiratory disease; oxytetracycline, tetracycline, or doxycycline added to the drinking water suppresses but does not eliminate disease. For individuals oral or parenteral doxycycline, enrofloxacin, or chloramphenicol may help.[32] Newer reports suggest that *M pulmonis* could be a potential zoonotic pathogen, with people exposed developing significant titers suggestive of active infection.[46]

Corynebacterium kutscheri (zoonosis)
Corynebacterium kutscheri is a gram-positive rod that is routinely isolated from the nasopharynx of rats; mice and hamsters can also be carriers.[1,25] The organism causes pneumonia only rarely, and in conjunction with debilitation and immunosuppression in older animals.[33] Abscesses may be found in many organs, hence its alternate name pseudotuberculosis. Transmission is through direct contact, and diagnosis through culture from the submandibular lymph nodes.[1] Antibiotic treatment includes ampicillin, chloramphenicol, and tetracycline but may not be efficacious in acute epizootics and can lead to a carrier state.[1,33] This organism has been isolated from a human case of chorioamnionitis so rodents should be considered a potential reservoir source.[25]

Cilia-associated respiratory bacillus
CAR bacillus is found between and parallel to the cilia of the respiratory epithelium. The organism is a notable pathogen in rats, rabbits, and mice and has been found in wild rats, hamsters, and guinea pigs.[1] In mice, the infection is opportunistic and frequently associated with other respiratory copathogens. Treatment with sulfamerazine or ampicillin has been reported to be efficacious in eliminating colonization of the organisms and reducing severity of clinical signs.[47] Infections in rats are usually asymptomatic but lifelong. Diagnosis is with histology or ELISA or PCR in screening colonies.[1]

Respiratory Pathogens of Ferrets

Bacterial
Pneumonia is not common in ferrets; viral causes include canine distemper virus (CDV) and influenza virus. It may appear as part of a systemic infection, such as with Aleutian disease and ferret systemic coronavirus.[48] Bacteria commonly associated with pneumonia in ferrets include: *S zooepidemicus* and other group C and G streptococci, *Escherichia coli*, *Klebsiella pneumoniae*, *Pseudomonas* spp, *B bronchiseptica*, *Listeria monocytogenes*, and numerous mycobacterial species.[48] Recently, a novel *Mycoplasma* sp was isolated from pet ferrets after an outbreak from a single source.[49]

Clinical signs in ferrets with pneumonia include: nasal discharge, labored breathing, dyspnea, lethargy, anorexia, increased lung sounds, cyanosis, and fever. Fulminant pneumonia may progress to sepsis and death.[48] Diagnosis is based on history, clinical signs, a complete blood cell count, culture or cytology of a tracheal or lung wash, and radiographs.[48,50]

Treatment of pneumonia includes antibiotics, supportive care, oxygen, fluids, force feeding, and managing husbandry to minimize stress and overcrowding.

Antimicrobials efficacious in the treatment of bacterial pneumonia include: amoxicillin/clavulanate, fluoroquinolones, trimethoprim-sulfamethoxazole, or a cephalosporin.[48]

Viral

Canine distemper. CDV is a paramyxovirus, of genus Morbillivirus, related to measles and rinderpest.[48,50,51] CDV is the most serious viral infection of ferrets because mortality approaches 100%; vaccination and appropriate husbandry are vital.[48,51] There are two phases of CDV: the catarrhal phase and then the fatal neurotropic phase. The catarrhal phase is associated with anorexia, pyrexia, photosensitivity, and serous nasal discharge. Skin lesions include an erythematous pruritic rash from the chin to inguinal region and hyperkeratosis of footpads. The central nervous system signs include: hyperexcitability, muscle tremors, ataxia, hypersalivation, seizures, and coma.[48,50,51]

CDV is transmitted by direct contact with conjunctival and nasal exudate, urine, feces, and skin.[51,52] Presumptive diagnosis is based on clinical signs, questionable vaccine history, and exposure. Diagnostic tests include: fluorescent antibody test or reverse transcriptase PCR. During outbreaks, affected animals should be isolated, and the remainder of the colony vaccinated. Vaccinate with modified live vaccine of chicken embryo tissue culture origin. Kits should be vaccinated every 2 to 3 weeks starting at 6 weeks, until 14 weeks, and annually thereafter.[52] Humane euthanasia of affected animals is recommended because of the invariably fatal disease.[51]

Human influenza virus (zoonosis). Ferrets are susceptible to influenza types A and B of the class Orthomyxovirus. Natural epizootics occur with human influenza type A, the human strain of pandemic H1N1 virus, and swine-origin H1N1 influenza virus.[48,53] Transmission is more likely from infected humans.[54] Generally influenza infection in ferrets is mild with pyrexia, respiratory signs (sneezing, oculonasal discharge, coughing), lethargy, anorexia, photophobia, and conjunctivitis.[50] Severe cases in older animals may progress to bronchitis, pneumonia, or central nervous system signs.[41] In adults, disease is usually self-limiting, with a 5- to 7-day course typical. Diagnosis is based on typical clinical presentation and short course of disease. The use of virus isolation or hemagglutinin-inhibiting antibody titers are not usually required for diagnosis.[48] An ELISA has been developed for rapid testing.[50] Treatment is with supportive care and if signs progress antibiotics, bronchodilators, cough suppressants, decongestants.

Fungal

Pulmonary mycoses in ferrets seem to be uncommon.[55] Several cases involving *Blastomyces*, *Coccidioides*, *Cryptococcus*, and *Histoplasma* have been described.[50] The reservoir of most of these fungi is the soil, so in production facilities, selection of source animals, appropriate sanitation, and control of pests, particularly birds is important. Prognosis for systemic mycotic infections is usually guarded and treatment mimics therapies used in dogs and cats (itraconazole).[50,55]

GASTROINTESTINAL PATHOGENS OF EXOTIC COMPANION MAMMALS

Enteric diseases are second only to pasteurellosis as a health problem in domestic rabbits.[56] Diarrhea and sometimes sudden death may be associated with a specific, well-defined etiologic agent, but in many cases the cause of disease is not obvious. Specific enteric diseases include coccidia (*Eimeria* spp), rotavirus, and such bacteria as Clostridia, Coliforms, and *Salmonella*.[2] Enterotoxemia refers to enteropathy caused by toxigenic clostridial organisms. Diseases with uncertain cause include colibacillosis

Table 4
Gastrointestinal bacterial pathogens of exotic companion mammals[9,10,12,24,27,28,33,35,39,43,47,50,59,60,63–65,80,86–90]

Organism Features	Species and Age Susceptibility	Clinical Signs/Lesions	Diagnosis	Treatment
Tyzzer disease *Clostridium piliforme* Pleomorphic, gram-negative, spore-forming, motile obligate intracellular rod-shaped bacteria	Rabbits: weanlings 6–12 wk of age, mortality can approach >50% Gerbils highly susceptible Outbreaks in hamsters more sporadic	Acute profuse watery diarrhea, sudden death (12–48 h) Necrosis of cecum, intestine, liver, and heart Chronic cases weight loss, cachexia, and intestinal fibrosis	Serology Histology	Generally unrewarding Reduce stress during weaning, removal of spores Tetracyclines or chloramphenicol are used to suppress infection but may be ineffective in outbreaks[26,29,43–46,48]
Enterotoxemia *Clostridium spiroforme* Gram-positive, spore-bearing, helically coiled, semicircular, anaerobic bacteria that produces iota toxin	Rabbits: weanlings age 4–8 weeks old, exposure alone is enough to induce disease	Acute diarrhea, anorexia, hypothermia, and moribund progressing to death in 24–48 h Petechial and ecchymotic hemorrhages on serosal surface of cecum	Gram-staining Anaerobic culture toxin detection assays PCR	Little evidence for antibiotic efficacy Vaccination with toxoid
Enterotoxemia *Clostridium difficile* Gram-positive, spore-forming, anaerobic bacillus	Newly weaned animals are most susceptible also secondary to antibiotic use	Anorexia, diarrhea, fecal staining of perineum, decreased fecal output, abdominal distention and peracute death without signs	Isolation and toxin assays	Largely supportive
Clostridium perfringens type A	Weanling ferrets; overeating or supplementation of liver mix was cause of bacterial overgrowth and toxin production	Abdominal distention, dyspnea, and cyanosis, sudden death	Isolation of organism or toxin identification	Good management and feeding practices; restricting feeding 2 twice daily rather than three times daily[49]

(continued on next page)

Table 4
(continued)

Organism Features	Species and Age Susceptibility	Clinical Signs/Lesions	Diagnosis	Treatment
Colibacillosis *Escherichia coli:* EPEC and STEC are associated with enzootic disease in rabbits EHEC is a subset of STEC Zoonosis	Rabbits: Weanlings (4–6 weeks old) more common than sucklings (1–2 weeks old) Guinea pigs, chinchillas, hamsters, mice	Sucklings: severe yellowish diarrhea and high mortality Weanlings: 2 types 1st profuse liquid diarrhea, dehydration, weight loss and high mortality within 5–14 d 2nd mild diarrhea, growth retardation, and minimal mortality Thickening of ileum, cecum, and colon; paintbrush hemorrhages on serosal surfaces; enterocolitis, nephropathy, and thrombotic microangiopathy in EHEC	Histology Culture microscopy serotyping biotyping PCR cELISA	Largely supportive care; severe cases unrewarding but mild diarrhea may respond
Proliferative bowel disease *Lawsonia intracellularis* Gram-negative, curved to spiral-shaped, obligate intracellular bacteria	Ferrets, rabbits, hamsters Rabbits: weanlings Hamsters: 3–10 wk of age Ferrets: 12–24 wk old	Hamsters: Unkempt hair coat; anorexia; fecal staining of perineum; fetid, watery diarrhea; and dehydration **(Fig. 6)** Ferrets: Green diarrhea of >6 wk duration, severe weight loss, rectal prolapse and dehydration Severe cases, ataxia and muscle tremors Occasional deaths	Gross and microscopic lesions, PCR or ELISA, culture Ferrets: palpably thickened colon, colonic biopsy, with silver stain or PCR	Fluid and nutritional support important Rabbits: treatment usually ineffective, decreasing food intake when shipping and for 48 h post Hamsters: Tetracycline or metronidazole in dw, oral or parenteral enrofloxacin (10 mg/kg q 12 h for 10 d), or trimethoprim-sulfa (30 mg/kg PO q 12 h for 5–7 d) Ferrets: Chloramphenicol 50 mg/kg q 12 h at least 10 d

Disease / Organism	Species affected	Clinical signs	Diagnosis	Treatment / Control
Salmonellosis *S enterica* serotypes Typhimurium or Enteritidis Gram-negative, facultative, anaerobic bacilli Zoonosis	Many mammals affected: rabbits, guinea pigs, hamsters, mice, rats, ferrets (rare), sugar gliders, hedgehogs Late pregnant, weanling, aged and malnourished guinea pigs most susceptible	Primarily septicemic condition (rapid death), can cause diarrhea, respiratory signs and abortion Guinea pigs may exhibit rough hair coats, weakness, conjunctivitis, abortion, and light-colored feces or intermittent diarrhea Vascular congestion of organs and petechial hemorrhages	Culture	Treatment not recommended because of zoonotic risk, antibiotic use causes subclinical infection, and leads to antibiotic resistance Control: depopulate and sanitize caging and equipment thoroughly, restocking with disease-free animals
Listeriosis *Listeria monocytogenes* Pleomorphic, motile, non-spore-forming, β-hemolytic, gram-positive bacillus that inhabits the soil Zoonosis	Chinchillas most susceptible Ferrets may serve as source for zoonotic infection	Anorexia, diarrhea, depression, ataxia, circling, convulsions, and paralysis The disease is usually peracute with death occurring within 48–72 h of signs	Clinical signs, culture and immunohisto-chemistry	Prevention and control: disinfection of cages, water and feed containers, and dust baths; removal of infected feed or hay Treatment of moribund animals is not recommended because of zoonosis
Yersinia spp *Yersinia pseudotuberculosis, Y enterocolitica* Ingestion of contaminated food, by inhalation, or through dermal lacerations Zoonosis	Chinchillas	Acute: septicemia, Chronic: anorexia, depression, weight loss, intermittent diarrhea, or sudden death Mesenteric lymphadenopathy is pathognomonic	Observation of organisms or culture	Treatment with tetracyclines can be attempted but is usually ineffective[32] Because of zoonosis and persistent carrier states, euthanasia is recommended
Plague *Yersinia pestis* Flea-borne vectors Zoonosis	Black-footed ferret, squirrels, chipmunks, prairie dogs, mice	3 forms: bubonic, pneumonic, and septicemic	Gram staining of abscesses, culture, fluorescent antibody test	No cases of plague have been associated with exotic companion mammals in the United States, but have been in guinea pigs in Andean countries (food production)[50]

(continued on next page)

Table 4
(continued)

Organism Features	Species and Age Susceptibility	Clinical Signs/Lesions	Diagnosis	Treatment
Campylobacter *Campylobacter jejuni* Zoonosis	Ferrets	Young, self-limiting, mild-watery mucinous diarrhea Abortion	Special culture requirements (microaerophilic) PCR of intestine	Isolate, provide supportive care and antibiotics based on culture and sensitivity Azithromycin and fluoroquinolones are commonly used in humans
Helicobacter spp *H cinaedi*, which is a significant pathogen of immunocompromised humans *H aurati*, significant in older hamsters *H mustelae*, ferrets Zoonosis	Hamsters Ferrets: 5–6 wk and prevalent in adult population, colonizes nearly 100% of ferrets after weaning	Hamsters usually asymptomatic Ferrets: gastritis, gastroduodenal ulcers Vomiting, chronic weight loss, low hematocrit, melena	Can be challenging, mucosal biopsy and endoscopy Culture	Ferrets: clarithromycin (12.5 mg/kg q 12 h) double therapy used with either omeprazole (1 mg/kg PO q 12 h) or ranitidine bismuth citrate (24 mg/kg) was found to be more effective than original amoxicillin-based triple therapy[26] ±Antacids and sucralfate
Tuberculosis *Mycobacterium bovis, M avium, M tuberculosis* Zoonosis	Ferret	Dependent on strain Diarrhea, weight loss, lymph node enlargement, conjunctival lesions, splenomegaly, and pneumonia	Isolation and identification of organism from tissues (retropharyngeal and mesenteric nodes), acid-fast staining, PCR, and culture	Because of zoonotic risk of *M bovis* and *M tuberculosis*, euthanasia is recommended *M avium* may pose a risk to immunocompromised people

Abbreviations: ETEC Enteropathogenic *E coli*; STEC, Shiga toxin producing *E coli*.

Table 5
Gastrointestinal viral pathogens of exotic companion mammals[51,77–79,91–94]

Organism Features	Species and Age Susceptibility	Clinical Signs/Lesions	Diagnosis	Treatment
Rabbit hemorrhagic disease virus Calicivirus *Lagovirus* genus	>2 mo, high morbidity and mortality	Acute death with tachypnea, cyanosis, abdominal distention, hepatic necrosis, CNS signs (convulsions, incoordination, prostration) DIC with hemorrhage of many organs, particularly lungs	ELISA, PCR	Vaccination Culling of infected colonies Quarantining and testing of new animals from endemic areas
Rotavirus Reoviridae	Rabbits: weanlings, older animals are more naturally resistant Rats; sucklings <2 wk of age Ferrets; neonatal diarrhea 2–6 week old kits	Variable pathogenicity in rabbits; anorexia, dehydration, watery-mucoid diarrhea and high mortality or mild, transient diarrhea High morbidity and mortality in ferrets Rats have stunted growth Congestion and distention of SI, petechiae in colon Villous atrophy and loss of epithelial cells in SI are characteristic	PCR, histology, viral detection, serology (cELISA)	Largely supportive Infection is acute and self-limiting Mortality is reduced if ferret kits continue nursing and are given supportive care
Epizootic catarrhal enteritis Coronavirus "Green slime disease"	Adult ferrets most susceptible with recent exposure from young asymptomatic carrier	100% morbidity, low mortality Dehydration, projectile vomiting, diarrhea, depression Acute: profuse, green Chronic: grainy "bird seeds"	Clinical signs, and histology	Supportive, aggressive fluid therapy, assist feeding, sucralfate

(continued on next page)

Table 5
(continued)

Organism Features	Species and Age Susceptibility	Clinical Signs/Lesions	Diagnosis	Treatment
Ferret systemic coronavirus	Generally younger, average age is 11 mo	Resembles dry form of feline infectious peritonitis Lethargy, weight loss, anorexia, diarrhea, vomiting, CNS signs Hypergammaglobulinemia, leukocytosis, anemia Palpable abdominal masses of mesenteric lymph nodes and viscera	Histology, immunohistochemistry and PCR	Poor prognosis, no effective treatment Immunosuppressive therapy and supportive care with nutritional support, GI protectants, antiemetics, and empirical antibiotic therapy
Aleutian disease Parvovirus	Ferrets	Wasting disease, nonspecific signs, hypergammaglobulinemia and glomerulonephritis at end stage	Serology, hyperproteinemia, postmortem lesions	Chemical disinfection (sodium hydroxide, formalin, and phenolics) Infected animals should be culled Control of Aleutian disease depends on testing, cessation of breeding, and isolation of seropositive ferrets

Abbreviations: CNS, central nervous system; DIC, disseminated intravascular coagulopathy.

Table 6
Endoparasites of exotic companion mammals[24,33,39,47,56,59,54,65,80,89,90,95–99]

Endoparasite	Species Affected	Clinical Signs	Diagnosis	Treatment
Protozoa *Spironucleus muris*	Mice, rat	Diarrhea and occasionally death in young mice	Fecal testing	0.1% dimetridazole to drinking water for 14 d
Protozoa *Toxoplasmosis gondii* Zoonosis	Chinchilla	Vulvar bleeding, abortion, still births, or encephalitis	Serology and histopathology	Limit access to feces or fomites contaminated with feces from cats. Oocysts are resistant to desiccation, temperature extremes, and disinfectants. Extensive cleaning of environment
Protozoa *Giardia* sp Zoonotic	Chinchilla, hamster, rat, mice	Typically, subclinical infection, stress, and poor husbandry can lead to increased numbers of *Giardia* organisms predisposing to opportunistic bacterial infections and death	Direct fecal cytology (trophozoites), zinc sulfate flotation (*Giardia* cysts), or PCR	Nitroimidazole drugs (metronidazole, tinidazole, ronidazole). Shedding will be reduced and clinical signs improve but treatment does not eliminate the infection. Dimetridazole is more effective in hamsters than metronidazole. Zoonosis
Protozoa Intestinal coccidiosis *Eimeria* sp *Eimeria furonis* or *Isospora* spp	Rabbits; postweanling (2–3 months old) most susceptible, sucklings are immune. Chinchillas, guinea pigs, hamsters, rats, mice. Ferrets	Depression, anorexia, diarrhea. Ferrets: diarrhea, rectal prolapse, and death	Fecal direct, flotation, or centrifugation with histopathology. PCR to identify species	Prevention with in water/feed sulfonamide. Ferrets: Sulfadimethoxine 50 mg/kg PO once then 25 mg/kg PO for 9 d

(continued on next page)

Table 6
(continued)

Endoparasite	Species Affected	Clinical Signs	Diagnosis	Treatment
Protozoa Hepatic coccidiosis Eimeria stiedae	Rabbits; young animals (2–3 mo of age) most affected with adult carriers	Hepatomegaly with potbellied appearance, icterus, anorexia, diarrhea, and death Adults asymptomatic Diffuse, multifocal white nodules on liver surface	Fecal direct, flotation or centrifugation Oocysts within the gallbladder exudate	Prevention with in water/feed sulfonamide
Protozoa Cryptosporidium sp Zoonosis	Rabbit, chinchilla	Rabbits; asymptomatic Chinchillas; severe diarrhea unresponsive to antimicrobials	Immunofluorescent tests, ELISA, PCR, and histology	Largely supportive Antibiotics are ineffective
Protozoa Sarcocystis sp (formerly Frankelia sp)	Chinchilla	Acute death with hepatic inflammation and necrosis	Necropsy	None described
Nematode (Pinworms) Syphacia obvelata, Aspiclaris tetraptera S obvelata S muris S mesocriceti	Mice, rat Mice, rat, gerbil Mice, rat, hamster, gerbil Gerbil	Clinical signs usually absent in mice, rat heavy burdens cause enteritis, pruritis, rectal prolapse, intestinal impaction or intussusception	Tape prep of perianal skin to identify eggs of S obvelata S muris Fecal examination or intestinal examination for A tetraptera	Fenbendazole in feed, ivermectin, piperazine Environmental decontamination
Nematode Trichosomoides crassicauda	Rat	Found in urinary bladder or renal pelvis, can cause uroliths and bladder cancer	Urinalysis	Ivermectin, selamectin
Nematode Pinworm Dentostomella translucida	Gerbil, hamster	No clinical signs	Fecal examination	Fenbendazole-medicated diet (150 ppm) fed for a total of 5 wk with or without ivermectin-supplemented drinking water (ivermectin dose 0.005 mg/mL)

	Species	Clinical signs	Diagnosis	Treatment/Control
Nematodes *Baylisascaris procyonis* (cerebral nematodiasis)	Chinchilla	Ataxia, torticollis, paralysis, incoordination, and death	Histology	Treatment is supportive and control is reducing access by raccoons
Other nematodes *Ostertagia* sp, *Trichostrongylus colubriforms,* *Haemonchus contortus*	Chinchilla	Emaciation; infection from ingestion of grass from pasture housing ruminants	Fecal examination	Limit access to grass contaminated by ruminants
Nematodes (rare) *Toxasacaris lenina,* *Toxocara cati,* *Ancylostoma* spp, *Dipylidium caninum,* *Mesocestoides* spp, *Filaroides* spp	Ferret	Diarrhea, weight loss	Fecal examination	Ivermectin and praziquantel
Nematode *Dirofilaria immitis*	Ferret	Coughing, weakness, dyspnea, ascites, pleural effusion, heart murmur, pale mucus membranes, and hypothermia	Clinical signs, radiographs, echocardiogram, and the detection of heartworm antigens or antibodies with assays	Ivermectin (50 µg/kg SC) q 30 d until clinical signs resolve and no microfilaria Prevention: Ivermectin (0.5 mg/kg) PO, SC, or selamectin year-round
Cestodes The dwarf tapeworm *Rodentolepsis nana* Zoonosis *R microstoma,* *Hymenolepsis diminuta*	Mice, rats, hamsters, gerbils Mice, hamsters Mice, rats, hamsters	Usually benign, impactions with large worm burdens	Ova or proglottid observed directly in feces	Praziquantel, thiabenazdazole, and niclosamide Usually requires depopulation for eradication
Cestode *Taenia taeniaformis* larval form *Cysticercus fasciolavis*	Mice, rats, hamsters	Liver cysts	Postmortem	Nonpathogenic, definitive host is cat

(continued on next page)

Table 6
(continued)

Endoparasite	Species Affected	Clinical Signs	Diagnosis	Treatment
Cestodes *Taenia serialis, T pisiformis, Echinococcus granulosus, Rodentolepsis nana* Zoonosis	Chinchilla	Postweaning listlessness and poor body condition Cystic subcutaneous masses caused by the intermediate stage of *T multiceps*, *T serialis* are occasionally seen	Fecal flotation	Praziquantel Surgical removal of cystic masses

and mucoid enteropathy.[10] Together, these diseases are often grouped under the designation "rabbit enteropathy complex" (**Tables 4–6**).[10,12,21]

Enteritis is a common cause of mortality in fur-farmed chinchillas. In one study,[57] captive chinchillas from two commercial ranches in Argentina were submitted for necropsy, and 35% (244 animals) died of enteric diseases. Among the causes of enteritis *E coli*, *Salmonella enterica* subsp. *typhimurium*, *Salmonella arizonae* and enteritidis, *P aeruginosa*, *Yersinia pseudotuberculosis*, *Yersinia enterocolitica*, *K pneumoniae*, and *Clostridium perfringens* were identified as the primary agents identified.[57] Yeast overgrowth with *Cyniclomyces guttulatus* is another common finding in chinchillas with soft stool. A normal inhabitant of the stomach lining, it is believed to proliferate secondarily and is treated with nystatin (100,000 IU/kg orally every 8 hours for 5 days).[35] Intestinal parasitism is generally uncommon in chinchillas but there are reports of infections with protozoa (*Toxoplasma gondii*, *Giardia duodenalis*), cestodes (*Taenia* spp, *Echinococcus granulosus*, and *Hymenolepis nana*), and nematodes (*Baylisascaris procyonis*) occurring in fur-ranched chinchillas.[39]

The most common causes of bacterial enteritis in guinea pigs are *Clostridium piliforme* and *Salmonella* spp. Less common causes include: *Y pseudotuberculosis*, *C perfringens*, *E coli*, *P aeruginosa*, *Citrobacter freundii*, and *L monocytogenes*.[27] These organisms are usually transmitted through contaminated food. Parasites that cause diarrhea in weanling guinea pigs include: *Eimeria caviae*, *Balantidium caviae*, and *Paraspidodera uncinate*.[27]

Diarrhea is one of the most common manifestations of disease in ferrets. Any disorder that disrupts their already short gastrointestinal transit time (4 hours), can lead to diarrhea.[58] Causes of diarrhea in ferrets range from noninfectious (sudden diet change and foreign bodies), to infectious with bacteria (*Lawsonia intracellularis*, *Salmonella* spp, *Campylobacter jejuni*, and *Helicobacter mustelae*), parasites (*Coccidia* spp), and viruses (rotaviruses, coronavirus, and distemper virus).[58]

Antibiotic Use in Rabbits, Guinea Pigs, Chinchillas, Hamsters, and Gerbils

Several antibiotics have been associated with the outbreaks of enterotoxemia in rabbits and rodents. The primary gastrointestinal flora in these species is gram-positive, thus antibiotics targeting this spectrum likely lead to overgrowth of gram-negative and clostridial organisms.[28] The antibiotics that should be avoided include: penicillins, including ampicillin and amoxicillin; lincomycin; clindamycin; erythromycin; bacitracin; streptomycin; and cephalosporins.[28,59] Gerbils, can generally be treated with a wide variety of antibiotics; however, they are particularly sensitive to dihydrostreptomycin.[60] These antibiotics can cause toxicity when administered parenterally, orally, and even topically.[28] *Clostridium difficile* seems to play a role in the development of enterotoxemia that follows antibiotic therapy. Treatment is generally unrewarding because disease is almost always fatal. Alternative antibiotics that are less hazardous include: fluoroquinolones, trimethoprim-sulfonamide combinations, tetracycline, and chloramphenicol.[28]

Management of Enteropathy Complex

The multifactorial enteropathy complex of juvenile rabbits is explained by factors that allow pathogenic bacteria to proliferate. These factors include stress, diet change, antibiotics, and genetic predisposition to gut dysfunction.[21] The first 14 days after weaning is a critical period in postnatal development and the time when rabbits are most susceptible to infectious diseases and consequently when enormous production losses occur.[10,16] Weaning is particularly stressful because of separation from the doe and deprivation of the mother's milk, waning maternal antibody levels, and the unstable and incompletely developed gastrointestinal microflora.[12,16,61] Frequently, during weaning animals are fed diets low in fiber, which inhibits gastrointestinal motility and leads to feed retention and alkalization of the stomach contents.[16] It is these changes in gastrointestinal pH that allows replication of microbial pathogens and toxin production. The enterotoxins cause damage to enterocytes, with diarrhea, dehydration, and death resulting.[10] In adults stress during parturition and lactation, antibiotic usage, and coinfection with other pathogens are factors that can lead to disease.[21]

General approaches to therapy include symptomatic treatment with fluids, electrolytes, gastric protectants (bismuth subsalicylate or sucralfate) providing heat support, and increasing fiber in the diet. A high-quality feed with up to 20% fiber should be fed and sudden changes in diet avoided.[10,12,16,56] For E coli infections reducing the amount of concentrates to less than 2 to 3 oz per day with added roughage is more effective than antibiotics.[10]

Other general supportive measures for enterotoxemia include the addition of copper sulfate (400 ppm added to diet)[12] to help reduce toxin production, or cholestyramine to bind toxins, fecal flora transplants with nonpathogenic Clostridium spiroforme or C difficile, oral probiotics, and vaccination with a toxoid.[10,12,16] Preventative measures for proliferative enteropathy include decreasing food intake when shipping and for 48 hours post-shipment.[10]

In severe cases of enteritis or enterotoxemia antibiotic use is questionable in treatment and generally unrewarding. The use of imidazoles (metronidazole) and tetracyclines have been shown to reduce number of deaths associated with clostridial diseases when added to drinking water or food in the face of an outbreak.[12,16] Similarly, the use of enrofloxacin parenterally before shipment reduced morbidity and mortality associated with endemic Enteropathogenic E coli (EPEC).[16]

Ensuring husbandry practices are optimal is important in the control and prevention of epizootics. These include frequent cage cleaning, changing of substrate, the use of nonsolid flooring, dust and temperature control, and the prevention of overcrowding.[12,21] Knowledge of pathogen resistance in the environment is important in choice of disinfectant. Clostridial spores, for example, require treatment with heat (70°C–80°C) for 30 minutes or with sodium hypochlorite (0.3%) for 5 minutes.[16] The use of vaccines where available (Eimeria sp), screening new animals by PCR or culture, and adequate quarantine before introduction are also important in controlling spread of disease.[16]

INTEGUMENTARY PATHOGENS OF SMALL MAMMALS
Bacterial

Staphylococcus aureus
Staphylococcus aureus is a gram-positive coccus that commonly infects the skin and mucus membranes of animals.[12] Abscess and ulcerative dermatitis are frequently caused by S aureus in hamsters and mice.[47,59] Diagnosis is usually by culture of the lesion and antibiotics recommended for treatment include systemic enrofloxacin, tetracycline, or ciprofloxacin.[59]

Rats are frequently infected with S aureus, which causes ulcerative dermatitis and pododermatitis (**Fig. 7**). Good sanitation and trimming the toenails helps minimize self-mutilation from scratching in ulcerative dermatitis cases.[33]

Facial eczema (nasal dermatitis) is a common skin condition seen in gerbils (**Fig. 8**). The skin around the nares becomes erythematous, then progresses to alopecia and ulcerative dermatitis.[62,63] Excessive porphyrin secretion by the Harderian gland is a

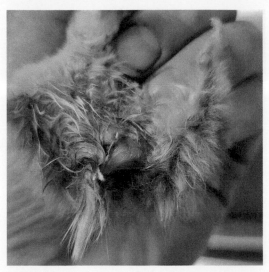

Fig. 6. Hamster with characteristic fecal staining of perineum from proliferative enteritis. (*Photo courtesy* of Dr Brent Couts, DVM.)

source of skin irritation, which may become secondarily infected by *S aureus* or *Staphylococcus xylosus*.[64] Stress from overcrowding or environmental humidity greater than 50% are underlying causes. Gerbils require sand baths to keep the fur from becoming oily, so provision of a soft clay or sand substrate helps in management of the disease. Topical or parenteral antibiotics and disinfectants may be used to treat the infection.[64]

Treponema paraluiscuniculi

Treponema paraluiscuniculi is a slender, spiral-shaped gram-negative spirochete organism that causes ulcerative and crusted lesions of the genitalia, lips, eyelids, and

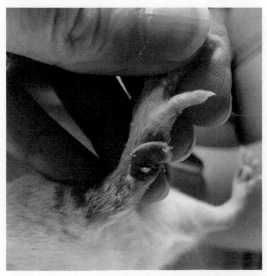

Fig. 7. Pododermatitis in a rat.

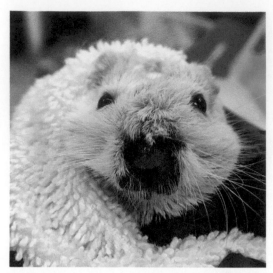

Fig. 8. Gerbil with facial eczema.

anus of rabbits.[10,65] Transmission occurs through direct contact with intact or damaged mucus membranes, usually venereally but also maternally during suckling. An ELISA for *Treponema pallidum* (human syphilis) is used to diagnose *T paraluiscuniculi* infections.[10] Treatment with benzathine procaine penicillin at a dosage of 42,000 to 84,000 U/kg subcutaneously every 7 days is effective at eliminating infection.[16]

Fungal

Dermatophytosis
Dermatophytosis of exotic companion mammals are important because of their zoonotic potential, and that they are often asymptomatic carriers.[66,67]

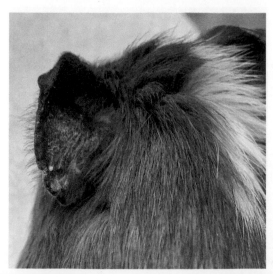

Fig. 9. Crusting of the pinna typical of dermatophytosis in a guinea pig.

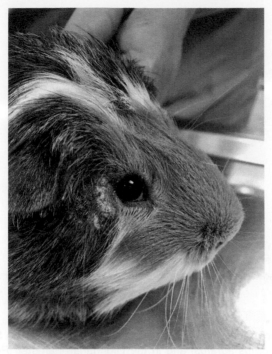

Fig. 10. Crusting and alopecia around the face of a guinea pig with dermatophytosis.

Dermatophytosis is most common in rabbits and guinea pigs, and uncommon in the ferret, rat, chinchilla, prairie dog (*Cynomys ludovicianus*), and mouse.[55,66–68] There are emerging reports of transmission of dermatophytes from the Central European hedgehog (*Erinaceus europaeus*) and the African Pygmy hedgehog (*Atelerix*

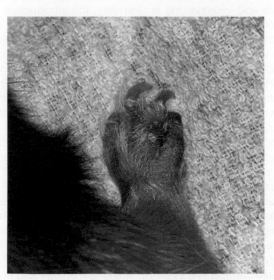

Fig. 11. Crusting, erythema and fur thinning of the digits in a guinea pig with dermatophytosis.

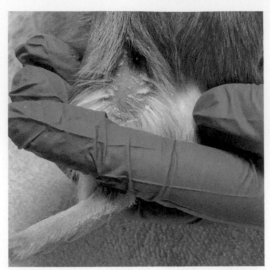

Fig. 12. Crusting, scale and alopecia on the ventral aspect of the leg of a guinea pig with dermatophytosis.

albiventris) to humans.[67] Ringworm seems to be extremely rare in Syrian or Golden hamster (*Mesocricetus auratus*) and in the Djungarian hamster (*Phodopus sungorus*).[9] There are no reports of naturally occurring disease in the Mongolian gerbil (*Meriones unguiculatus*).[64]

Exotic companion mammals are infected with a variety of dermatophytes that inhabit the fur, skin, nails, and spines and the environment, cage, and soil.[67] Humans are susceptible to infection; however, it is usually younger or immunocompromised people or those that have close contact with these animals. In one study surveying guinea pig owners and veterinarians in Germany, the introduction of a new guinea pig to a household preceded the onset of clinical signs in 43% of cases.[66] One-third of the affected guinea pigs had lived in the household for less than 3 months. In approximately one-quarter of the guinea pig cases, humans also showed clinical signs of dermatophytosis, and in half the households only children were affected.

The most important dermatophyte species for small animals are: *Trichophyton mentagrophytes*, *Trichophyton erinacei*, *Trichophyton quinckeanum*, *Arthroderma benhamiae*, *Arthroderma vanbreuseghemii*, *Microsporum gypseum*, and *Microsporum persicolor*.[69] Young animals seem to be most susceptible to disease and other predisposing factors include pregnancy, high temperatures and humidity, health status, overcrowding, ectoparasites, and genetics.[9] Trichophyton mentagrophytes was found in 97% of cases in the aforementioned study in Germany.[66] *M gypseum* is a less frequent cause of disease in rodents.[68]

Lesions are seen on the nose, eyelids, pinna, and legs of the animal with occasional spread to the nailbed (**Figs. 9–12**).[9] There is patchy alopecia, erythema, and crustiness with an underlying inflammatory reaction.[9,67,70] Diagnosis is made through microscopy and culture. Because *T mentagrophytes* does not fluoresce with Wood lamp, this test frequently produces false-negative results in guinea pigs.[9]

Treatment requires topical and systemic antifungal agents and environmental control. Infected animals should be removed and the environment thoroughly decontaminated and disinfected with sodium hypochlorite (1:10 dilution), benzalkonium chloride,

Table 7
Viral skin diseases of rabbits[16,75,77–79,100]

Organism Features	Route of Transmission	Clinical Signs	Diagnosis	Treatment
Myxomatosis Myxoma virus, genus *Leporipoxvirus*	Insect vectors (fleas and mosquitoes), or direct contact (uncommon)	Swelling of the eyelids, ear margins, progressing to general swelling of the face and genitalia with ocular discharge. Pyrexia, lethargy and systemically ill with skin nodules. Septicemia with death at 10–12 d. In southern California a peracute and acute form occurs where rabbits die within 5–7 d of infection, with minimal clinical signs; periocular edematous swelling, or no signs at all.	Clinical signs and serology	Vector control and vaccination (UK and Europe). Supportive treatment with nonsteroidal anti-inflammatories, fluid therapy, assisted feeding, systemic antibiotics for cases with attenuate virus strain. No effective treatment of acute or peracute form.
Shope fibroma virus *Leporipoxvirus*	Insect vectors	Benign, self-limiting disease in wild rabbits. Domestic rabbits develop subcutaneous fibromas over the legs, feet, muzzle, periorbital, and perineal areas. Young or immunocompromised animals can develop generalized disease that is fatal.	Histopathology and virus isolation	Vector control. Supportive care and systemic antibiotics. A live-attenuated Shope fibroma virus is used as a myxomatosis vaccine because it provides cross-immunity.
Shope papilloma virus, Cottontail rabbit papillomavirus *Kappapapillomavirus* genus, oncogenic	Insect vectors (including ticks)	Multiple hyperkeratotic hornlike lesions around ears, eyelids, neck, and shoulders.	Histopathology	Vector control or surgical removal of papillomas. In wild rabbits, manual removal is curative but experimental infection in domestic rabbits led to malignant transformation into squamous cell carcinoma.

Table 8
Ectoparasites of exotic companion mammals[24,39,64,65,76,84,85,89,90,97,98]

Ectoparasite	Species Affected	Clinical Signs	Diagnosis	Treatment
Fleas *Ctenocephalides canis* or *C felis* (wild rabbit flea) *Spilopsyllus cuniculi* (wild rabbit flea) *Nosopsylla* spp or *Xenopsylla* spp (wild rat and mice)	Rabbit, chinchilla, gerbil, ferret, hedgehog, mice, rats Rabbit Rodents	Intense pruritis, allergic dermatitis	Visualization of fleas and/or feces in fur	Imidacloprid or selamectin Treat in contact animals (dogs and cats) Role in transmission of myxomatosis, Rocky Mountain spotted fever, *Trypanosoma* spp, and RHDV
Ear mite *Psoroptes cuniculi*	Rabbit	Intense pruritis, shaking, or scratching ears Copious brown exudate builds up on the inner aspect of the pinna and ear canal (**Fig. 13**)	Clinical signs, visual or otoscopic examination of the ears Observation of exudate can be pathognomonic	Selamectin, ivermectin, moxidectin Do *not* remove these crusts because they are painful and can cause damage to the thin and delicate structures of the ears
Ear mite *Otodectes cynotis*	Ferret	Brown-black discharge, pruritis, head shaking, alopecia, can spread to face and tail	Microscopic visualization or mites or eggs	Ivermectin
Sarcoptic mites *Sarcoptes scabiei*, Zoonotic *Notoedres* spp	Ferret, rabbit Rabbit, rat, hamster	Pruritis, alopecia, lichenification, paw inflammation, "foot rot," nail deformation, nail sloughing Intense pruritis, alopecia, white-yellow crusting	Multiple skin scrapings	Ivermectin, selamectin
Fur mite *Cheyletiella parasitovorax* ("walking dander") Zoonotic *Leporacarus gibbus* *Cheyletiella* spp	Rabbit Rabbit Chinchilla	Flakey, dandruff to large crusts and patchy alopecia along the back, tail, and base of neck, broken hairs Scaly alopecia, sometime self-mutilation from hypersensitivity reaction	Visualization from skin brushings or pluckings	Maybe associated with inability groom with obesity, arthritis, spinal disorders, or dental disease Ivermectin, selamectin, permethrin, carbaryl products

Parasite	Species	Clinical signs	Diagnosis	Treatment
Fur mite *Trixacaris caviae*, *Chirodiscoides caviae*, rarely *Demodex caviae*	Guinea pig	*T caviae* worse skin lesions than *C caviae*; alopecia, crusting and pruritis. Animals may scratch so intently they seem to be seizuring (**Fig. 14**)	Microscopy or direct visualization of mites or eggs	Ivermectin (0.4 mg/kg SC every 10–14 d for 4 treatments) or selamectin (15 mg/kg single topical dose)[25]
Fur mite *Myocoptes musculinus* and *Myobia musculi*	Mice	Localized pruritis, alopecia, ulcerative dermatitis, lymphadenopathy, weight loss	Skin scrapes	Ivermectin, selamectin, moxidectin
Fur mite *Radfordia* spp	Mice > rats	*M musculi* (head), *M musculinus* (along the back)	Skin scrapes	Ivermectin, selamectin, moxidectin
Demodectic mite *Demodex* spp	Ferret, gerbils, hamsters	Pruritis, alopecia, dermatitis	Deep skin scrapes	Ivermectin. May be related to age and underlying disease, immunosuppression
Tropical rat mite *Ornithonyssus bacoti* Zoonosis	Rats, mice, gerbil, hamster, degus, African pygmy hedgehogs	Pruritis, excoriation, head, ears, nose	Visualization of mites or microscopy	Selamectin. Transmission of Q fever, plague, Hantaan viruses, WEE
Mite *Acarus farris*	Gerbil, hamster	Alopecia, scaling, thickening of skin around tail	Microscopy	Selamectin or ivermectin
Mite *Atricholaelaps chinchillae*	Chinchilla	Described in free-ranging chinchillas in Peru	Microscopy or direct visualization of mites or eggs	No treatment recommendation
Louse *Hemodipsus ventricosus*	Rabbit	Heavy parasite loads are associated with anemia, weight loss, alopecia, pruritis, and papules	Visualization of lice or eggs	Ivermectin, may act as a vector for myxomatosis and *Rickettsia*
Louse *Gliricola porcelli*, *Gyropus ovalis*	Guinea pig	Pruritic alopecia, crusts, unthrifty coat	Microscopy or direct visualization of louse or eggs (**Fig. 15**)	Ivermectin

(continued on next page)

Table 8
(continued)

Ectoparasite	Species Affected	Clinical Signs	Diagnosis	Treatment
House mouse louse *Polyplax* spp	Mice, rats	Severe pruritis, alopecia, dermatitis, anemia	Visualization of lice or eggs	Ivermectin, permethrin dust
Ticks Europe: *Ixodes ricinus, Ripicephalus* sp, *Haemaphysalis* sp North Eastern United States: *Ixodes scapularis, I dentatus, Haemaphysalis leporisplalustris, Dermacentor variabilis*	Rabbits, ferrets, hedgehogs	No clinical cases of Lyme disease in rabbits	Visualization on skin	Ivermectin May serve as biologic vector for *Borrelia* sp, and potential zoonosis
Myiasis (Fly strike) *Calliphoridae* spp *Lucilia* spp	Rabbit	Lay eggs on soiled skin Moist dermatitis, severe cases with shock and bacterial infection	Visualization of larvae	Removal of larvae, treating tissue damage and infection, manage underlying cause Treatment with ivermectin, systemic antibiotics, wound care, and environmental management to control flies
Warble flies *Cuterebra* spp	Rabbit	2–3 cm subcutaneous masses around the head, neck, back with a painful fistula	Finding of a fistula in the skin with the larva inside	Mechanical removal of the warble and treatment of concurrent infection

Abbreviation: RHDV, rabbit hemorrhagic disease virus; WEE, western equine encephalomyelitis virus.

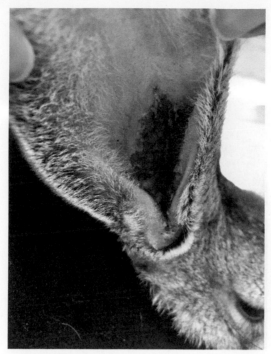

Fig. 13. Rabbit with otitis externa crusting typical of *Psoroptes cuniculi*.

glutaraldehyde, or 0.2% enilconazole solution.[9,71] For colony outbreaks, weekly application of lime sulfur dip, or enilconazole spray/fogger may be applied for 6 weeks.[9] In chinchillas, the addition of antifungal powders to dust bathes has been shown to be effective in treating dermatophytosis. These include one teaspoon of captan (Orthocaptan) with two cups of dust or clotrimazole powder added to dust. Topical creams and lotions must be used with caution because of the risk of ingestion after grooming. Currently, oral itraconazole (50–10 mg/kg every 24 hours) (noncompounded) and oral

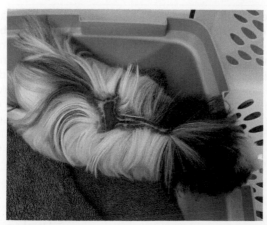

Fig. 14. Guinea pig severe dermatitis caused by the fur mite *Trixacarus caviae*.

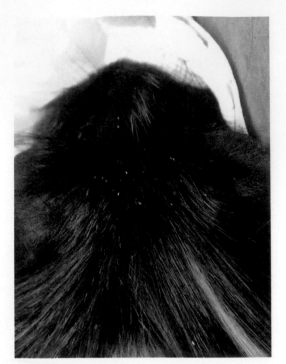

Fig. 15. Guinea pig with nits (louse eggs).

terbinafine (20 mg/kg every 24 hours) are the most effective and safest therapeutics for treatment of dermatophytosis.[69,72–74] Powdered griseofulvin is added to food at a dose of 0.825 mg/kg of food; however, this may be cost prohibitive and not without side effects (hepatotoxicity).[71] Prevention is aimed at reducing exposure to infected animals and contaminated environments. Environmental management includes limiting overcrowding, parasite control, and proper temperature and humidity regulation.[9,24]

Viral and Parasitic

Management of the viral and parasitic skin diseases in exotic companion mammals is focused largely on control of the environment and insect vectors (**Tables 7** and **8**). This includes physical means, such as insect screens and netting; ultraviolet fly killers; keeping animals inside; and preventing contact with wild rabbits and rodents, dogs, and cats.[75] Insecticidal treatment with ivermectin, selamectin, imidaclopramid, and permethrin should cover against most arthropods.[75] Fipronil should not be used in rabbits because of toxicity and potentially fatal seizures.[65,76] None of the viral infections of rabbits are known to be of public health importance because there are no reports of the definitive spread of viruses from rabbits to humans; however, myxomatosis is a severe and invariably fatal systemic disease of domestic rabbits that could lead to enormous production losses.[75,77–79]

SUMMARY

Management of epizootics of exotic companion mammal herds relies on careful observance of animals, proper management and husbandry, adequate nutrition, and stress reduction. Many diseases occur because of the stress of weaning so anticipating this and maximizing sanitation and ventilation, minimizing overcrowding and concurrent disease, and providing enough fiber for herbivores is prudent. The choice to use antibiotics in small herbivores must be weighed against whether antibiotics will help in the treatment course versus the risk of development of enterotoxemia. Insect and pest control are of paramount importance because of the risk of disease introduction in naive populations. Distemper and rabies vaccination of ferrets is highly recommended because of high fatality and potential zoonoses of these diseases. An appropriate response when faced with an epizootic includes separation of affected animals, rapid diagnostic testing, and implementation of treatment and supportive care to help minimize losses. Animals should be obtained from reputable vendors or quarantined and screened before entry.[1] Finally, knowledge of potential zoonotic pathogens is important for veterinarians and any staff working closely with these species.

CLINICS CARE POINTS

- Disease outbreaks are often the result of stress from weaning, transport, overcrowding, or concurrent diseases.
- The use of culture and sensitivity, virus isolation, PCR, and serology are important tools in elucidating etiologic agents and deciding appropriate antimicrobial therapy.
- For small herbivores, because of their primarily gram-positive gastrointestinal flora, avoidance of antibiotics with this spectrum is recommended because of the risk of gram-negative overgrowth and clostridial enterotoxemia.
- For many of the gastrointestinal pathogens of herbivores, reducing stress, providing a high-fiber diet (20%), and optimal husbandry practices, such as appropriate disinfection and judicious use of antibiotics, help control and prevent disease outbreaks.
- Some forms of pasteurellosis and pneumonia may not respond well to antimicrobials.
- Control of insects and pest rodents help reduce spread of disease and minimize dermatitis lesions caused by external parasites.

ACKNOWLEDGMENTS

The author thanks Dr Nick St. Erne for help with planning this article.

DISCLOSURE

The author has nothing to disclose.

REFERENCES

1. Kling MA. A review of respiratory system anatomy, physiology, and disease in the mouse, rat, hamster, and gerbil. Vet Clin North Am Exot Anim Pract 2011; 14(2):287–337.
2. Bivolarski BL, Vachkova EG. Morphological and functional events associated to weaning in rabbits. J Anim Physiol Anim Nutr 2014;98(1):9–18.
3. Thrusfield M, Brown H. Surveys. In: Thrusfield M, editor. Veterinary epidemiology. 4th edition. Hoboken, NJ: Wiley-Blackwell; 2018. p. 270–94.
4. Evers EG, Nauta MJ. Estimation of animal-level prevalence from pooled samples in animal production. Prev Vet Med 2001;49(3–4):175–90.

5. Christensen J, Gardner IA. Herd-level interpretation of test results for epidemiologic studies of animal diseases. Prev Vet Med 2000;45(1–2):83–106.
6. Cowling DW, Gardner IA, Johnson WO. Comparison of methods for estimation of individual-level prevalence based on pooled samples. Prev Vet Med 1999;39(3): 211–25.
7. Laurin E, Thakur K, Mohr PG, et al. To pool or not to pool? Guidelines for pooling samples for use in surveillance testing of infectious diseases in aquatic animals. J Fish Dis 2019;42(11):1471–91.
8. Muñoz-Zanzi C, Thurmond M, Hietala S, et al. Factors affecting sensitivity and specificity of pooled-sample testing for diagnosis of low prevalence infections. Prev Vet Med 2006;74(4):309–22.
9. Pollock C. Fungal diseases of laboratory rodents. Vet Clin North Am Exot Anim Pract 2003;6(2):401–13.
10. Hrapkiewicz K, Colby L, Denison P. Introduction to disease of rabbits. In: Clinical laboratory animal medicine. 4th ed. Wiley-Blackwell; 2013. p. 249–89.
11. Kannangara DW, Pandya D, Patel P. *Pasteurella multocida* infections with unusual modes of transmission from animals to humans: a study of 79 cases with 34 nonbite transmissions. Vector Borne Zoonotic Dis 2020;20(9):637–51.
12. DeLong D. Bacterial diseases. In: Suckow MA, Stevens KA, Wilson RP, editors. The laboratory rabbit, Guinea pig, hamster, and other rodents. 1st edition. Waltham, MA: Elsevier; 2012. p. 322–48.
13. Holmes HT, Matsumoto M, Patton NM, et al. A method for culturing the nasopharyngeal area of rabbits. Lab Anim 1987;21(4):353–5.
14. Holmes HT, Matsumoto M, Patton NM, et al. Serologic methods for detection of *Pasteurella multocida* infections in nasal culture negative rabbits. Lab Anim Sci 1986;36(6):640–5.
15. Deeb BJ, DiGiacomo RF, Bernard BL, et al. *Pasteurella multocida* and *Bordetella bronchiseptica* infections in rabbits. J Clin Microbiol 1990;28(1):70–5.
16. Nowland MH, Brammer DW, Garcia A, et al. Biology and diseases of rabbits. In: Fox JG, Anderson LC, Otto GM, et al, editors. Laboratory animal medicine. 3rd ed. Elsevier; 2015. p. 864–97.
17. Kawamoto E, Sawada T, Sato T, et al. Comparison of indirect haemagglutination test, gel-diffusion precipitin test, and enzyme-linked immunosorbent assay for detection of serum antibodies to *Pasteurella multocida* in naturally and experimentally infected rabbits. Lab Anim 1994;28(1):19–25.
18. Kumar AA, Shivachandra SB, Biswas A, et al. Prevalent serotypes of *Pasteurella multocida* isolated from different animal and avian species in India. Vet Res Commun 2004;28(8):657–67.
19. Rougier S, Galland D, Boucher S, et al. Epidemiology and susceptibility of pathogenic bacteria responsible for upper respiratory tract infections in pet rabbits. Vet Microbiol 2006;115(1–3):192–8.
20. Quinton JF, Lennox A, Guillon L, et al. Results of bacterial culture and sensitivity testing from nasolacrimal duct flushes in one hundred and three both healthy and clinically ill pet rabbits (oryctolagus cuniculus). Int J Appl Res Vet Med 2014;12(2):107–20.
21. Delong D. Section II rabbits. In: Suckow MA, Stevens KA, Wilson RP, editors. The laboratory rabbit, Guinea pig, hamster, and other rodents. 1st edition. Waltham, MA: Academic Press; 2012. p. 303–63.
22. Suckow MA, Martin BJ, Bowersock TL, et al. Derivation of *Pasteurella multocida*-free rabbit litters by enrofloxacin treatment. Vet Microbiol 1996;51(1–2):161–8.

23. Lennox AM, Mancinelli E. Respiratory diseases. In: Quesenberry KE, Orcutt CJ, Mans C, et al, editors. Ferrets, rabbits, and rodents: clinical medicine and surgery. 4th edition. St Louis, MO: Elsevier; 2020. p. 188–200.

24. Brabb T, Newsome D, Burich A, et al. Infectious diseases. In: Suckow MA, Stevens KA, Wilson RP, editors. The laboratory rabbit, Guinea pig, hamster, and other rodents. 1st edition. Waltham, MA: Elsevier; 2012. p. 638–76.

25. Mitchell MA, Tully TN Jr. Zoonotic diseases associated with small mammals. In: Quesenberry KE, Orcutt CJ, Mans C, et al, editors. Ferrets, rabbits, and rodents: clinical medicine and surgery. 4th edition. St Louis, MO: Elsevier; 2020. p. 609–18.

26. Shomer NH, Holcombe H, Harkness JE. Biology and diseases of guinea pigs. In: Fox JG, Anderson LC, Otto GM, et al, editors. Laboratory animal medicine. 3rd edition. Cambridge, MA: Elsevier; 2015. p. 247–77.

27. Pignon C, Mayer J. Guinea pigs. In: Quesenberry KE, Orcutt CJ, Mans C, et al, editors. Ferrets, rabbits, and rodents: clinical medicine and surgery. 4th edition. St Louis, MO: Elsevier; 2020. p. 271–95.

28. Introduction to diseases of guinea pigs. In: Hrapkiewicz K, Colby L, Denison P, editors. Clinical laboratory animal medicine. 4th edition. Ames, IA: John Wiley & Sons, Ltd; 2013. p. 195–243.

29. Yarto-Jaramillo E. Respiratory system anatomy, physiology, and disease: guinea pigs and chinchillas. Vet Clin North Am Exot Anim Pract 2011;14(2):339–55.

30. Tamura Y. Current approach to rodents as patients. J Exot Pet Med 2010;19(1): 36–55.

31. Maguire S, Hawk CT. Formulary. In: Suckow MA, Stevens KA, Wilson RP, editors. The laboratory rabbit, Guinea pig, hamster, and other rodents. 1st edition. Waltham, MA: Elsevier; 2012. p. 1193–225.

32. Frolich J. Rats and mice. In: Quesenberry KE, Orcutt CJ, Mans C, et al, editors. Ferrets, rabbits, and rodents: clinical medicine and surgery. 4th edition. St Louis, MO: Elsevier; 2020. p. 357–65.

33. Introduction to diseases of rats. In: Hrapkiewicz K, Colby L, Denison P, editors. Clinical laboratory animal medicine. 4th ed. Wiley-Blackwell; 2013. p. 123–43.

34. Mitchell CM, Johnson LK, Crim MJ, et al. Diagnosis, surveillance and management of Streptococcus equi subspecies zooepidemicus infections in Chinchillas (Chinchilla lanigera). Comp Med 2020;70(4):370–5.

35. Mans C, Donnelly TM. Chinchillas. In: Quesenberry KE, Orcutt CJ, Mans C, et al, editors. Ferrets, rabbits, and rodents: clinical medicine and surgery. 4th edition. St Louis, MO: Elsevier; 2020. p. 308–20.

36. Berg CC, Doss GA, Mans C. Streptococcus equi subspecies zooepidemicus infection in a pet chinchilla (Chinchilla lanigera). J Exot Pet Med 2019;31:36–8.

37. Martel A, Donnelly T, Mans C. Update on diseases in chinchillas: 2013–2019. Vet Clin North Am Exot Anim Pract 2020;23(2):321–35.

38. Ramakers BP, Heijne M, Lie N, et al. Zoonotic Chlamydia caviae presenting as community-acquired pneumonia. N Engl J Med 2017;377(10):992–4.

39. Norton JN, Reynolds RP. Diseases and veterinary care. In: Suckow MA, Stevens KA, Wilson RP, editors. The laboratory rabbit, Guinea pig, hamster, and other rodents. 1st edition. Waltham, MA: Elsevier; 2012. p. 993–1006.

40. Mans C, Donnelly TM. Update on diseases of chinchillas. Vet Clin North Am Exot Anim Pract 2013;16(2):383–406.

41. Hirakawa Y, Sasaki H, Kawamoto E, et al. Prevalence and analysis of Pseudomonas aeruginosa in chinchillas. BMC Vet Res 2010;6(52):1–10.

42. Ozawa S, Mans C, Szabo Z, et al. Epidemiology of bacterial conjunctivitis in chinchillas (Chinchilla lanigera): 49 cases (2005 to 2015). J Small Anim Pract 2017;58(4):238–45.

43. Introduction to diseases of chinchillas. In: Hrapkiewicz K, Colby L, Denison P, editors. Clinical laboratory animal medicine. 4th edition; 2013. p. 239–44.

44. Graham JE, Schoeb TR. Mycoplasma pulmonis in rats. J Exot Pet Med 2011; 20(4):270–6.

45. Weisbroth SH, Kohn DF, Boot R. Bacterial, mycoplasmal and mycotic infections. In: Suckow MA, Weisbroth SH, Franklin CL, editors. The laboratory rat. 2nd edition. Cambridge, MA: Elsevier; 2006. p. 339–96.

46. Piasecki T, Chrzastek K, Kasprzykowska U. Mycoplasma pulmonis of rodents as a possible human pathogen. Vector Borne Zoonotic Dis 2017;17(7):475–7.

47. Introduction to diseases of mice. In: Hrapkiewicz K, Colby L, Denison P, editors. Clinical laboratory animal medicine. Fourth. Wiley-Blackwell; 2013. p. 80–102.

48. Perpinan D. Respiratory diseases of ferrets. In: Quesenberry KE, Orcutt CJ, Mans C, et al, editors. Ferrets, rabbits, and rodents: clinical medicine and surgery. 4th edition. St Louis, MO: Elsevier; 2020. p. 71–5.

49. Kiupel M, Desjardins DR, Lim A, et al. Mycoplasmosis in ferrets. Emerg Infect Dis 2012;18(11):1763–70.

50. Mayer J, Marini RP, Fox JG. Biology and diseases of ferrets. In: Fox JG, Anderson LC, Otto G, et al, editors. Laboratory animal medicine. 3rd edition. Ames, IA: Elsevier; 2015. p. 587–616.

51. Langlois I. Viral diseases of ferrets. Vet Clin North Am Exot Anim Pract 2005;8(1): 139–60. https://doi.org/10.1016/j.cvex.2004.09.008.

52. Quesenberry KE, de Matos R. Basic approach to veterinary care of ferrets. In: Quesenberry KE, Orcutt CJ, Mans C, et al, editors. Ferrets, rabbits, and rodents: clinical medicine and surgery. 4th edition. St Louis, MO: Elsevier; 2020. p. 14–6.

53. Wyre NR, Michels D, Chen S. Selected emerging diseases in ferrets. Vet Clin North Am Exot Anim Pract 2013;16(2):469–93.

54. Swenson SL, Koster LG, Jenkins-Moore M, et al. Natural cases of 2009 pandemic H1N1 influenza A virus in pet ferrets. J Vet Diagn Invest 2010; 22(5):784–8.

55. Greenacre CB. Fungal diseases of ferrets. Vet Clin North Am Exot Anim Pract 2003;6(2):435–48.

56. Oglesbee B, Lord B. Gastrointestinal diseases of rabbits. In: Quesenberry KE, Orcutt CJ, Mans C, et al, editors. Ferrets, rabbits, and rodents: clinical medicine and surgery. 4th edition. St Louis, MO: Elsevier; 2020. p. 174–85.

57. Martino PE, Bautista EL, Gimeno EJ, et al. Fourteen-year status report of fatal illnesses in captive chinchilla (chinchilla lanigera). J Appl Anim Res 2017; 45(1):310–4.

58. Veterinary care. In: Matchett CA, Marr R, Berard FM, et al, editors. The laboratory ferret. 1st edition. Boca Raton, FL: CRC Press; 2012. p. 29–61.

59. Introduction to diseases of hamsters. In: Hrapkiewicz K, Colby L, Denison P, editors. Clinical laboratory animal medicine. 4th edition. Ames, IA: Wiley-Blackwell; 2013. p. 182–9.

60. Introduction to diseases of gerbils. In: Hrapkiewicz K, Colby L, Denison P, editors. Clinical laboratory animal medicine. 4th edition. Ames, IA: Wiley-Blackwell; 2013. p. 156–61.

61. Paul-Murphy J. Critical care of the rabbit. Vet Clin North Am Exot Anim Pract 2007;10(2):437–61.

62. Batchelder M, Keller LS, Ball Sauer M, et al. Gerbils. In: Suckow MA, Stevens KA, Wilson RP, editors. The laboratory rabbit, Guinea pig, hamster, and other rodents. 1st ed. Elsevier; 2012. p. 1144–6.
63. Miwa Y, Mayer J. Hamsters and gerbils. In: Quesenberry KE, Orcutt CJ, Mans C, et al, editors. Ferrets, rabbits, and rodents: clinical medicine and surgery. 4th ed. Elsevier; 2020. p. 372–83.
64. Donnelley TM, Bergin I, Ihrig M. XIII Gerbils and Jirds: Meriones. In: Fox JG, Anderson LC, Otto GM, et al, editors. Laboratory animal medicine. 3rd ed. Elsevier; 2015. p. 318–20.
65. Lennox AM, Kelleher S. Bacterial and parasitic diseases of rabbits. Vet Clin North Am Exot Anim Pract 2009;12(3):519–30.
66. Kraemer A, Hein J, Heusinger A, et al. Clinical signs, therapy and zoonotic risk of pet guinea pigs with dermatophytosis. Mycoses 2013;56(2):168–72.
67. Fehr M. Zoonotic potential of dermatophytosis in small mammals. J Exot Pet Med 2015;24(3):308–16.
68. Kraemer A, Mueller RS, Werckenthin C, et al. Dermatophytes in pet guinea pigs and rabbits. Vet Microbiol 2012;157(1–2):208–13.
69. Moriello KA, Coyner K, Paterson S, et al. Diagnosis and treatment of dermatophytosis in dogs and cats: clinical consensus guidelines of the World Association for Veterinary Dermatology. Vet Dermatol 2017;28(3):266–8.
70. Canny CJ, Gamble CS. Fungal diseases of rabbits. Vet Clin North Am Exot Anim Pract 2003;6(2):429–33.
71. Brock K, Gallaugher L, Bergdall VK, et al. Mycoses and non-infectious diseases. In: Suckow MA, Stevens KA, Wilson RP, editors. The laboratory rabbit, Guinea pig, hamster, and other rodents. 1st edition. Waltham, MA: Elsevier; 2012. p. 504–23.
72. Pollock C. Fungal diseases of columbiformes and anseriformes. Vet Clin North Am Exot Anim Pract 2003;6(2):351–61.
73. Petranyi G, Meingassner JG, Mieth H. Activity of terbinafine in experimental fungal infections of laboratory animals. Antimicrob Agents Chemother 1987, 31(10):1558–61.
74. Uchida K, Yamaguchi H. Effectiveness of oral treatment with terbinafine in a guinea pig model of tinea pedis. Jpn J Antibiot 1994;47(10):1401–6.
75. Meredith AL. Viral skin diseases of the rabbit. Vet Clin North Am Exot Anim Pract 2013;16(3):705–14.
76. Fehr M, Koestlinger S. Ectoparasites in small exotic mammals. Vet Clin North Am Exot Anim Pract 2013;16(3):611–57.
77. Brabb T, di Giacomo RF. Viral diseases. In: Suckow MA, Stevens KA, Wilson RP, editors. The laboratory rabbit, Guinea pig, hamster, and other rodents. 1st edition. Waltham, MA: Elsevier; 2012. p. 365–401.
78. Kerr PJ, Donnelly TM. Viral infections of rabbits. Vet Clin North Am Exot Anim Pract 2013;16(2):437–68.
79. Krogstad AP, Simpson JE, Korte SW. Viral diseases of the rabbit. Vet Clin North Am Exot Anim Pract 2005;8(1):123–38.
80. Introduction to diseases of ferrets. In: Hrapkiewicz K, Colby L, Denison P, editors. Clinical laboratory animal medicine. 4th ed. Wiley-Blackwell; 2013. p. 312–30.
81. Wheler CL. Antimicrobial drug use in rabbits, rodents, and ferrets. In: Giguere S, Prescott JF, Dowling PM, editors. Antimicrobial therapy in veterinary medicine. 5th edition. Ames, IA: Wiley-Blackwell; 2013. p. 601–21.

82. Fisher P, Graham J. Rabbit. In: Carpenter JW, Marion CJ, editors. Exotic animal formulary. Fifth. Elsevier; 2018. p. 494–531.

83. Mayer J, Mans C. Rodents. In: Carpenter JW, Marion CJ, editors. Exotic animal formulary. Fifth. Elsevier; 2018. p. 459–93.

84. Whary MT, Baumgarth N, Fox JG, et al. Biology and diseases of mice. In: Fox JG, Anderson LC, Otto GM, et al, editors. Laboratory animal medicine. 3rd ed. Elsevier; 2015. p. 73–137.

85. Otto GM, Franklin CL, Clifford CB. Biology and diseases of rats. In: Fox JG, Anderson LC, Otto GM, et al, editors. Laboratory animal medicine. 3rd ed. Elsevier; 2015. p. 166–96.

86. Delong D, Manning P. Bacterial diseases. In: Manning P, Newcomer C, Ringler D, editors. The biology of the laboratory rabbit. 2nd ed. Academic Press; 1994. p. 131–62.

87. Frisk CS. IV hamsters. In: Suckow MA, Stevens KA, Wilson RP, editors. The laboratory rabbit, Guinea pig, hamster, and other rodents. 1st ed. Elsevier; 2012. p. 798–813.

88. Ruiz A. Plague in the Americas. In: Emerging infectious diseases, Vol 7. Centers for Disease Control and Prevention (CDC); 2001. p. 539–40. https://doi.org/10.3201/eid0707.017718.

89. Souza MJ. Bacterial and parasitic zoonoses of exotic pets. Vet Clin North Am Exot Anim Pract 2009;12(3):401–15.

90. Powers LV. Bacterial and parasitic diseases of ferrets. Vet Clin North Am Exot Anim Pract 2009;12(3):531–61.

91. Porter HG, Porter DD, Larsen AE. Aleutian disease in ferrets. Infect Immun 1982; 36(1):379–86.

92. Wade LL. Vaccination of ferrets for rabies and distemper. Vet Clin North Am Exot Anim Pract 2018;21(1):105–14.

93. McIntosh MT, Behan SC, Mohamed FM, et al. A pandemic strain of calicivirus threatens rabbit industries in the Americas. Virol J 2007;4:96.

94. Capucci L, Scicluna MT, Lavazza A. Diagnosis of viral haemorrhagic disease of rabbits and the European brown hare syndrome. Rev Sci Tech 1991;10(2): 347–70.

95. Szkucik K, Pyz-ŁUkasik R, Szczepaniak KO, et al. Occurrence of gastrointestinal parasites in slaughter rabbits. Parasitol Res 2014;113(1):59–64.

96. Reusch B. Rabbit gastroenterology. Vet Clin North Am Exot Anim Pract 2005; 8(2):351–75.

97. Pritt S, Cohen K, Sedlacek H. Parasitic diseases. In: Suckow MA, Stevens KA, Wilson RP, editors. The laboratory rabbit, Guinea pig, hamster, and other rodents. 1st edition. Waltham, MA: Elsevier; 2012. p. 415–43.

98. Burr HN, Paluch L-R, Roble GS, et al. IV hamsters. In: Suckow MA, Stevens KA, Wilson RP, editors. The laboratory rabbit, Guinea pig, hamster, and other rodents. 1st edition. Waltham, MA: Elsevier; 2012. p. 830–63.

99. Sasai H, Kato K, Sasaki T, et al. Echocardiographic diagnosis of dirofilariasis in a ferret. J Small Anim Pract 2000;41(4):172–4.

100. Kashuba C, Hsu C, Krogstad A, et al. Small mammal virology. Vet Clin North Am Exot Anim Pract 2005;8(1):107–22.

APPENDIX TABLE 1: ANTIMICROBIALS AND ANTIPARASITIC AGENTS USED IN EXOTIC COMPANION MAMMALS

Drug	Dosage	Comments
Amoxicillin	0.25 mg/mL dw for 7 d	Mice, only effective against highly susceptible bacteria
Ampicillin	500 mg/mL dw	Mice only
Amprolium (9.6%)	0.5 mL/500 mL dw for 10 d 5 mL/gal dw for 5 d 100 mg/kg in food or water for 7 d	Rabbits Ferrets
Chloramphenicol	1 mg/mL 0.5 mg/mL dw 0.83 mg/mL	Guinea pigs Mice Gerbils
Decoquinate (Deccox, Rhone-Poulenc)	62.5 ppm in feed	Rabbit
Diclazuril	1 ppm in feed	Rabbit
Dimetridazole	1 g/L dw for 40 d 4 g/L dw for 7 d 500 mg/L dw	Chinchillas Rats, mice Hamsters, degus
Enrofloxacin	200 mg/L dw for 30 d 0.05–0.2 mg/mL dw ×14 d	Rabbits Guinea pig, hamsters, gerbils, rats, mice
Erythromycin	0.13 mg/mL (500 mg/gal) dw continuously, use with caution can cause enterotoxemia 220 g/ton feed	Hamsters Ferret; *Campylobacter*
Fenbendazole	50 ppm in feed for 2–6 wk	Rabbits
Furazolidone	5.5 g/L dw	Rabbits
Ivermectin	8 mg/L dw for 4 d on, 3 d off, for 5 wk 25 mg/L dw for 4 d on, 3 d off, for 5 wk	Mice Rats
Lasalocid	120 ppm in feed	Rabbits
Mebendazole	1 g/kg of feed	Rabbits
Metronidazole	2.5 mg/mL dw for 5 d 2 mg/mL dw	Rats, mice Hamsters
Monensin	0.002%0.004% in feed	Rabbits
Neomycin	0.5 mg/mL dw 2.6 mg/mL dw	Hamsters Gerbils, rats
Oxytetracycline	1 mg/mL dw 8 g/L dw 0.25–1 mg/mL dw 400 mg/L dw for 10 d	Rabbits Guinea pigs, chinchillas, Hamsters, gerbils, rats, mice Rat; curative

(continued on next page)

Drug	Dosage	Comments
(continued)		
Piperazine	2–5 mg/mL dw for 7 d	Rabbits
	4–7 mg/mL dw for 3–10 d	Guinea pigs, mice, rats
	35 mg/mL dw for 7 d, off 7 d, repeat	Hamster, gerbils, rats, mice
Praziquantel	140 ppm in feed for 5 d	Mice
Ronidazole	400 mg/L dw	Rats, mice, gerbils
Spectinomycin	1 g/L	Rabbit
Sulfadimethoxine/ ormetoprim (RofenAid 40, Roche)	62.5–250 ppm in feed	Rabbit
Sulfadimethoxine	0.5 mL/kg of a 12.5% solution in dw	Ferret
Sulfadimidine	100–233 mg/L dw	Rabbit
Sulfamerazine	1 mg/mL dw q 24 h	Guinea pigs,
	0.8 mg/mL dw q 24 h	hamsters,
	500 mg/L dw	rats, mice
		Gerbil
		Mouse
Sulfamethazine	0.77 g/L dw	Rabbits
	1 mg/mL dw	Ferrets, rabbits,
	0.8 mg/mL dw q 24 h	guinea pigs,
	5–10 g/kg feed	chinchillas,
		hamsters, rats, mice
		Gerbils
		Rabbits
Sulfaquinoxaline	1 mg/mL dw	Rabbits, guinea pigs,
	0.6 g/kg feed	hamsters, gerbils
		Rabbits
Sulfaquinoxaline	0.04%0.1% in drinking water	Rabbits
	125–250 ppm in feed	
Tetracycline	250–1000 mg/L dw q 24 h	Rabbits
	0.32 mg/mL dw q 24 h	Chinchillas
	0.4 mg/mL dw q 24 h	Hamsters
	2–5 mg/mL dw q 24 h	Gerbils, rats, mice
	0.1%0.5% feed for 14 d	Rats
Thiabendazole	0.1% in feed × 3 mo	Rabbits
	0.3% in feed for 7–10 d	Mice
Tinidazole	2.5 g/L dw	Rats, mice, gerbils
Toltrazuril (Baycox, Bayer)	25–50 ppm dw	Rabbits
	25 mg/L dw	Most species
Tylosin	0.5 mg/mL dw	Hamsters
		Gerbils, rats, mice
		Toxicity in hamsters reported

Abbreviation: dw, drinking water.
Adapted from Ref. [10,28,33,43,47,59,60,80–83]

Managing the Health of Captive Groups of Reptiles and Amphibians

Trent Charles van Zanten, BSc (Hons), DVM[a],*,
Shane Craig Simpson, BVSc (Hons), GCM(VP), CMAVA[b]

KEYWORDS

- Amphibian • Diagnostics • Examination • Fecal • Husbandry • Nutrition
- Quarantine • Reptile

KEY POINTS

- The health of large herpetological collections is heavily centered on maintaining species-appropriate environmental parameters and husbandry techniques.
- Dietary provisions for each species must be evidence-based, provide adequate macronutrients and micronutrients, and use clean and fresh ingredients provided in a practical manner.
- Reducing disease transmission relies on careful collection planning, experienced staff, controlled entry into the collection, and awareness of potential zoonoses.
- Quarantine is focused on clearing pathogens through diagnostic testing rather than holding animals for a specified period.
- Veterinarians are required to assess new acquisitions, perform routine diagnostics, treat medical cases, and provide guidance on husbandry and collection management.

INTRODUCTION

Reptiles and amphibians have been maintained in large collections with increasing frequency over the last 20 years, which is due to their popularity in the pet trade, increased study of their wild ecology, recognition of the need for species-focused conservation programs, and the need to supply the meat and skin trade with captive-bred animals and eliminate the demand for wild stock. Herpetological collections can range from private keepers who house several of their favorite species at home, to zoos exhibiting hundreds of animals from a diverse range of species, as

[a] Conservation, Research and Veterinary Services, Wildlife Reserves Singapore, Jurong Bird Park, 2 Jurong Hill, Singapore 628925; [b] The Unusual Pet Vets, 210 Karingal Drive, Frankston, Victoria 3199, Australia
* Corresponding author.
E-mail address: trent.vanzanten@wrs.com.sg

Vet Clin Exot Anim 24 (2021) 609–645
https://doi.org/10.1016/j.cvex.2021.05.005
1094-9194/21/© 2021 Elsevier Inc. All rights reserved.

vetexotic.theclinics.com

well as to a farming operation rearing several thousand American bullfrogs for slaughter. In all scenarios, a linking factor in the success and health of herptiles is providing species-appropriate environmental conditions, nutrition, and husbandry scaled to the size and demands of the collection. Clinicians and keepers face similar challenges when managing herpetological captives: each taxon is reliant on specific conditions that can be challenging to consistently provide, their progression of disease is often slow and insidious, they display limited signs of illness, and many unknowns remain regarding their optimal husbandry, disease prevention, and treatment. Veterinary wellness programs catered by experienced clinicians have the most value in large collections; however, these principles can be applied equally to smaller menageries frequently encountered in private practice. Veterinarians managing large herpetological collections must have a sound understanding of what influences the health of a reptile or amphibian ("herptile"), the physiology and husbandry of the species kept, how to assist with collection management decisions, and implement disease surveillance protocols for new acquisitions and long-term captives.

THE TRIFECTA OF HERPETOLOGICAL HEALTH

Maintaining the health of a herpetological collection is dependent on 3 separate but related factors: the condition of the animals, their captive environment, and the management techniques they experience (**Fig. 1**). For ectothermic species where internal homeostasis depends on external physical factors,[1,2] environmental and husbandry conditions have more impact than animal-related factors. Under optimal conditions, most species are incredibly hardy. Thus, maintaining the health of a large collection shifts from focusing on individual animals during acquisition to ensuring appropriate care and conditions for the species after entering the collection.[3,4]

SOURCING THE COLLECTION

Selecting healthy foundation stock is essential to any animal enterprise and an important point of contact for the client and veterinarian. New additions should be sourced from reputable breeders/dealers and preferably physically assessed before purchase. Captive-bred stock are preferred; wild-caught animals should be avoided because of the infectious disease risk they pose to the existing collection, poor welfare during capture and transportation, low rates of acclimation to captivity, and the impact of unsustainable harvesting on wild populations.[5,6] Rare exceptions include sourcing species unavailable from other institutions where the need for captive repopulation is identified by a taxon-advisory group,[7] and appropriate permits and documentation for the process are obtained. Evidence demonstrates that wild-caught herptiles suffer far greater mortalities than captive-bred animals and cause greater difficulty and disappointment for surveyed keepers.[4,8] Wild-caught herptiles also represent considerable biosecurity and zoonotic risks to existing collections, local wildlife, and keepers by introducing exotic pathogens directly or through foreign parasitic vectors.[9,10] The importation of wild-caught animals has declined significantly (−70% over a 12-year period) because of increased regulation and CITES protection of coveted species, while the importation of "ranched" animals (hatched and sold from wild-caught adults) from Africa, Asia, and South America has seen a 50-fold increase in recent years.[11] Ranching systems can be readily overexploited as a front for wild-caught operations because of limited oversight and trade regulation.[11,12]

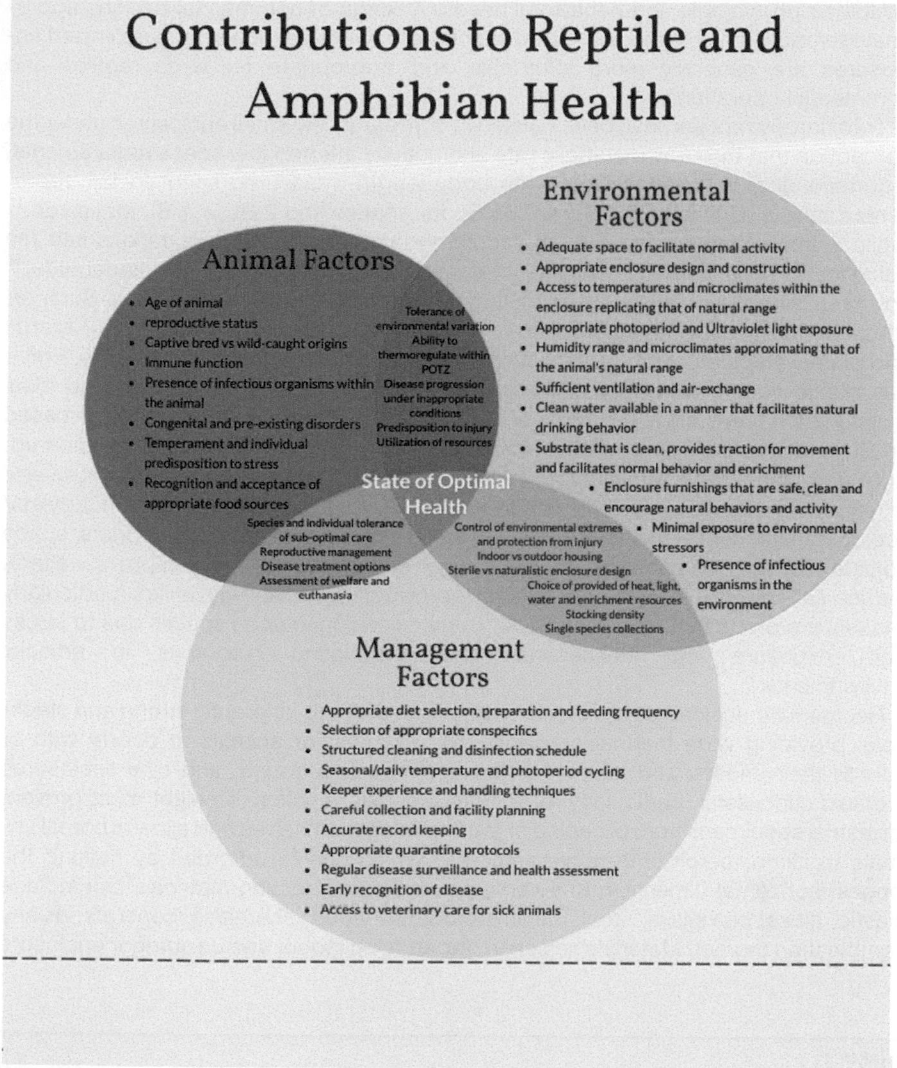

Contributions to Reptile and Amphibian Health

Environmental Factors

- Adequate space to facilitate normal activity
- Appropriate enclosure design and construction
- Access to temperatures and microclimates within the enclosure replicating that of natural range
- Appropriate photoperiod and Ultraviolet light exposure
- Humidity range and microclimates approximating that of the animal's natural range
- Sufficient ventilation and air-exchange
- Clean water available in a manner that facilitates natural drinking behavior
- Substrate that is clean, provides traction for movement and facilitates normal behavior and enrichment
  - Enclosure furnishings that are safe, clean and encourage natural behaviors and activity
  - Minimal exposure to environmental stressors
  - Presence of infectious organisms in the environment

Animal Factors

- Age of animal
- reproductive status
- Captive bred vs wild-caught origins
- Immune function
- Presence of infectious organisms within the animal
- Congenital and pre-existing disorders
- Temperament and individual predisposition to stress
- Recognition and acceptance of appropriate food sources

Tolerance of environmental variation
Ability to thermoregulate within POTZ
Disease progression under inappropriate conditions
Predisposition to injury
Utilization of resources

State of Optimal Health

Species and individual tolerance of sub-optimal care
Reproductive management
Disease treatment options
Assessment of welfare and euthanasia

Control of environmental extremes and protection from injury
Indoor vs outdoor housing
Sterile vs naturalistic enclosure design
Choice of provided of heat, light, water and enrichment resources
Stocking density
Single species collections

Management Factors

- Appropriate diet selection, preparation and feeding frequency
- Selection of appropriate conspecifics
- Structured cleaning and disinfection schedule
- Seasonal/daily temperature and photoperiod cycling
- Keeper experience and handling techniques
- Careful collection and facility planning
- Accurate record keeping
- Appropriate quarantine protocols
- Regular disease surveillance and health assessment
- Early recognition of disease
- Access to veterinary care for sick animals

Fig. 1. Representation of the relative importance and interactions between animal, environment, and management factors contributing to the health of individual animals and the sustainability of a herpetological collection.

ENVIRONMENTAL CONDITIONS AND HUSBANDRY
Enclosure Size, Design, and Construction

Enclosure design should suit the species' needs and purpose of the collection. Pets and animals exhibited for education are often afforded more space and naturalistic furnishings aimed at appealing aesthetics and providing environmental stimulation. By contrast, specimens kept for research, breeding, and commercial industries are generally given more spartan conditions to maximize cleanliness, ease of maintenance, and the number of animals per unit area.[13,14] Neither approach is inappropriate; however, all animals must receive adequate space and sanitary conditions to fulfill their physiologic and behavioral needs. A range of commercial designs appropriate for most small to medium-sized species are available; however, customized enclosures are generally more affordable and appropriate for large reptiles and commercial operations.

Traditionally reptiles have been housed in comparatively small enclosures under the perception that their low metabolic rate and activity inferred low space requirements, recommending floor dimensions (with body length, measured snout to tail, represented by BL) as little as 0.5 BL × 0.33 BL for snakes and 2 BL × 1 BL for lizards.[15] While animals may survive in such accommodations, recent investigations into the behavior of wild herptiles indicate that such dimensions may be inadequate,[16] compromising their welfare by restricting normal movement and activities. Such restrictions are particularly relevant to large athletic species such as monitor lizards and diurnal elapids/colubrids, indicating species-specific spatial requirements. Previous publications have suggested successful maintenance areas (SMAs) and ideal maintenance areas (IMAs) in terms of floor space for reptiles and amphibians based on BL, described in **Table 1**.[13] For arboreal species, height must also be considered. SMA floorplans provide minimum dimensions geared toward breeders/wholesalers/research conditions, while the larger IMA floorplans are intended for hobbyists/zoologic institutions—the area between these values indicating appropriate space adjusted for species and size. Although larger enclosures generally improve welfare, reduce self-inflicted injuries, and bolster reproductive activity—juveniles (particularly snakes) are prone to anorexia and poor body condition in open spaces due to stress from exposure and inexperience thermoregulating resources in artificial environments.[17]

Rectangular enclosures are common because they are inherently strong and stackable, providing wide thermal gradients, few corners for animals to collide with or abrade their snouts, and improved viewing.[18] Square, round, and oval enclosures are also successful, particularly for aquatic species. Enclosure height must prevent terrestrial specimens from escaping or traumatizing themselves and allow arboreal animals to climb, perch, and move vertically, which can be afforded by making the longest horizontal dimension to a vertical one.[18] Construction materials can include plastic, glass, plexiglass, steel, melamine coated wood, fiberglass, concrete, or any combination thereof. Materials selection depends on indoor versus outdoor enclosure

Table 1
Comparison of successful maintenance area (SMA) and ideal maintenance area (IMA) recommendations for various herpetological taxa[5,11,19]

Species	SMA	IMA
Terrestrial snakes	0.6 m²/m BL	1.2 m²/m BL
Arboreal snakes	0.6 m³/m BL	1.2 m³/m BL
Terrestrial lizards	0.2 m²/0.1 m BL	0.5 m²/0.1 m BL
Arboreal lizards	0.2 m³/0.1 m BL	0.5 m³/0.1 m BL
Tortoises and semiaquatic turtles	0.2 m²/0.1 m BL	0.5 m²/0.1 m BL
Purely aquatic turtles	0.2 m³/0.1 m BL	0.5 m³/0.1 m BL
Crocodilians	0.2 m²/0.1 m BL	0.5 m²/0.1 m BL
Terrestrial amphibians	0.2 m³/0.1 m BL	0.5 m³/0.1 m BL
Arboreal amphibians	0.2 m³/0.1 m BL	0.5 m³/0.1 m BL

Abbreviation: BL, body length from snout to tail.

placement, local climate, maintenance of specific temperature and humidity, security, ease of disinfection, providing nonabrasive surfaces, enrichment requirements, and human viewing.[19] Ventilation should be adequate to prevent microbial overgrowth in stagnant air, which can be achieved using air vents or mesh screens on opposite sides of the enclosure to create cross-current airflow.[20] Adequate ventilation is difficult to achieve in traditional glass aquariums without significant modification.

Outdoor housing is possible where the local climate reflects an animal's native range or can be similarly approximated with modification (eg, greenhouses in temperate regions to stabilize higher temperatures for crocodilians). Outdoor enclosures (typically open-topped pits or enclosed aviaries) are often larger than indoor setups and can afford more naturalistic furnishings to create conditions conducive to group housing and incite natural behaviors that improve breeding success (**Fig. 2**).[13] Increased reproductive activity, reduced ongoing expenses, and space for group housing make outdoor systems are very popular with large-scale hobbyists

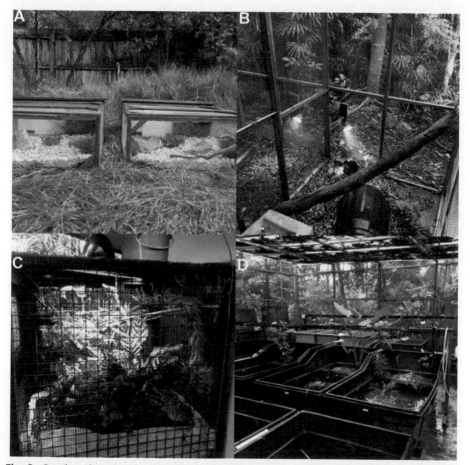

Fig. 2. Outdoor housing for reptiles. (*A*) Lockable outdoor housing for temperate elapids and blue-tongued lizards made from converted rabbit hutches. (*B*) Converted aviary for temporary reptile housing with a supplemental heat source. (*C*) Outdoor breeding enclosure for chameleons with supplemental heating and water dripper system. (*D*) Outdoor breeding facility for semiaquatic turtles within a protective aviary to prevent predation.

and commercial industries.[3] "Wild" conditions bring about "wild" problems—enclosures require predator proofing, and access of noxious pests such as rodents, metaldehyde baited snails, or cane toads (Rhinella marina) should be prevented.[21,22] Weather extremes, inappropriate population dynamics (competition, bullying, starvation), and parasitism can have a greater impact in poorly managed outdoor enclosures than either wild or indoor conditions. Setups must be secure and protected against natural disasters. Most problems can be managed or eliminated with careful enclosure design, making outdoor accommodation optimal for large collections and displays.

All facilities should have hospital housing for unwell animals separate from the main collection and quarantine facilities where possible. Hospital enclosures prioritize cleaning and monitoring the occupant. Thus, they should be minimalistic (water bowl, newspaper or water substrate, hide, heat and light source, perch for arboreal species) and made from easily disinfected surfaces (eg, HDPE plastic).[13,23] Racking systems designed for breeding snakes/lizards are ideal for this situation; however, any suitably sized plastic tub with adequate ventilation holes can be used, providing they can maintain the temperature and with humidity requirements needed for recovery.[19]

Temperature Regulation and Heating

Ectothermy dictates that herptiles rely on environmental temperatures for physiologic and behavioral functions. These body temperatures are typically maintained within a narrow range above ambient temperature through behavioral thermoregulation.[1,24] Many amphibians experience thermoregulatory constraints from preventing evaporative water loss at higher temperatures, selecting cooler preferred body temperatures (PBTs) with higher moisture content.[24–26] The measurement of PBT and establishment of a preferred optimal temperature range (POTR) maintain the PBT has been evaluated in many species using combined analyses of temperatures during field studies, coelomic temperature logging, thermal shuttle boxes, peak temperature survival times, physiologic processing, and protein denaturation studies.[27–29] Swaths of published references for commonly available species are available describing temperature ranges in captivity. For species where the POTR is unknown, inferences are made based on temperatures within their wild distribution, altitude, habitat, and ecological niche as well as data from similar species. Understanding a species' unique microclimate requirements is essential, as temperatures can vary significantly among fossorial, aquatic, terrestrial, and arboreal strata in the same location.[30] These temperatures are best provided as a gradient from the upper optimal temperature (UPOT) to lower optimal temperature (LPOT) ends of the animal's POTR either horizontally or vertically, depending on the animal's ecology.[13] Providing a uniform constant temperature can reduce growth and inhibit normal behavior patterns in Leopard geckos and other species.[31] Diurnal heliothermic species such as monitors and most agamids are more reliant on basking than ambient temperature to achieve PBT (relying on radiant heat sources), and larger species can maintain a core PBT under cooler ambient conditions when provided a warm basking site or direct sunlight because of thermal inertia.[32,33] By contrast, thigmothermic or poikilothermic species are more dependent on ambient temperature and conduction of heat (often from ventrally derived heat sources).[34] Temperature gradients are created based on the species and scale of operation. Sunlight, heat lights, radiant panels, heat cord, aquarium heaters, pool heating, and greenhouses have all been successfully used. Smaller collections housing a range of species may utilize individually controlled enclosures, while background room heating or cooling to keep ambient conditions at the LPOT combined with a small enclosure basking site can improve power efficiency in large establishments and provides supplemental heat if enclosure heating fails.[3] Semiaquatic species often require heated water and basking sites to adequately thermoregulate.[30,35] By contrast, depending on the surrounding climate, most Urodeles and herptiles with ranges of high latitude/altitude may require aquarium chillers or air-conditioning to maintain their lower POTR.[36,37] Animals housed outdoors must be afforded shaded or sheltered areas to prevent overheating.

Daily and seasonal temperature variations affect the diel activity and reproductive patterns of many species, which should be reflected in captivity. Variation exists between even closely related taxa regarding circadian temperature preferences; nocturnal Australian geckos do not display differences in thermoregulation between day and night,[38] while tokay geckos demonstrate peaked metabolism and seek warmer temperatures during the night.[39] Most diurnal reptiles reduce thermoregulatory efforts and utilize cooler temperatures at night.[38] This nightly temperature drop is recommended when simulating environmental conditions to promote natural physiologic behavior and development in zoologic settings; however, for meat and skin production systems, maintaining temperatures at the UPOT together with increased feeding is utilized to accelerate growth rates in juveniles prior to slaughter.[40,41] Temperature changes over the course of the year to induce seasonal dormancy in nontropical reptiles are natural processes and recommended in healthy animals because of correlations with reduced rates of preovulatory dystocia, hepatic disease, and obesity when practiced.[42,43] Gonadal development, sex steroid/sperm production, follicular cycling, and breeding behavior in many herptiles (particularly those from temperate or subtropical climates) are associated with seasonal temperature variation upregulating hypothalamic–pituitary–gonadal axis activity and thyroid hormone production as well as directly stimulating gonadal cells.[44–46] These seasonal changes often improve the breeding success of captive situations and can be artificially manipulated to increase clutch number and minimize nonproductive periods in some species.[47,48]

When artificial heat sources are used, the heat output should be regulated via a thermostat to prevent excessive heat load, and animals should be prevented from directly accessing heat sources with physical barriers or careful placement of heaters out of reach from occupants to prevent thermal burns.[49] Recording of temperatures at different locations in all enclosures should be performed regularly to confirm the appropriate thermal gradient.[13] Electrical elements near water or with risk of breakage should employ ground fault circuit interrupters to prevent electrocution, and an uninterrupted power supply should be considered to reduce the effects of power outages on the collection.

Lighting and Photoperiod

Providing ultraviolet (UV) lighting and regular photoperiod creates great discussion in herpetocultural industries. Light serves important physiologic functions in herptiles. Visible light (400–750 nm) permits vision, thermoregulation, and immune function and influences seasonal reproductive activity and other neuroendocrine responses through circadian melatonin production.[50,51] UV-A (320–400 nm) composes the visible light range for many reptiles and affects social interactions between conspecifics.[30,52] UV-B (290–320 nm) is required for cutaneous vitamin D3 synthesis, contributes to calcium metabolism, and can stimulate appetite.[50] Wild reptiles and amphibians are exposed to a daily and seasonal photoperiod in addition to variable visible/UV light exposure each day depending on shade/cover, activity, elevation, and the time of year. UV and visible light exposure thus depends on species ecology.[53] Many nocturnal geckos and frogs demonstrate basking behavior for short periods during the morning/evening and experimentally can maintain higher systemic vitamin D3 concentrations when given access to UV-B radiation.[54–56] Herpetoculturists agree that diurnal reptiles (agamids/iguanids, monitors, chelonians, skinks, some frogs) require UV-B to avoid syndromes of metabolic bone disease, but many argue nocturnal species (snakes, geckos, crocodilians, most amphibians) do not require artificial light supplementation to thrive in captivity. Lighting is forgone because of added expense and maintenance. Although these animals can survive without light provisions, increasing evidence demonstrates improved health, development, and welfare when light sources are added. Corn snakes demonstrate normal behavior patterns and increased vitamin D3 synthesis when provided with UV-B,[57] crocodiles and caiman experience better growth and improved immune function when exposed to natural light,[40,58] and frogs raised without UV-B and given only oral vitamin D3 supplementation have reduced bone density compared with wild counterparts.[59] In Panther chameleons, adequate maternal UV-B provision reduced the incidence of full-term dead embryos in clutches,[60] and reduced rates of postovulatory dystocia are observed when females are supplied UV-B to facilitate calcium metabolism for oviposition.[13,47] Further research is required to investigate the light requirements in a greater range of species, but all evidence indicates that providing captive reptiles and amphibians full-spectrum lighting should be recommended because of the potential benefits for their health, welfare, reproductive function, and behavior.

The light intensity, wavelength, and duration of exposure required are dependent on species ecology. Herptiles of higher latitudes should experience seasonal variations in day length and light intensity compared with equatorial species, where photoperiod light exposure is more consistent. In some chelonians, a period of shortened day length is demonstrated to trigger reproductive behavior, and seasonal photoperiod (and temperature) shifts are recommended as an adjunct breeding stimulus.[61,62] The UV requirements for over 250 species have been determined based on observations in their natural range, microhabitat, basking behavior, and measured ranges of UV exposure and temperature requirements, categorizing animals into 4 Ferguson zones according to the UV index (UVI).[53,63] Examples of species from this list are included in **Table 2**, and requirements for species not yet determined can be estimated from related and ecologically similar taxa on the list.[53] Not all related species are alike in terms of preferred UVI: 2 chameleons from Madagascar (*Calumma brevicorne* and *C nasutum*) are Ferguson zone 1 reptiles, whereas *C parsonii* is a Ferguson zone 3 species requiring much higher exposure.[53,64]

A wide range of UV-B lighting options exist, and suitable choices for each Ferguson zone are provided in **Table 2**. These lights vary considerably in output wavelength and intensity allowing keepers to select an appropriate option for their species. Mercury vapor and metal halide lamps and can produce considerable heat, and this should be factored into the selection process if other heat sources are to be used. Any mesh placed between the light and the animal can reduce the visible and UV light output by as much as 50%, and glass/most plastics between the light filter almost all UV-B and UV-A, preventing access by the animal.[50] Conversely, aluminum reflectors can increase the irradiance of a lamp 218% compared with its standard output, increasing the functionality of low output lamps for higher Ferguson zones.[53] UV production should be measured monthly in-situ with a quality UVI meter, and most lights require replacement every 6 to 12 months from progressive UV output decay through solarization—even if the light is apparently working.[20]

Natural light should be used wherever possible to provide the greatest wavelength range and intensity and is ideal for facilities where the climate is appropriate for the species—for both reduced cost to the keeper and optimized light exposure to the animal. Herptiles kept outdoors should be offered both exposed and shaded areas

Table 2
Ferguson zone divisions, UV index (UVI) estimates, and appropriate methods of provision for various herpetological taxa in captivity[52,62]

Ferguson Zone	Characteristics	UVI Zone Range	Maximum Recorded UVI	Method of UV Provision[a]	Example Species
1	Crepuscular/ shade dweller	0–0.7	0.6–1.4	Shade method	Fire salamander, blue dart frog, spiny hill turtle, emerald tree boa, crocodile skink
2	Partial sun/ occasional basker	0.7–1.0	1.1–3.0	Shade method (in large cages, gentle sunbeam can be used)	White's tree frog, eastern box turtle, western hognose snake, angle-headed dragon sp, spectacled caiman
3	Open/partial sun basker	1.0–2.6	2.9–7.4	Sunbeam method	Amazon milk frog, leopard tortoise, diamond python, Argentine tegu
4	"Midday" open sun basker	2.6–3.5	4.5–9.5	Sunbeam method	Galapagos tortoise, Komodo dragon, chuckwalla, Cunningham's skink

[a] Shade method: a lower UV level over the entire enclosure → fluorescent tube ideal sunbeam method: higher UVI focused on basking site; lower background UV level → mercury vapor, metal halide, or T5-HO fluorescent tube.

providing an ultraviolet gradient. Indoor-housed specimens can be placed outside for short periods (15–30 minutes) on a regular basis ensuring these setups be monitored, well ventilated, and partially shaded; glass/plastic can create dangerous heat build-up in confined spaces. Further investigation is required into the minimum time and frequency of sunlight exposure required for maintaining normal systemic vitamin D concentrations.

Care must be taken with the placement of enclosure lighting to adhere to recommended distances from animals and prevent direct access to the light, particularly with mercury vapor and metal halide lamps, where the risk of burn injuries is high; however, even fluorescent tubes can be dangerous if broken by strong lizards or snakes.[49] Some lights produce very short wavelength UV-B and UV-C (below 290 nm), both of which are toxic to epithelial cells at close range and can result in photokeratoconjunctivitis, severe photodermatitis, and death with prolonged exposure.[65,66]

Humidity and Water

The sensible and insensible fluid loss of captive herptiles must be compensated for to prevent dehydration. Drinking water alone is insufficient without creating an appropriate microclimate to replace cutaneous and respiratory losses.[67] Water balance is essential to kidney health, ecdysis, growth, reproduction, and digestion.[33] Establishing a humidity gradient that replicates an animal's native habitat can be challenging because of the inverse relationship between humidity and ventilation. Rainforest and semiaquatic species are provided high (70%–100%) relative humidity (RH) through limited enclosure ventilation, a moisture-laden substrate, and a substantial water source—combined, this creates a stagnant environment that promotes bacterial and fungal overgrowth—predisposing inhabitants to respiratory and dermatologic infections.[68] The accessory saccular lung lobe extending from the cervical trachea of some chameleons is suspected to predispose chameleons to pneumonia in poorly ventilated environments.[69,70] Amphibians have high requirements for humidity owing to their permeable skin; however, stagnant conditions with excessive environmental pathogens will result in bacterial, fungal, or algal dermatosepticemia.[71,72] Better means for providing rainforest species high humidity involve creating humid microclimates using hides filled with moist sphagnum, substrates with drainage layers to remove excess moisture, timed misting systems to allow cages to periodically dry out, and IV-line drip systems as a water source for arboreal species.[13] If very high humidity is required (eg, tree boas, dendrobatids, *Abronia*, *Tribolonotus*), increased moisture can be paired with increased ventilation using screen top/sided enclosures or axial fans to increase airflow.[49] The RH of entire rooms can be raised using vaporizers or humidifiers, allowing features like drip systems in each enclosure to be used without excessively wetting every surface. For arid-adapted species, a lower RH (20%–60%) can be provided by limiting access to water over the course of the week and using nonabsorbent or desiccating substrates. Even arid animals that require humid microclimates periodically can suffer dysecdysis without a humid retreat or brief misting approaching shedding.[73] Regularly soaking tortoises and providing a higher RH to juveniles during periods of growth is demonstrated to have a greater impact on preventing pyramiding than diet, lighting, and temperature.[74]

Water should be kept clean, preferably being replaced daily except for large, filtered sources. Arboreal herptiles can be provided elevated bowls or misting, terrestrial species can be given water bowls or puddles, and aquatic species can be given water sources large enough to swim in and maintain PBT. Water receptacles must be appropriately sized (ideally large enough for soaking), readily disinfected, and shaped to permit escape and avoid accidental drowning. Dechlorination by aging tap water or adding dechlorinator is recommended for amphibians and aquatic reptiles, and the use of reverse osmosis/deionized (RO/DI) water with reconditioning salts will remove toxins, impurities, and infectious agents (including *Batrachochytrium*).[75] RO water also appears to reduce the incidence of spindly leg syndrome in Harlequin toads, the reason for this is unknown.[76] Aquatic systems can be supplied via constant influx-efflux of fresh, clean water (open systems) or the periodically changing a percentage of the total water volume (semiclosed systems); the former being a challenge to maintain except in the largest facilities.[75] Appropriate biological filtration, temperature, aeration, water changing, and water testing (for pH, ammonia, nitrite, nitrate, GH, KH) should be provided and factored into the maintenance of aquatic semiclosed systems.

Substrate and Furnishings

Substrate choice is a major determinant of collection health and is decided by the purpose of the collection and the species kept. In large facilities, substrates that are easily cleaned take priority over aesthetics and enrichment; however, providing for behavioral needs like burrowing, foraging, and hiding and furnishing a comfortable surface with enough traction for locomotion are required. Quarantine, laboratory, and farming facilities may elect no substrate at all for frogs, crocodiles, lizards, or chelonians in plastic, fiberglass, or smooth concrete pens, with the transition from land to water surfaces provided by sloping the tub, using plumbed drainage systems for continuous cleaning.[4,19,41] Snakes and lizards in intensive industries are maintained on newspaper, butcher paper, or wood shavings such as aspen or cypress, which facilitates hiding and burrowing of these animals.[77] In zoos or private collections, shredded/ground coconut husk, washed river sand, sterilized soil, or sphagnum moss are excellent choices when paired with appropriate maintenance. Cedar and treated pine products contain a resin that is potentially toxic to herptiles affecting the brain, liver, and respiratory tract and should not be used.[77,78] Similarly, substrates that are dusty or form a powder should be avoided because of irritation of the airways, eyes, and scales.[13] Crushed walnut or pecan shells cause impactions when ingested and promote *Aspergillus* spp spore growth and are not recommended.[13,20] Artificial compacting sands, fine gravel, and clay-based cat litters should also not be used because of the risk of gastrointestinal impaction.[49] Stones larger than the animal's head are safe but are difficult to keep clean. Moisture-retentive substrates affect the microclimates within the enclosure and minimize insensible water loss by increasing both local and enclosure-wide humidity, and this is particularly important to fossorial species or juvenile reptiles with a high surface area/volume ratio, where chronic dehydration from the use of desiccating substrates can cause mortalities.[4,79,80] Persistently wet, warm substrate without top-down ventilation to replace the warm moist air with cool, dry air will promote rapid bacterial overgrowth; therefore, moisture-retentive substrates are not recommended for closed plastic tubs or racking systems without adequate top ventilation.[13,18,79] Bioactive substrates utilizing a "cleanup crew" of nitrifying bacteria, fungi, plants, and invertebrate detritivores (eg, springtails and isopods) to break down fecal and food waste have become incredibly popular as they reduce pathogenic bacteria in the environment, stabilize humidity and reduce stress to the animal through less frequent cleaning.[79,81] Bioactive systems require a deep substrate base (bottom drainage layer, mesh separation, nutrient-rich/aerated loam, and often a surface cover of leaf litter/stones) in addition to live plants, natural furnishings, and regular water supply to thrive, and depend on a stable population of "janitors" to aerate the soil, preventing saturation, impaction, and toxic anaerobic conditions.[13,82] Such arrangements are very successful and have revolutionized keeping dendrobatids; however, their initial expense and ongoing maintenance can prove challenging to apply to large-scale production industries. Additionally, during an infectious disease outbreak, the substrate must be discarded and replaced regularly, which is expensive and time-consuming.

Minimalist enclosure furnishings should include a dark hide for cover, a water bowl, a haul-out area for semiaquatics, and a basking surface for "sun-worshippers." Animals without hiding places demonstrate overt stress and higher cortisol levels and are prone to illness through stress-induced immunosuppression.[14,83–85] The "bare-minimum" approach to herpetoculture should be considered only in quarantine, research, or large-scale production facilities. Enrichment options such as ground cover, wood/branches, rocks, live plants, and artificial backgrounds should be considered for all captive herptiles to fulfill normal ecological activities and simulate their natural habitat (**Fig. 3**). Arboreal species have an innate need to climb, perch, and be off the ground and fail to thrive without these provisions.[17] Furnishings should be fixed in position to prevent collapse and injury to the animal. Natural furnishings from wild sources require disinfection prior to use—wood and rocks can be scrubbed with dilute bleach, and soil and leaf litter may be sterilized by baking in a dry oven.[13,79] Doing so

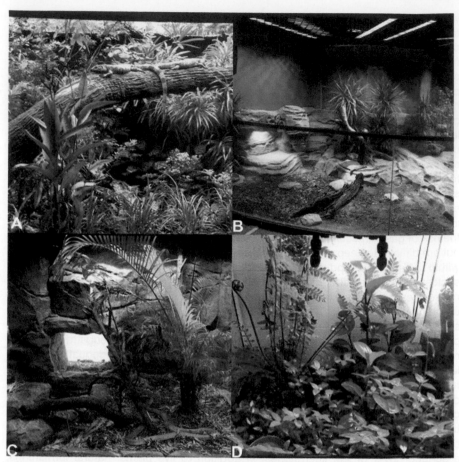

Fig. 3. Naturalistic enclosures. (*A*) Larger enclosures afford more opportunities for cohabitation, increased enrichment opportunities, and improved aesthetics for onlookers. (*B*) Arid-themed setup incorporating multiple focused basking sites and multiple feeding opportunities for inhabitants. (*C*) Naturalistic housing for venomous species should include trap boxes, as shown in the rear of the image. (*D*) Dart frog vivarium with copious growth of live plants over a bioactive substrate.

removes parasites, fungi, bacteria, and viruses that may be potentially pathogenic, permitting recolonization with beneficial microbiota.

DIETARY REQUIREMENTS

The nutritional needs for reptiles and amphibians is highly understudied; thus, dietary inadequacy remains a leading cause of disease in herpetoculture.[13] Captive diets should always be based on studies of wild observations, yet this can be both challenging and conflicting—1 study in wild adult bearded dragons identified animal matter constituting 61% DM (dry matter) of the total diet, whereas a second demonstrated that insects are comprised in only 10% of DM.[86,87] Food items should be freshly prepared; however, freezing or partial cooking of foods is acceptable and may release some nutrients locked in plant cell walls.[13,88] Frozen food items should be disposed of within 6 months if not used, and uneaten food should be removed from enclosures within 6 hours to reduce ingestion of rancid material. Ontogenetic shifts in dietary requirements are common and should be accounted for when feeding juveniles versus adults.[89] Despite the psychological stimulation it provides, feeding live vertebrate prey is not considered acceptable, and hunting behavior can be replicated with forceps or tong feeding; additionally, prey items can seriously wound disinterested predators when confined together.[90] Food is a potential vector for parasites, bacteria, fungi, and viruses. Animal prey should be frozen for 4 weeks and plant matter thoroughly washed before feeding, wild-caught food items should be avoided, and transferal of unwanted items from 1 enclosure to the next should never be practiced.[68,88] Preparation of carnivorous and herbivorous diets should be performed separately to reduce potential cross-contamination of pathogens like *Salmonella, Campylobacter,* and *Escherichia coli.*[91] The vitamin and mineral requirements of most herptiles remain undetermined, and overprovision can be toxic; however, supplementation in captivity is required in most cases for insectivores, omnivores, and less so, herbivores. Some general rules apply:

1. Herpetocultural supplements have little oversight, and composition varies greatly. Many available options are not complete multivitamins.[88] Selection is based on careful analysis of labeling and species needs. Human multivitamins are not recommended. Ca and vitamin supplements should not be premixed.
2. Calcium is required in almost all cases but should not be supplied with a phosphorus-based salt (negates the calcium supplement) or iron and zinc (Ca reduces absorption). Ca supplements containing phosphorus require a Ca:$P>20:1$ to overcome the poor Ca:P of commercially available insects.[88]
3. Not all species metabolize dietary vitamin D efficiently, and many iguanids and chameleons preferentially synthesize vitamin D when provided with ample UV-B radiation.[60,92,93]
4. Vitamin A is frequently not provided in supplements but traded for a stable precursor β-carotene, which many reptiles cannot convert.[88]

Commercially formulated diets are increasingly popular; however, these also suffer poor oversight in their production, and buyers must carefully assess options to ensure guaranteed analysis and appropriate nutrient analysis on a DM basis from the product label.[94] Formulated diets have great potential in herpetoculture, and continued research into species-specific requirements for complete nutrition and maximal growth is required.

The known requirements for captive herptiles are summarized:

Insectivores

This group includes nearly all amphibians, most lizards, some turtles, and a few snakes.[88] Specific nutritional requirements are unknown for most species and are extrapolated from NRC requirements for laboratory insectivores.[95] Larval insects (except silkworms) contain excessive fat, but all invertebrates have adequate protein to support growth.[95,96] Commercially raised insects are severely Ca-deficient, whereas annelids and crustaceans have positive (yet still inadequate) Ca/P ratios.[97] Ca and vitamins A/D require supplementation for captive insectivores.[95,97] Gut-loading insects with a quality dry, nutrient-dense, Ca-fortified diet containing greater than 8% Ca for 12 hours to 5 days prior to feeding can overcome these deficits[98,99] and should be augmented through the use of regular calcium and multivitamin dusting of feeders, though this is less effective for aquatic animals and inadequate after 4 to 5 hours if not eaten.[100,101] Improved growth and nutrient availability are obtained from feeding a variety of invertebrates instead of a monoculture diet.[88,102] The risk of pesticide ingestion in animals fed wild invertebrate sources is exceedingly rare. All insectivores should be provided with UV-B to promote vitamin D uptake. Fireflies are toxic to many reptiles and amphibians and should never be fed.[103]

Carnivores

Carnivores include most snakes, all crocodilians, some lizards and amphibians, and many aquatic turtles.[88] Carnivorous reptile nutritional requirements are based on laboratory analyses of mammalian predators that require high protein (25%–60% DM), high fat (30%–60% DM) and low carbohydrates (<10% DM) with a species-appropriate amino acid profile.[104,105] Dietary deficiencies are rare when fed whole prey, as most choices represent a balanced nutrient base.[88] Prey should be fed a commercial formulated diet; not seed/scraps/dog food creating poor nutritional quality. Muscle and viscera has a low Ca/P ratio and should not be fed exclusively.[68] Very specific dietary requirements (eg, ophiophagy in King cobras) can either be accommodated in captivity or attempts can be made to convert to more conventional diets without apparent ill effect.[106] Some fish are thiamine and vitamin E deficient after freezing because of activation of thiaminase and oxidation of lipids, warranting supplementation.[107] Feeding a range of fish species will circumvent this. Crocodile farms commonly use by-products of other animal industries, which is acceptable for animals to be culled but not for long-term use.[108]

Omnivores

Includes some lizards (eg, bearded dragons, sailfin dragons, blue-tongued skinks) and turtles (sliders, box turtles, sea turtles, Australian short-necked turtles). Variable, adaptable nutritional requirements of 15% to 40% protein, 5% to 40% fat, 20% to 75% carbohydrates DMB.[109] Fruits should be avoided because of low overall nutritional content, otherwise a mix of plant, insect and animal material can be offered in addition to a large proportion of commercial dragon/turtle pelleted diet, with calcium and multivitamin supplementation required less frequently than for insectivores. The juveniles of omnivorous species typically consume far more insect and animal protein than adults.[88]

Herbivores

Herbivores include most iguanids, some agamids, monkey-tailed skinks, some sea turtles, and most tortoises. They require a dietary composition of approximately 15% to 35% protein, greater than 10% fat, 50% to 75% carbohydrates (containing 15%–45% crude fiber) DMB.[109] Herbivore diets are challenging to accommodate in captivity. Reptile herbivores are hindgut fermenters receiving proteins, vitamins, and volatile fatty acids for digestion from symbiotic gut flora.[110] All herbivores require appropriate UV-B to synthesize vitamin D and allow dietary Ca absorption.[88,93] Natural diets are very diverse and offering variety in captivity is more important than 1 "best choice" as few captive options are similar to what these animals naturally feed on.[88] Salad greens and vegetables are typically too low in fiber, Ca, trace minerals/vitamins and high in simple carbohydrates; fed in large volumes these predispose herbivores to hepatic lipidosis and intestinal dysbiosis.[88,111] It is difficult to provide a balanced diet with only greens, vegetables, and fruit, and providing Ca/vitamin supplements with green-foods often remains insufficient.[92] Commercial herbivore diets vary greatly in suitability, but several brands closely match the needs of herbivorous chelonians/lizards and can account for 40% to 50% of the diet. Timothy and grass hays closely match the nutrient profile of wild desert tortoises, and together with fresh grasses and native vegetation should contribute 40% (as fed) to tortoise diets.[112,113] Fresh greens, vegetables, flowers, and weeds can be comprised in 20% of the chelonian diet and in 50% of the iguanid diet.[92] When fed predominantly balanced commercial diets, limited Ca/vitamin supplementation is required for herbivores.[88]

CONSIDERATIONS REGARDING STRESS AND WELFARE IN HERPETOLOGICAL COLLECTIONS

Animals under human care should be afforded the 5 domains of animal welfare (physical related factors such as adequate/balanced nutrition and water, a comfortable physical environment, maintenance of a healthy/fit physical state, the ability to express rewarding behaviors, and opportunities to maximize positive experiences while minimizing aversive ones) to ensure physical and mental wellbeing, regardless of their reason for captivity.[114,115] At a minimum, for herptiles this translates to having choice when accessing required environmental parameters within their enclosure, providing food/water based on their natural history, and providing enrichment through features in their setup or interactions with conspecifics where appropriate.[81] Regular rearrangement of furnishings, creating social complexity through cohabitation, training and interaction with caretakers, and controlled low level "stressors" (eg, male combat, seasonal temperature cycling, seasonal dietary restriction) add intrinsic psychological value for many taxa and should be accounted for (**Fig. 4**).[81,116] Naturalistic exhibits frequently support these requirements; however, basic setups that are species-appropriate and well maintained can provide good welfare (**Fig. 5**).[117] Reptile welfare and cognition studies are identifying many inconsistencies and inadequacies in previously accepted mantra. Space provisions for captive reptiles are currently being questioned: snakes are frequently denied the opportunity for rectilinear motion or positioning in small enclosures, and monitor lizards with extensive wild ranges and active diurnal behavior are routinely confined to cages twice their total length.[16,118] There is a movement away from keeping reptiles in small, barren setups toward housing them in ways that better fulfill their enrichment and cognitive needs.[119] Another contended issue is stocking density and communal housing. For commercially farmed species (crocodiles, alligators, soft-shelled turtles, bullfrogs) ideal stocking rates are known,[41,120,121] but these can rarely be applied to similar animals (eg, snapping turtles are more aggressive than soft-shelled turtles, increased territoriality of dendrobatids compared with bullfrogs).[5,122] Many species in the pet trade, zoos, and conservation programs have no published data on stocking density and may be subjected to unnecessary social stress in captivity. Breeders must balance providing for these physiologic and psychological needs with maximizing animals per unit area for peak production. Clinicians must be able to recognize signs of stress in herptiles and potential stressors and advise on how these can be controlled.[81]

PLANNING THE COLLECTION

Successful herpetological enterprises require clear definable goals and adequate curatorial input to ensure such targets are attained. Institutions should budget for proposed financial inputs/outputs to prevent overexpenditure and compromised welfare. Thought should be given to maintaining population sustainability and counteracting unexpected losses or repopulation costs. Zoologic and conservation facilities must select species based on regional biodiversity, conservation and educational value, and are guided by the needs and recommendations of governing zoologic organizations to promote genetic diversity, meet population targets, repatriation goals, and prevent surplus breeding.[3,123] Where species recovery or reintroduction is the primary

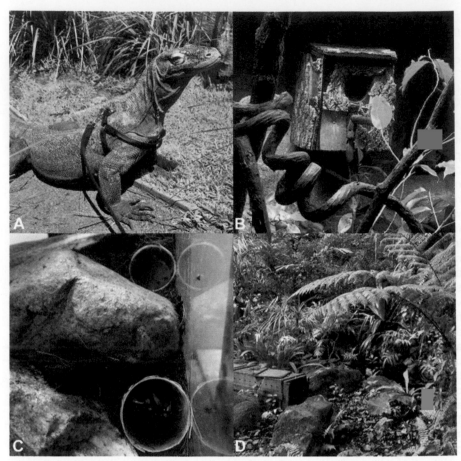

Fig. 4. Enrichment and training. (*A*) Young Komodo dragon taken on a controlled walk around a zoo for regular enrichment. (*B*) Raised nest box for egg deposition and hiding in arboreal reptiles. (*C*) Artificial humid tunnels for amphibians. (*D*) Acclimation and training of an African Dwarf crocodile (bottom left of image) to transport container prior to shipping.

output, planning is required to maintain genetic diversity; however, for taxa threatened with imminent extinction, increasing the global metapopulation takes priority. Controlled short-term inbreeding may be required, with few long-term consequences for wild populations based on genetic analysis of previously fragmented populations.[124,125] Skilled, educated, experienced staff are invaluable to provide daily assessment of both animals and equipment, and less experienced team-members should receive ongoing opportunities for continuous education.[3] Staff dedicated to particular roles (food preparation, general husbandry, quarantine) are preferred and reduce disease transmission versus 1 staff member performing all these tasks.

Facility design heavily influences husbandry and maintenance (**Fig. 6**). Species from different biogeographical regions (temperate, tropical, arid) can be maintained in separate rooms that are temperature, photoperiod, and humidity controlled, allowing background regulation of conditions corresponding to each climatic zone, with individual cages offering species-specific microclimates more effectively.[3] Utilizing

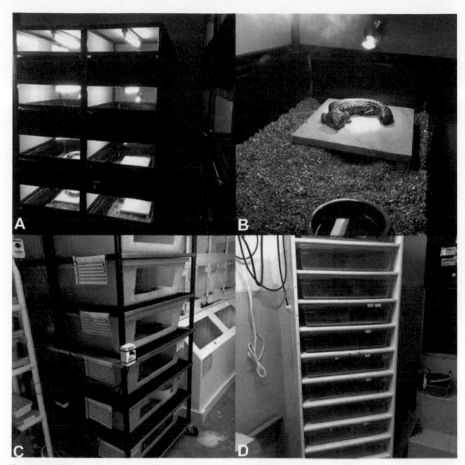

Fig. 5. Racking systems. (*A + B*) Racking design at the Author's facility for housing Tiliqua skinks; each tub provides ample space, basking, UV, digging, hiding, and foraging opportunities required for this species. (*C*) Modified racking system for elapids with cutout viewing panels to allow inspection prior to enclosure access. (*D*) Racking system to house nocturnal lizards.

natural sunlight with minimal filtering provides an accessible, beneficial and aesthetic background light source in enclosures.[125] Water supply, electrical access, adequate storage, and waste disposal in all rooms will greatly improve workflow.[13] Colder locations require insulated or heated flooring to prevent the "heat-sink" effect on concrete enclosures at ground level, which can negatively affect thermoregulation and basking behavior.[3]

Interspecific and intraspecific cohabitation of herptiles is possible. Inappropriate cohabitation is stressful for captives, and pairing cannibalistic or territorial species can be unacceptably dangerous.[81] Successful cohabitation requires increased space (adding half the minimum enclosure dimensions for each additional animal),[18] multiple additional resources such as basking sites/hides/feed bowls/perches (*n+1* resources at a minimum, where *n* = number of animals), providing visual barriers, closely monitoring the group (with fortnightly weight/condition scoring) and removing problem individuals.[3,125,126] Specimens are matched on size and behavioral traits, and species

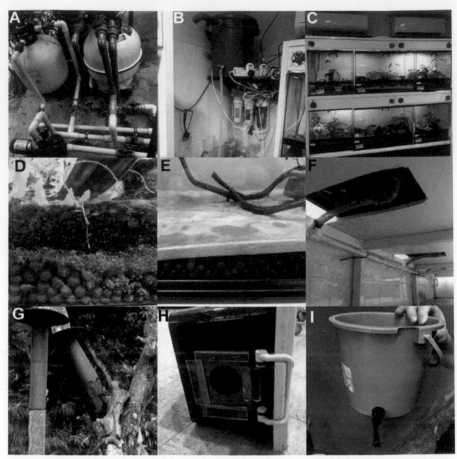

Fig. 6. Enclosure design features. (*A*) Sand and charcoal filtration system for aquatic display located external to building to improve access and reduce heat accumulation. (*B*) RO/DI filtration system for amphibian water supply to remove contaminants and stabilize water conditions. (*C*) Dual air-conditioning system running at alternate times to reduce overload on a single unit and act as a backup in the event of failure. (*D* + *E*) Example of drainage, separation, substrate and surface layering in a bioactive substrate, and modification of a bioactive media during medical treatment using a sponge for easy cleaning and replacement. (*F*) Multilayered water draining to prevent fluid accumulation in substrates of a semi-aquatic setup. (*G*) Guard poles around natural tree trunks in outdoor setup allowing controlled access to climbing resources while preventing escape. (*H*) Quarantine trap box design for venomous species. (*I*) modified bucket-drip system for simple, cost-effective water supply and humidity control in a chameleon breeding facility.

capable of predating on another should not be paired. Males often cannot be cohabited because of territorial aggression, and although male–female and female–female groups are often successful, this is not always the case (eg, most female chameleons are intolerant of males outside breeding and will not accept other females except in very large cages).[69] Species from different geographic locations should not be paired because of increased pathogen susceptibility in an immunologically naïve population.[13] Some species asymptomatically carry organisms that cause disease in others, such as chelonians and crocodilians harboring commensal proto-zoa like *Entamoeba* causing severe gastrointestinal disease in squamates—mixing of these taxa (particularly snakes with chelonians) should be avoided (**Fig. 7**).[111]

Maintaining accurate records of an individual's identification, physical state, prior history, husbandry conditions, daily observations, reproductive events, and medical interventions is crucial in large collections.[127] Individual identifiers (microchips, photo-graphs, scale/toe cuttings, cage cards, scute tags) are recommended for all animals. Records should be stored electronically with duplicate copies maintained off-site,[3] and this can be done using excel spreadsheets or through an online database service for animal collections.[128]

REDUCING DISEASE TRANSMISSION

Different collections have differing biosecurity requirements and disease risks. In closed collections with no new animals entering the collection under any means, dis-ease prevention is the focus of biosecurity and veterinary work. By comparison, open collections (most operations, particularly wholesalers and retailers) focus on detecting new diseases, although prevention must still be considered.[4,129] Written biosecurity protocols should be available to all staff and reviewed regularly for currency. Daily workflow should ensure vulnerable groups (neonates, delicate species) are fed/cleaned first, followed by mature/hardy animals; those with medical conditions are handled last.[3] Feeding and cleaning facilities should be physically separated, and gloves worn/changed between cages (washing hands thoroughly between animals is acceptable). Each room should contain separate, labeled, nontransferable equip-ment. Footbaths between large enclosures (or at a minimum between quarantine and hospital) is recommended; however, these must be well maintained to prevent inactivation of disinfectant with organics.[3,4,41] Daily, weekly, monthly, quarterly, and annual cleaning schedules should be developed; these requirements vary but at a minimum, feces, food waste and other unsanitary materials should be removed daily, and soiled substrate or furnishings that cannot be disinfected disposed of.[130] Disin-fecting bioactive substrates will kill beneficial microorganisms; instead feces can be removed and substrate changed in sections if needed. Naturalistic enclosures should be reserved for collections (or parts thereof) where infectious disease prevalence is low, as clearing pathogenic organisms established in these enclosures is diffi-cult.[13,18,79] Organic matter must be removed from enclosures using detergent and hot water for effective disinfection.[130] Cleaning items should be disposable and not reused between enclosures. Disinfectants should be chosen based on disease risk analysis and requirements; chlorhexidine, iodophors, and phenolic compounds have demonstrated fatal toxicities when in contact with amphibians, and chlorhexidine bathing has previously caused 2 turtle mortalities.[130–133] Quaternary ammonium com-pounds such as F10 represent a safe choice for most situations and have a broad effective spectrum against bacteria (may be limited against *Pseudomonas*), bacterial spores, mycobacterium, fungi, and enveloped and nonenveloped viruses.[130,131,134] All disinfectants require a contact time of 10 to 30 minutes depending on the compound, and some are more effective when not rinsed off after use.[130]

Stress can be reduced by minimizing unwanted disruptions, keeping changes to enclosure furnishings/keepers/routines to a minimum, creating appropriate social groups, and providing optimal microclimates and nutrition. These steps will help pre-vent chronic corticosterone elevation, which negatively affects growth, reproduction, and immune function.[81] Pest species that can pose a direct threat to captives, intro-duce diseases, or consume captive diets include birds, rodents, insects, small

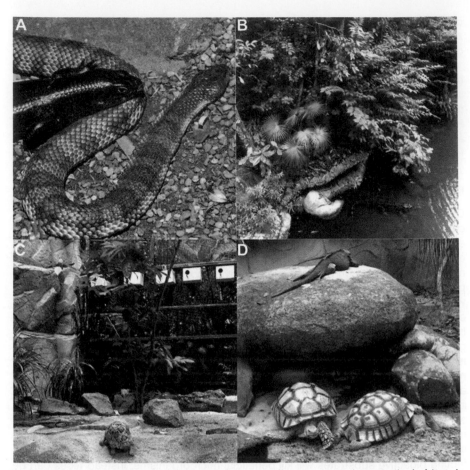

Fig. 7. Multispecies enclosures. (*A*) Species that naturally co-occur and use similar habitats in the wild (such as this land mullet and tiger snake) and are of similar size make appropriate cohabitants; however, housing snakes with other species always presents some degree of risk. (*B*) Large outdoor enclosure cohousing Tomistoma and Siamang; both species naturally never share the same space in these enclosures and have adequate provisions to avoid each other. (*C*) Birds can be safely cohoused with some reptiles, such as tortoises, with few chances of predation or disease spread. (*D*) Squamates and chelonians should not be cohabited in enclosures unless the health status of both species is thoroughly investigated prior to introduction to reduce disease transmission.

carnivores and wild reptiles/amphibians.[3,135] Establishing an integrated pest management program targeting indirect suppressive control measures (eliminate desirable pest resources and improve sanitation in animal facilities) is the cornerstone of pest control, with direct suppression (baiting, repellents, removal) being used adjunctively.[135] Routine epidemiologic evaluation of disease events will aid the control of future outbreaks, identify areas of inadequate husbandry, and provide guidelines for collection management. Doing so requires evaluation of husbandry notes, veterinary records, pathology reports, collection plans, and enclosure designs on a regular basis.[136] Facilities housing high densities of reptiles and amphibians should practice strict personal hygiene to minimize zoonotic disease potential. A list of zoonotic genera linked to herptile-transmitted cases is provided in **Table 3**.[137,138] Preventing zoonotic infections entails prohibiting immunocompromised individuals from working with reptiles, avoiding using live foods, keeping human kitchen areas away from animal facilities, washing hands and wearing gloves during maintenance, draining water into toilets instead of the sink, using face-masks/shields when cleaning, and screening for zoonotic pathogens as a part of collection health management.[9,138,139]

QUARANTINE

Quarantine is essential to prevent the entry of infectious diseases into collections, monitor recovery after shipment, and allow animals to adjust to new husbandry measures. Stressed reptiles are more susceptible to infectious disease and increase pathogen shedding; thus, quarantine is required to avert this increased transmission risk.[140,141] Quarantine facilities should be physically separated from the main collection, utilize a separate ventilation system, and ideally employ separate staff (at a minimum, tend to quarantined animals on alternate days to or after working with the main collection).[141,142] Enclosures should accommodate the needs of the animal and minimize stress during acclimation, containing minimal furnishings that can be either disinfected or disposed of.[140] Newspaper, water, no substrate, or thin replaceable sponge (for amphibians) are all ideal substrate choices.[19] Dedicated quarantine equipment should not leave the facility. Accurate health and husbandry records before and after transfer from isolation are essential and often required as a part of international standards for zoologic and farming industries.[125,142]

Disease risk analysis (DRA) involves estimating the current presence, exposure, and consequences of introducing a pathogen to a collection and should be performed for all major infectious diseases for the species being acquired and for other species currently held in the collection.[141,143] Steps to performing DRA include (1) hazard identification, (2) risk assessment, (3) risk management, and (4) risk communication.[143] To complete this, the animal's origins, medical records, disease pathophysiology, recommended transmission controls, and ways the disease risk can be communicated to relevant parties should be identified. A list of pathogens to be considered for DRA in herpetocultural facilities is provided in **Table 4**.[141] The preexistence of these pathogens in a collection, and the function of those animals can greatly influence the decision matrix of a DRA. Where the collection is aimed at displaying animals and not focused on breeding and distribution, preexisting chronic viral or bacterial disorders

Table 3	
Zoonotic pathogens causing disease in humans with confirmed or suspected links to reptile/amphibian-transmitted cases[136-138]	
Bacteria	*Salmonella, Aeromonas, Plesiomonas, Campylobacter, Clostridium, Mycobacterium, Coxiella burnetii, Leptospira, Chlamydia, Rickettsia, Borrelia,*
Fungi	*Entomophthorales, Metarhizium, Beauveria*
Viruses	Western equine encephalitis virus, Eastern equine encephalitis virus, West Nile virus
Protozoa	*Sarcocystis, Cryptosporidia*
Pentatomidae	*Armillifer, Kiricephalus, Porocephalus, Raillietiella sp.*
Helminths	*Spirometra, Diphyllobothrium, Trichinella, Gnathostoma, Alaria, Echinostoma,*
Arthropods	Ticks (Spreading vector-borne diseases), trombiculid mites, snake mites

Table 4
Pathogens to be considered in disease risk analyses for different herpetological species[140]

Amphibians	Chelonians	Crocodilians	Lizards	Snakes
Ranavirus	Herpesvirus	Pox Virus	Adenovirus	Paramyxovirus
Chytridiomycosis	Iridovirus	West Nile Virus	Nidovirus	Reptarenavirus
Chlamydiosis	Picornavirus	Chlamydiosis	*Nannizziopsis* +	Nidovirus
Helminthiasis	Amebiasis	Mycoplasmosis	*Paranannizziopsis*	Bornavirus
	Helminthiasis	Helminthiasis	Cryptosporidiosis	Adenovirus
	Intranuclear		Helminthiasis	*Ophidiomyces*
	Coccidiosis		Mites	Cryptosporidiosis
	Mycoplasmosis		Ticks	Helminthiasis
	Ticks			Amebiasis
				Mites
				Ticks

that can otherwise be managed on a case-by-case basis without euthanasia of asymptomatic individuals may preclude the need to screen for these organisms during quarantine or the elimination of specimens testing positive. Conversely, a refuge population maintained in a conservation program would typically aim to remain free of infectious diseases, necessitating screening for all major pathogens during quarantine and euthanasia of confirmed positives for contagious disorders.

Quarantine protocols entail a sequence of key disease-rule outs. Entering quarantine, all specimens must be thoroughly examined, their reference weights recorded, and their obvious disorders identified and addressed on arrival.[140] Permanent identification should be established on entry. Transport boxes should be discarded or disinfected prior to reuse.[142] Animals are ideally quarantined individually to allow better assessment of behavior, appetite, and fecal output.[140] Any problems identified in quarantine require extension of the predetermined quarantine period until the condition is resolved.[141] Ectoparasites must be screened for on multiple occasions; mites are easily missed, and ticks, which represent clinically significant vectors of disease, are commonly shipped from the country of origin on wild-caught or outdoor-housed animals.[140,144,145] Internal parasite screening (direct smear, flotation, and sedimentation) should not be performed on arrival—instead, waiting 1 to 2 weeks for animals to begin feeding and shedding more parasites after the stress of transport results in better detection.[141,146] A second fecal exam is performed 2 to 4 weeks later. Wellness bloodwork, fungal skin cytology, viral PCR, serologic testing, radiographs, or ultrasound can be taken as required, keeping the contact time with quarantining animals to a minimum. PCR for snake viruses (particularly in python/boid collections) and *Batrachochytrium* in amphibians are valuable during quarantine because of their high sensitivity/specificity.[147,148] PCR and serologic testing of some diseases (*Cryptosporidium, Mycoplasma*) have limited value in healthy animals not currently shedding, and negative serologic results will not exclude early infections.[141] Many novel pathogens cannot be tested for, warranting a consistent quarantine structure for every shipment. The quarantine period depends greatly on the DRA of incoming animals; wild-caught specimens require longer a quarantine and more rigorous testing than animals with well-documented health records and no identified disease risks.[149] Thus, quarantine periods can range from as little as 14 to 90 days, with 3 months being standard in most collections.[141] *Sunshinevirus* and tortoise picornavirus can be shed from asymptomatic animals for several years, indicating that we cannot "out-quarantine" some viral diseases; clearing these pathogens requires testing prior to entering a collection.[147,150] Ideally, no new animals should enter quarantine until the previous batch has completed its duration, and an "all-in/all-out" policy is recommended if new animals must enter beforehand—quarantine for all animals is extended until the last group has completed its duration.[141,142]

VETERINARY INVOLVEMENT: WHY, WHERE, WHEN, AND HOW OFTEN?

Veterinarians have a role in collection management when acquiring and sexing new stock, during quarantine, and for annual health assessment, reproductive assessment, disease treatment, and end-of-life care. All new animals require physical assessment and history collection pertaining to prior husbandry, diet, their origins, breeding, and medical history.[142] During quarantine, veterinarians perform diagnostics and analyze samples to identify infectious agents or investigate other health concerns identified at initial examination.

Annual health assessment is ideally performed on all animals in the collection, and this is often timed prior to the onset of breeding season (or immediately before brumation) to assist with management decisions through the year.[129,151] Annual health assessment may not be feasible when working with thousands of animals or dangerous species (**Fig. 8**).[129] In these cases, examining a percentage of the collection can be planned annually based on specimen value, population size, the disease prevalence, and the sensitivity/specificity of diagnostic tests using epidemiologic services such as Epitools to calculate the number of samples required to diagnose and control a disease.[152] Performing annual examinations more or less frequently depends on the collection's disease status, the species held, and the purpose for which they are kept.[4] Annual examinations can include bloodwork, reproductive ultrasound, radiographs for periodontal disease/progressive conditions, fecal parasite, fungal, and viral screening.[129] Ultrasonographic reproductive evaluation is sometimes required.[4,47] Veterinarians may be hired to develop health management programs requiring regular visitation or permanent contracts; in other cases, they may be called on only to treat clinical cases and assess new acquisitions.[4]

Euthanasia and quality-of-life evaluations are critical to the humane treatment of all animals. Veterinarians must ensure that slaughter practices in farming operations are appropriate and follow current standards. Multimodal (2-step or 3-step) euthanasia or slaughter techniques are recommended entailing inducing anesthesia, chemical/physical euthanasia, followed by pithing or freezing for assurance of death.[153] International euthanasia guidelines through the AVMA and Swiss FVO are available for animals kept for pet/conservation/research purposes and those bred for food.[153–155] Currently, no standardized quality-of-life assessment exists for geriatric or chronically ill herptiles, and some facilities adopt scoring systems used for mammalian species as a basis for the decision to euthanize (Douay G, personal communication, 2020). Such decisions are based on the animal medical status, deterioration in behavior, and the level of long-term care required. Necropsies should be performed in all specimens after death or euthanasia, preferably within 24 to 48 hours of death if refrigerated.[156] Postmortem sample submission is case-based, and histopathology on all gross abnormalities is recommended at a minimum; however, a definitive diagnosis is rarely obtained from gross examination, and specific ancillary testing is generally required.[156]

PREVENTIVE HEALTH

Diagnostic tests are essential when managing the health of large herpetological collections. Protocols should be customized for each facility, as differing geography and species kept will ultimately affect the recommended testing. A variety of

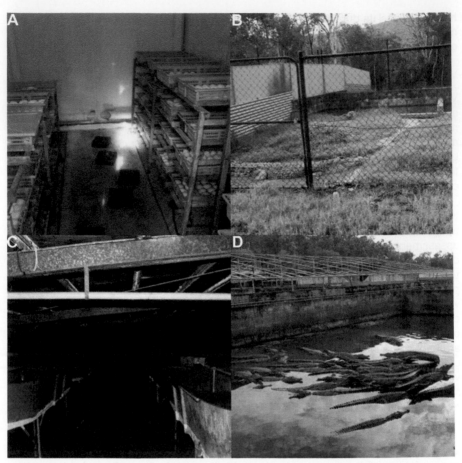

Fig. 8. Saltwater crocodile farming. (*A*) Incubator room for crocodile eggs is temperature-controlled and humidity-controlled and requires complete disinfection prior to entry. (*B*) Breeding pen design for adult crocodiles. (*C*) Crocodile facilities commonly raise hatchlings in water tanks in total darkness to reduce stress and competition without the provision of any light. (*D*) Grow-out pens for subadult crocodiles prior to slaughter.

diagnostics are available, with the challenge being selecting the correct tests to perform, with the correct time and frequency to perform them. Testing can be divided into 2 broad groups, screening diagnostics and targeted diagnostics.

SCREENING DIAGNOSTICS

These tests are not designed to look for a specific problem but rather to check animals for a range of potential issues. The results of these tests may then indicate whether further investigation is required.

Fecal Testing

The collection and analysis of fecal samples for internal parasites should be considered routine, if not mandatory, for all reptiles and amphibians entering a collection and during quarantine. Because of the intermittent shedding of many parasites and their eggs, serial sampling should be conducted to ensure the animals are clear before release into the main collection. The actual frequency and duration that fecal testing is performed will depend on the species being tested, the known parasitic pathogens for that species, the housing method (ie, the likelihood of reinfestation), and the original source of the animal (eg, captive-bred vs wild-caught). As a rule, ascarids, strongyles, cestodes, trematodes, pentastomids, acanthocephalans (more so amphibians), microsporidia (*Cryptosporidium*), and *Entamoeba* are always pathogenic and should be cleared from the collection. Fecal samples must be as fresh as possible, free from contaminants, and not dry when examined.[111] Gross examination of the sample can be conducted, noting the volume, color, and consistency and the presence of blood, mucous, or obvious parasites. Direct fecal smears should be made and examined shortly after obtaining the sample unless it has been refrigerated or is large enough such that the center of the sample remains moist. Fecal smears are particularly useful at detecting protozoans and motile bacteria. Just as with small-animal medicine, fecal flotation is an important diagnostic tool. This technique is useful to detect parasites such as coccidia, nematodes, cestodes, and pentastomids; sedimentation can be used to detect trematodes.[157,158] Fecal cytology, particularly using acid-fast stains to detect Cryptosporidia, can be used in collections where this is a known concern. Many "parasites" found on fecal examinations may in fact constitute normal gastrointestinal flora of the reptile or amphibian. The decision to treat is often subjective and based on an appreciation for the normal flora seen in each species and the presence of clinical signs attributable to the parasite's presence. Fecal culture as a screening test in herptiles is of limited value, particularly in relation to the presence of *Salmonella* sp. All reptiles should be considered as potentially carrying Salmonella, and a positive culture should therefore not necessarily be interpreted as that animal harboring a pathogen.

Blood Testing

The routine analysis of hematological and biochemical data is extremely useful as a screening tool to detect illness. Sample collection in the animal's normal environment, after it has had a chance to settle (not at import/purchase), will reduce stress leukocytosis. There can be considerable variation in blood values between individuals depending on their physiologic state, so routine blood screening allows the development of baseline values for individual animals that can be used as comparisons with later samples. Additionally, normal reference ranges may not be readily available for the species in question. Hematological assessment can range from packed cell volume measurement (often all that is available in small patients) to complete blood counts based on examination of prepared blood smears. Total white cells count can be conducted along with cell morphology and assessment for the presence of blood parasites such as *Hemogregaria,* assorted microfilaria, and bacterial/viral inclusions.[147] Biochemical analysis is most useful in clinically ill animals, though establishing baseline data for animals shortly after entry into collections can be invaluable.

PCR and Viral Screening

Several key viral diseases can be prevented from entering a collection via appropriate testing while animals are in quarantine. Examples of these infections include paramyxoviruses (eg, *Ferlavirus, Sunshinevirus*), Bornavirus, Reptarenavirus, Nidovirus, Adenovirus, Herpesvirus, and Ranavirus; most of which require oro-cloacal swabs or fresh-frozen tissues.[147] It is vital that the appropriate tests for the species in question be performed. Testudidae herpesvirus and mycoplasmosis of chelonians can be screened using PCR or virus isolation (for herpesvirus); however, false negatives are common in clinically well animals, and given their high prevalence in captive populations, results are unlikely to add value unless required for export/conservation/ex situ release purposes or when clinical cases are frequent.[159] When combined with endoscopic gastric/intestinal mucosal biopsy or lavage samples, *Cryptosporidium* can be identified readily via PCR and differentiated from species derived from prey items.[157] *Chytridiomycosis* in amphibians is readily identified from skin swab PCR and is recommended for all recent acquisitions; however, screening via cytologic examination of stained/unstained skin smears may be preferred for annual assessment.[148] The fungal pathogens *Ophidiomyces* and *Nannizziopsis sp.* can be screened for using PCR from lesions on the arrival of new imports (particularly bearded dragons + snakes collected from the wild in the United States).[160] Systemic amebiasis caused by *Entamoeba invadens* and intranuclear coccidiosis and can be screened for via qPCR; however, sensitivity is poor (trichrome staining is more effective), and given that *Entamoeba* is a commensal organism in many chelonians, annual screening for this pathogen is normally required only where other reptiles are housed with or alongside chelonians, particularly in collections with previous clinical cases.[157]

TARGETED DIAGNOSTICS

These tests are used when an animal develops clinical signs of disease or when assessing for a specific condition.

Diagnostic Imaging

Various diagnostic imaging modalities can be used to assess animals with clinical disease or incorporated into the annual health assessment for many species. Ultrasonography can be incorporated into routine reproductive evaluations on breeding operations, particularly for female snakes, varanids, agamids, and chelonians. It is used to evaluate follicular size prior to pairing animals, detect ovulation, confirm the formation of developed eggs/embryos, and assess reproductive pathology, all of which assist reproductive decision-making over the course of a season.[161] Radiographs can be used for several screening purposes. Geriatric animals can be assessed for spinal and long bone abnormalities annually. Dental radiography can be performed regularly on lizards with acrodont dentition to assess for the development of periodontal disease (though CT provides greater detail for lesion severity). Radiographs can provide postoviposition evaluation in chelonians (not applicable to snakes/most lizards because of lower calcification of shells) and for assessment of urinary calculi in tortoises in regions where high silicates predispose this disorder.[162]

Serology

Serologic evaluation is infrequently used as a stand-alone diagnostic in reptiles either as a component of annual health assessment in collections or as a part of import screening. Evidence of an immune response on its own is not enough to indicate active infection and requires either quantification of increased immune response or pairing with evidence of the pathogen's presence with the animal (eg, PCR). Exceptions to this are conditions that persistently infect animals, such as chelonian mycoplasmosis and testudinid herpesvirus—ELISA serology for *Mycoplasma agassizii* and *M testudineum* may detect subclinical, intermittent shedders, and chronically infected animals.[159] Similar reports exist for ophidian paramyxovirus in snakes; however, limited availability and poor reliability (a negative result does not exclude early infection, requiring second-round testing for the 6-week to 9-week period to develop a twofold increase in antibody titers) means these techniques are rarely used in quarantine assessment.[141] May be considered in extremely valuable collections as a means of annual screening for such chronic disorders.

Endoscopy

Cryptosporidia can be detected via endoscopic biopsy of gastric mucosa, or alternately from gastric lavage samples (followed by subsequent PCR, or acid-fast staining and histology) and is more sensitive than fecal cytology, but could be time-consuming for large imports and should be considered only for at-risk species or specimens showing GI abnormalities at the time of acquisition.[157] In populations considered at risk of mycobacteriosis, chlamydiosis, or other hepato-centric infections, coelioscopic hepatic biopsy followed by tissue-PCR is considered a sensitive method of screening for these disorders and may be considered for use in large collections as a part of annual screening and prior to transfer between exhibits containing prior positive cases or to other facilities.[163]

Fecal Testing

Just as fecal testing is an important screening diagnostic; it can be just as important as a targeted diagnostic when investigating clinical disease. Those tests already discussed above can be performed should the clinical signs warrant them.

Blood Testing

Bloodwork is critical to investigating disease in most species. In reptiles and amphibians, having baseline values to compare with disease-state samples is critical because of their individual variations.

THE FUTURE OF PREVENTIVE MEDICINE

Prophylactic medicine is a developing area in exotic animal management and continues to evolve as new diseases (and technologies to manage them) are continuously discovered. There is a tremendous scope for the development of new techniques and preventive health programs in herpetoculture. However, prophylactic management should still focus on optimizing husbandry practices for the health of the species being kept.

Vaccination is currently being explored in some herpetocultural industries, and an inactivated vaccine is currently in production against West Nile Virus in crocodilians—this product is licensed for use in the USA for alligators from 1 month in age.[164] Once vaccinated, uninfected animals can become PCR positive and cannot be differentiated from those that are truly infected.[165] An autogenous poxvirus vaccine developed from skin lesions in crocodilians sped healing and reduced scar formation in affected animals.[164] A similar autogenous vaccine has been used to manage Mycoplasma crocodyli outbreaks in Nile crocodiles; however, a trial using an inactivated vaccine proved unsuccessful.[166,167] Vaccine development has been investigated for ophidian Ferlavirus; however, to date, a positive antibody response has been inadequate and commercial options are not viable or recommended.[164] Similarly, an inactivated herpesvirus vaccine for use in chelonians showed no antibody response when delivered subcutaneously.[164]

SUMMARY

The cornerstone of effective preventive health in large herpetological collections is an in-depth knowledge of the ecology and husbandry of the species being kept, followed by designing effective screening and control measures for potential pathogens. When this is understood and provided for, reptiles and amphibians can prove hardy, long-lived captives and breed readily. Developing health programs requires trust and open communication between the veterinarian and the client; without this, most protocols will not be maintained. As more is learned about emerging reptile and amphibian disease, preventive health represents an important area of research and development for clinicians, presenting new opportunities for its application in a variety of collections when adhering to these key principles.

CLINICS CARE POINTS

- The environmental conditions under which a reptile or amphibian collection is maintained, followed by the management techniques used to care for the animals, collectively have a far greater impact on the success and health of captive herptiles than the disease status of individual animals. Detailed knowledge of the natural history and subsequent application to the husbandry of the species being kept will significantly reduce the incidence of illness in the collection.
- The understanding of welfare in captive reptiles and amphibians is continually evolving, and a transition away from bare, cramped, "sterile" housing to larger and more naturalistic setups (even at a large scale) is currently in effect. Bioactive enclosures come with their own set of challenges, and veterinarians should be aware of these potential problems and how to mitigate them.
- Herptile nutrition can be generally subdivided into carnivore, insectivore, omnivore, and herbivore diets, with carnivores being the least complicated and herbivores often proving the most challenging to successfully establish long term. Limited regulatory oversight in the production of formulated reptile diets means a careful review of the product label is required prior to using them in large collections, despite their potential perks and ease of use.
- Quarantine alone is insufficient to prevent the introduction of pathogens to an established collection, yet the decision to test for every known disorder on an acquisition of specimens is not realistic. Performing a DRA on all incoming animals encourages appropriate disease screening based on species, place of origin, and consequences of pathogen introduction and will result in optimized decisions on quarantine duration and lab expenditure.
- Large collections will benefit greatly from the development of an annual health calendar for veterinary involvement under which individual health assessment, assistance with husbandry planning, and decisions on screening and targeted diagnostics can be made for all specimens based on epidemiologic principles.

DISCLOSURE

The authors have nothing to disclose.

REFERENCES

1. Pough FH. The advantages of ectothermy for tetrapods. Am Naturalist 1980; 115:92–112.
2. Bennett AF. The energetics of reptilian activity. 1982.
3. Gibbons PM. 178 - Large zoo and private collection management. In: Divers SJ, Stahl SJ, editors. Mader's reptile and amphibian medicine and surgery. 3rd Edition. St. Louis, MO: W.B. Saunders; 2019. p. 1398–405.e1391.
4. Stahl SJ. Reptile production medicine. Semin Avian Exot Pet Med 2001;10(3): 140–50.

5. Pasmans F, Martel A. 28 - Amphibians. In: Divers SJ, Stahl SJ, editors. Mader's reptile and Amphibian medicine and surgery. 3rd Edition. St. Louis, MO: W.B. Saunders; 2019. p. 224–34.e221.
6. Gascon C. Amphibian conservation action plan: proceedings IUCN/SSC Amphibian Conservation Summit 2005. Gland, Switzerland: IUCn; 2007.
7. Auliya M, Altherr S, Ariano-Sanchez D, et al. Trade in live reptiles, its impact on wild populations, and the role of the European market. Biol Conservation 2016; 204:103–19.
8. Robinson JE, John FAV St, Griffiths RA, et al. Captive reptile mortality rates in the home and implications for the wildlife trade. PLoS One 2015;10(11):e0141460.
9. Mendoza-Roldan JA, Modry D, Otranto D. Zoonotic parasites of reptiles: a crawling threat. Trends Parasitol 2020;36(8):677–87.
10. Warwick C. The morality of the reptile "pet" trade. J Anim Ethics 2014;4(1):74–94.
11. Robinson JE, Griffiths RA, St. John FAV, et al. Dynamics of the global trade in live reptiles: shifting trends in production and consequences for sustainability. Biol Conservation 2015;184:42–50.
12. Nijman V, Shepherd CR, Sanders KL. Over-exploitation and illegal trade of reptiles in Indonesia. Herpetological J 2012;22(2):83–9.
13. Rossi JV. 16 - general husbandry and management. In: Divers SJ, Stahl SJ, editors. Mader's reptile and amphibian medicine and surgery. 3rd Edition. St. Louis, MO: W.B. Saunders; 2019. p. 109–30.e101.
14. Warwick C, Steedman C. Naturalistic versus clinical environments in husbandry and research. Dordrecht, Netherlands: Springer; 1995. p. 113–30.
15. Howell TJ, Warwick C, Bennett PC. Self-reported snake management practices among owners in Victoria, Australia. Vet Rec 2020;187(3):114.
16. Warwick C, Arena P, Steedman C. Spatial considerations for captive snakes. J Vet Behav 2019;30:37–48.
17. Warwick C, Frye FL, Murphy JB. Health and welfare of captive reptiles. London: Springer Science & Business Media; 2013.
18. Enclosure design. In: Reptile medicine and surgery in clinical practice. Hoboken, NJ: John Wiley & Sons Ltd; 2017. p. 61–73.
19. Browne RK, Odum RA, Herman T, et al. Facility design and associated services for the study of amphibians 2007;48(3):188–202.
20. Brown D. A guide to Australian lizards in captivity. Burleigh, QLD Australia: Reptile Publications; 2014.
21. Morafka DJ, Berry KH, Spangenberg EK. Predator-proof field enclosures for enhancing hatching success and survivorship of juvenile tortoises: a critical evaluation. In: Paper presented at: proceedings of the international conference on conservation, restoration, and management of tortoises and turtles. New York: New York Turtle and Tortoise Society; 1997.
22. Blackett T, Morgan D, Groves G. Core fundamental standard of practice for captive wild animals. London: Wild Welfare; 2019.
23. Ziegler T, Rauhaus A, Mutschmann F, et al. Building up of keeping facilities and breeding projects for frogs, newts and lizards at the Me Linh Station for biodiversity in northern Vietnam, including improvement of housing conditions for confiscated reptiles and primates. Zoologische Garten 2016;85(3–4):91–120.
24. Durso AM, Maerz JC. 13 - natural behavior. In: Divers SJ, Stahl SJ, editors. Mader's reptile and amphibian medicine and surgery. 3rd Edition. St. Louis, MO: W.B. Saunders; 2019. p. 90–9.e94.
25. Lillywhite HB, Licht P, Chelgren P. The role of behavioral thermoregulation in the growth energetics of the Toad, Bufo Boreas. Ecology 1973;54(2):375–83.

26. Spotila JR. Role of temperature and water in the ecology of lungless salamanders. Ecol Monogr 1972;42(1):95–125.

27. Dawson WR. On the physiological significance of the preferred body temperatures of reptiles. In: Gates DM, Schmerl RB, editors. Perspectives of biophysical ecology. Berlin, Heidelberg: Springer Berlin Heidelberg; 1975. p. 443–73.

28. Cloudsley-Thompson JL. Thermal regulation and control. In: Ecophysiology of desert arthropods and reptiles. Berlin, Heidelberg: Springer Berlin Heidelberg; 1991. p. 52–79.

29. Berk ML, Heath JE. An analysis of behavioral thermoregulation in the lizard, Dipsosaurus dorsalis. J Therm Biol 1975;1(1):15–22.

30. Oonincx D, van Leeuwen J. Evidence-based reptile housing and nutrition. Vet Clin North Am 2017;20(3):885–98.

31. Autumn K, De Nardo DF. Behavioral thermoregulation increases growth rate in a Nocturnal Lizard. J Herpetol 1995;29(2):157–62.

32. Frank S, Shine R. Evaluating thermoregulation in reptiles: the fallacy of the inappropriately applied method. Physiol Biochem Zool 2004;77(4):688–95.

33. Anatomy and physiology of reptiles. In: Reptile medicine and surgery in clinical practice. Hoboken, NJ: John Wiley & Sons Ltd; 2017. p. 15–32.

34. Garrick D. Body surface temperature and length in relation to the thermal biology of lizards. Biosci Horizons 2008;1(2):136–42.

35. Tamplin JW, Moran VF, Riesberg EJ. Response of juvenile diamond-backed terrapins (Malaclemys terrapin) to an aquatic thermal gradient. J Therm Biol 2013; 38(7):434–9.

36. Trochet A, Dupoué A, Souchet J, et al. Variation of preferred body temperatures along an altitudinal gradient: a multi-species study. J Therm Biol 2018;77:38–44.

37. Novarro AJ, Gabor CR, Goff CB, et al. Physiological responses to elevated temperature across the geographic range of a terrestrial salamander. J Exp Biol 2018;221(18):jeb178236.

38. Angilletta MJ, Werner YL. Australian geckos do not display diel variation in thermoregulatory behavior. Copeia 1998;1998(3):736–42.

39. Sievert LM, Hutchison VH. Light versus heat: thermoregulatory behavior in a nocturnal lizard (Gekko gecko). Herpetologica 1988;44(3):266–73.

40. Zilber A, Popper DN, Yom-Tov Y. The effect of direct sunlight and temperature on growth and survival of captive young Nile crocodiles, Crocodilus Niloticus. Aquaculture 1991;94(4):291–5.

41. Mustin W, Nevarez JG. 177 - commercial reptile farming. In: Divers SJ, Stahl SJ, editors. Mader's reptile and Amphibian medicine and surgery. 3rd Edition. St. Louis, MO: W.B. Saunders; 2019. p. 1389–97.e1381.

42. Diseases of the gastrointestinal system. In: Reptile medicine and surgery in clinical practice. Hoboken, NJ: John Wiley & Sons Ltd; 2017. p. 273–85.

43. Disorders of the reproductive system. In: Reptile medicine and surgery in clinical practice. Hoboken, NJ: John Wiley & Sons Ltd; 2017. p. 307–21.

44. Paniagua R, Fraile B, Sáez FJ. Effects of photoperiod and temperature on testicular function in amphibians. Histol Histopathol 1990;5(3):365–78.

45. Kang H, Kenealy TM, Cohen RE. The hypothalamic-pituitary-gonadal axis and thyroid hormone regulation interact to influence seasonal breeding in green anole lizards (Anolis carolinensis). Gen Comp Endocrinol 2020;292:113446.

46. Norris DO, Lopez KH. Hormones and reproduction in amphibians and reptiles. In: Skinner MK, editor. Encyclopedia of reproduction. 2nd Edition. Oxford: Academic Press; 2018. p. 374–84.

47. Reproduction. In: Reptile medicine and surgery in clinical practice. Hoboken, NJ: John Wiley & Sons Ltd; 2017. p. 91–103.
48. Peterson KH, Lazcano D, Galván RDJ. Captive reproduction in the Mexican milksnake Lampropeltis triangulum annulata. Litteratura Serpentium 1995; 15(5):128–32.
49. Wilkinson SL. Reptile wellness management. Vet Clin North America: Exot Anim Pract 2015;18(2):281–304.
50. Baines FM, Cusack LM. 17 - environmental lighting. In: Divers SJ, Stahl SJ, editors. Mader's reptile and amphibian medicine and surgery. 3rd Edition. St. Louis, MO: W.B. Saunders; 2019. p. 131–8.e131.
51. Tosini G, Bertolucci C, Foà A. The circadian system of reptiles: a multioscillatory and multiphotoreceptive system. Physiol Behav 2001;72(4):461–71.
52. Alberts AC. Ultraviolet visual sensitivity in desert iguanas: implications for pheromone detection. Anim Behav 1989;38(1):129–37.
53. Baines FM, Chattell J, Dale J, et al. How much UVB does my reptile need? The UV-tool, a guide to the selection of UV lighting for reptiles and amphibians in captivity. J Zoo Aquarium Res 2016;4(1):42–63.
54. Carman EN, Ferguson GW, Gehrmann WH, et al. Photobiosynthetic opportunity and ability for UV-B generated vitamin D synthesis in free-living house geckos (Hemidactylus turcicus) and Texas Spiny Lizards (Sceloporus olivaceous). Copeia 2000;2000(1):245–50.
55. Gould A, Molitor L, Rockwell K, et al. Evaluating the Physiologic effects of short duration ultraviolet B radiation exposure in leopard geckos (Eublepharis macularius). J Herpetol Med Surg 2018;28(1–2):34–9.
56. Tapley B, Rendle M, Baines FM, et al. Meeting ultraviolet B radiation requirements of amphibians in captivity: a case study with mountain chicken frogs (Leptodactylus fallax) and general recommendations for pre-release health screening. Zoo Biol 2015;34(1):46–52.
57. Acierno MJ, Mitchell MA, Zachariah TT, et al. Effects of ultraviolet radiation on plasma 25-hydroxyvitamin D3concentrations in corn snakes (Elaphe guttata). Am J Vet Res 2008;69(2):294–7.
58. Siroski PA, Poletta GL, Fernandez L, et al. Ultraviolet radiation on innate immunity and growth of broad-snouted caiman (Caiman latirostris): implications for facilities design. Zoo Biol 2012;31(5):523–33.
59. Antwis RE, Browne RK. Ultraviolet radiation and Vitamin D3 in amphibian health, behaviour, diet and conservation. Comp Biochem Physiol A Mol Integr Physiol 2009;154(2):184–90.
60. Ferguson GW, Jones JR, Gehrmann WH, et al. Indoor husbandry of the panther chameleon Chamaeleo [Furcifer] pardalis: Effects of dietary vitamins A and D and ultraviolet irradiation on pathology and life-history traits. Zoo Biol 1996; 15(3):279–99.
61. Mendonça MT. Timing of reproductive behaviour in male musk turtles, Sternotherus odoratus: effects of photoperiod, temperature and testosterone. Anim Behav 1987;35(4):1002–14.
62. Lighting. In: Reptile medicine and surgery in clinical practice. Hoboken, NJ: John Wiley & Sons Ltd; 2017. p. 75–90.
63. Ferguson GW, Brinker AM, Gehrmann WH, et al. Voluntary exposure of some western-hemisphere snake and lizard species to ultraviolet-B radiation in the field: how much ultraviolet-B should a lizard or snake receive in captivity? Zoo Biol 2010;29(3):317–34.

64. Edmonds D, Razaiarimahefa T, Kessler E, et al. Natural exposure to ultraviolet-B radiation in two species of chameleons from Madagascar. Zoo Biol 2018;37(6): 452–7.

65. Gardiner DW, Baines FM, Pandher K. Photodermatitis and Photokeratoconjunctivitis in a Ball Python (Python regius) and a Blue-Tongue Skink (Tiliqua spp.). J Zoo Wildl Med 2009;40(4):757–66, 710.

66. Baines F. Photo-kerato-conjunctivitis in reptiles. In: Paper presented at: ARAV 1st Int conference on reptile and amphibian medicine; March 2010. 2010. Association of Reptile and Amphibian Veterinarians, Munich.

67. Lillywhite HB, Gatten RE. Physiology and functional anatomy. In: Warwick C, Frye FL, Murphy JB, editors. Health and welfare of captive reptiles. Dordrecht: Springer Netherlands; 1995. p. 5–31.

68. Husbandry and nutrition. In: Reptile medicine and surgery in clinical practice. Hoboken, NJ: John Wiley & Sons Ltd; 2017. p. 45–60.

69. Chameleons. In: Handbook of exotic pet medicine. Hoboken, NJ: John Wiley & Sons Ltd; 2020. p. 263–81.

70. Diaz RE, Anderson CV, Baumann DP, et al. Captive care, raising, and breeding of the veiled chameleon (Chamaeleo calyptratus). Cold Spring Harbor Protoc 2015;2015(10):943–9.

71. Wright KM, Whitaker BR. Amphibian medicine and captive husbandry. Malabar: Krieger Publishing Company; 2001.

72. Whitaker BR, Wright KM. 89 - amphibian medicine. In: Divers SJ, Stahl SJ, editors. Mader's reptile and amphibian medicine and surgery. 3rd Edition. St. Louis, MO: W.B. Saunders; 2019. p. 992–1013.e1013.

73. Harkewicz KA. Dermatologic problems of reptiles. Semin Avian Exot Pet Med 2002;11(3):151–61.

74. Wiesner CS, Iben C. Influence of environmental humidity and dietary protein on pyramidal growth of carapaces in African spurred tortoises (Geochelone sulcata). J Anim Physiol Anim Nutr 2003;87(1-2):66–74.

75. Odum RA, Zippel KC. Amphibian water quality: approaches to an essential environmental parameter. Int Zoo Yearb 2008;42(1):40–52.

76. Camperio Ciani JF, Guerrel J, Baitchman E, et al. The relationship between spindly leg syndrome incidence and water composition, overfeeding, and diet in newly metamorphosed harlequin frogs (Atelopus spp.). PLoS One 2018; 13(10):e0204314.

77. Pough FH. Recommendations for the care of amphibians and reptiles in Academic Institutions. ILAR J 1991;33(4):S1–21.

78. Platt SR. 77 - Neurology. In: Divers SJ, Stahl SJ, editors. Mader's reptile and amphibian medicine and surgery. 3rd Edition. St. Louis, MO: W.B. Saunders; 2019. p. 805–26.e803.

79. de Vosjoli P. Designing environments for captive amphibians and reptiles. Vet Clin North Am 1999;2(1):43–68.

80. Boyer DM. Providing adequate hydration in neonate arboreal snakes. In: Bulletin of the Association of Reptilian and Amphibian Veterinarians, 5 1995;. p. 5.

81. Hunt CJG. 15 - stress and welfare. In: Divers SJ, Stahl SJ, editors. Mader's reptile and amphibian medicine and surgery. 3rd Edition. St. Louis, MO: W.B. Saunders; 2019. p. 105–8.e101.

82. Poole V, Grow S. Amphibian husbandry resource guide, Edition 2.0. 2012.

83. Clayton LA, Tynes VV. Keeping the exotic pet mentally healthy. Vet Clin North Am 2015;18(2):187–95.

84. Warwick C. Reptilian ethology in captivity: observations of some problems and an evaluation of their aetiology. Appl Anim Behav Sci 1990;26(1):1–13.

85. Kalliokoski O, Timm JA, Ibsen IB, et al. Fecal glucocorticoid response to environmental stressors in green iguanas (Iguana iguana). Gen Comp Endocrinol 2012;177(1):93–7.

86. Oonincx DGAB, van Leeuwen JP, Hendriks WH, et al. The diet of free-roaming Australian Central Bearded Dragons (Pogona vitticeps). Zoo Biol 2015;34(3): 271–7.

87. MacMillen RE, Augee ML, Ellis BA. Thermal ecology and diet of some xerophilous lizards from western New South Wales. J Arid Environments 1989;16(2): 193–201.

88. Boyer TH, Scott PW. 27 - Nutrition. In: Divers SJ, Stahl SJ, editors. Mader's reptile and amphibian medicine and surgery. 3rd Edition. St. Louis, MO: Elsevier; 2019. p. 201–23.e202.

89. Vitt LJ, Caldwell JP. Herpetology: an introductory biology of amphibians and reptiles. Burlington, MA: Academic Press; 2013.

90. Cooper JE, Williams DL. The feeding of live food to exotic pets: issues of welfare and ethics. J Exot Pet Med 2014;23(3):244–9.

91. Schmidt DA, Travis DA, Williams JJ. Guidelines for creating a food safety HACCP program in zoos or aquaria. Zoo Biol 2006;25(2):125–35.

92. Allen ME, Oftedal OT. Nutrition in captivity. In: Husbandry and veterinary management of the green Iguana. Malabar, USA: Krieger Publishing Company; 2003.

93. Lemm J, Alberts AC. Cyclura: natural history, husbandry, and conservation of West Indian rock iguanas. San Diego, CA: Academic Press; 2011.

94. Using pet food labels and product guides. In: Applied veterinary clinical nutrition. Hoboken, NJ: John Wiley & Sons Ltd; 2012. p. 69–74.

95. Finke MD. Complete nutrient composition of commercially raised invertebrates used as food for insectivores. Zoo Biol 2002;21(3):269–85.

96. Bernard JB, Allen ME, Ullrey DE. Feeding captive insectivorous animals: nutritional aspects of insects as food. East Lansing, MI, 1997.

97. Latney LT, Clayton LA. Updates on amphibian nutrition and nutritive value of common feeder insects. Vet Clin Exot Anim Pract 2014;17(3):347–67.

98. Finke MD, Dunham SU, Kwabi CA. Evaluation of four dry commercial gut loading products for improving the calcium content of crickets, Acheta domesticus. J Herpetol Med Surg 2005;15(1):7–12.

99. Finke MD, Dunham SU, Cole JS III. Evaluation of various calcium-fortified high moisture commercial products for improving the calcium content of crickets, acheta domesticus. J Herpetol Med Surg 2004;14(2):17–20.

100. Livingston S, Lavin SR, Sullivan K, et al. Challenges with effective nutrient supplementation for amphibians: a review of cricket studies. Zoo Biol 2014;33(6): 565–76.

101. Michaels C, Antwis R, Preziosi R. Manipulation of the calcium content of insectivore diets through supplementary dusting. J Zoo Aquarium Res 2014;2(3): 77–81.

102. Vogel P, Hettrich W, Ricono K. Weight growth of juvenile lizards, anolis lineatopus, maintained on different diets. J Herpetology 1986;20(1):50–8.

103. Knight M, Glor R, Smedley SR, et al. Firefly toxicosis in lizards. J Chem Ecol 1999;25(9):1981–6.

104. Murphy JB, Adler K, Collins JT. Captive management and conservation of amphibians and reptiles. Ithaca, NY: Society for the Study of Amphibians and Reptiles; 1994.

105. Dierenfeld E, Alcorn HL, Jacobsen KL. Nutrient composition of whole vertebrate prey (excluding fish) fed in zoos. Beltsville, Maryland: U.S. Department of Agriculture, Agricultural Research Service, National Agricultural Library, Animal Welfare Information Center; 2002.

106. Pfaff CS. Taxon management account for King Cobra Ophiophagus hannah. Zoo Print 2008;23(5):13–6.

107. Bernard J, Allen M. Feeding captive piscivorous animals: nutritional aspects of fish as food. In: Nutritional Advisory Group Handbook, Fact Sheet 005. Silver Spring, MD: American Zoo and Aquarium Association; 1997.

108. Webb G, Reynolds S, Brien M, et al. Improving Australia's Crocodile Industry Productivity: nutritional requirements, feed ingredients and feeding systems for farmed crocodile production. Barton, ACT: Rural Industries Research and Development Corporation; 2013.

109. Rendle M. Nutrition. In: BSAVA manual of reptiles. Quedgeley, UK: British Small Animal Veterinary Association; 2019.

110. Baer DJ. Nutrition in the wild. In: Biology, husbandry, and medicine of the green iguana. Malabar, USA: Krieger Publishing Company; 2003. p. 38–46.

111. Eatwell K, Richardson J. 74 - gastroenterology—small intestine, exocrine pancreas, and large intestine. In: Divers SJ, Stahl SJ, editors. Mader's reptile and amphibian medicine and surgery. 3rd Edition. St. Louis, MO: W.B. Saunders; 2019. p. 761–74.e763.

112. Ullrey DE, Crissey SD, Edwards MS, et al. Hay quality evaluation. In: Nutrition advisory group handbook fact sheet. Brookfield, IL: Chicago Zoological Society; 1997.

113. Van Devender TR. The sonoran desert tortoise: natural history, biology, and conservation. Tuscon, AZ: University of Arizona Press; 2006.

114. Mellor DJ. Updating animal welfare thinking: moving beyond the "five freedoms" towards "a life worth living". Animals 2016;6(3):21.

115. Whitham JC, Wielebnowski N. New directions for zoo animal welfare science. Appl Anim Behav Sci 2013;147(3):247–60.

116. Skurski ML, Fleming GJ, Daneault A, et al. 14 - behavioral training and enrichment of reptiles. In: Divers SJ, Stahl SJ, editors. Mader's reptile and amphibian medicine and surgery. 3rd Edition. St. Louis, MO: W.B. Saunders; 2019. p. 100–4.e101.

117. Fàbregas MC, Guillén-Salazar F, Garcés-Narro C. Do naturalistic enclosures provide suitable environments for zoo animals? Zoo Biol 2012;31(3):362–73.

118. Warwick C, Arena P, Lindley S, et al. Assessing reptile welfare using behavioural criteria. In Pract 2013;35(3):123–31.

119. Burghardt GM. Environmental enrichment and cognitive complexity in reptiles and amphibians: concepts, review, and implications for captive populations. Appl Anim Behav Sci 2013;147(3):286–98.

120. Rodríguez-Serna M, Flores-Nava A, Olvera-Novoa MA, et al. Growth and production of bullfrog Rana catesbeiana shaw, 1802, at three stocking densities in a vertical intensive culture system. Aquacultural Eng 1996;15(4):233–42.

121. Manolis SC, Webb GJ. Best management practices for crocodilian farming. In: Group I-SCS, ed. Darwin, AUS 2016.

122. Mayeaux MH, Culley DD Jr, Reigh RC. Effects of dietary energy: protein ratio and stocking density on growth and survival of the common snapping turtle chelydra serpentinal. J World Aquaculture Soc 1996;27(1):64–73.

123. Committee AAPM. Association of zoos and aquariums. In: Species survival Plan® (SSP) program Handbook. Association of Zoos and Aquariums; 2020. Available at: https://assets.speakcdn.com/assets/2332/aza_species-survival-plan-program-handbook.pdf. Accessed November 26, 2020.

124. Rivera-Ortíz FA, Aguilar R, Arizmendi MDC, et al. Habitat fragmentation and genetic variability of tetrapod populations. Anim Conservation 2015;18(3):249–58.

125. Rees PA. Collection planning and captive breeding. In: An introduction to zoo biology and management. West Sussex, UK: John Wiley & Sons Ltd; 2011. p. 247–99.

126. Brereton SR, Brereton JE. Sixty years of collection planning: what species do zoos and aquariums keep? Int Zoo Yearb 2020;54(1):131–45.

127. Norton TM, Andrews KM, Smith LL. Chapter 29 - techniques for working with wild reptiles. In: Mader DR, Divers SJ, editors. Current therapy in reptile medicine and surgery. St. Louis: W.B. Saunders; 2014. p. 310–40.

128. Schwartz KR, Parsons ECM, Rockwood L, et al. Integrating in-situ and ex-situ data management processes for biodiversity conservation. Front Ecol Evol 2017;5:120.

129. Reavill DR, Griffin C. 179 - breeders, wholesalers, and retailers. In: Divers SJ, Stahl SJ, editors. Mader's reptile and Amphibian medicine and surgery. 3rd Edition. St. Louis, MO: W.B. Saunders; 2019. p. 1406–13.e1401.

130. Hunt CJG. 18 - Disinfection. In: Divers SJ, Stahl SJ, editors. Mader's reptile and Amphibian medicine and surgery. 3rd Edition. St. Louis, MO: W.B. Saunders; 2019. p. 139–41.e131.

131. Traverse M, Aceto H. Environmental cleaning and disinfection. Vet Clin North Am Small Anim Pract 2015;45(2):299–vi.

132. Diana SG, Beasley VB, Wright KM. Clinical toxicology. Malabar: Krieger Publishing Company; 2001.

133. Lloyd M. Chlorhexidine toxicosis from soaking in red-bellied short-necked turtles, emydura subglobosa. Bull Assoc Reptilian Amphibian Vet 1996;6(4):6–7.

134. de Jong MS, Weldon C. Efficacy of the product F10 against amphibian chytrid fungus/Effektiwiteit van die produk F10 teen Chytrid-fungus by amfibiee. Suid Afrik Tydskr Nat Tegnol 2014;33.

135. Langan JN. Chapter 8 - integrated pest management. In: Miller RE, Fowler M, editors. Fowler's zoo and wild animal medicine. Saint Louis: W.B. Saunders; 2012. p. 51–9.

136. Lloyd ML. Chapter 6 - disaster preparation for captive wildlife veterinarians. In: Miller RE, Fowler M, editors. Fowler's zoo and wild animal medicine. Saint Louis: W.B. Saunders; 2012. p. 38–46.

137. Ebani VV. Domestic reptiles as source of zoonotic bacteria: a mini review. Asian Pac J Trop Med 2017;10(8):723–8.

138. Johnson-Delaney CA, Gal J. 174 - zoonoses and public health. In: Divers SJ, Stahl SJ, editors. Mader's reptile and Amphibian medicine and surgery. Third Edition. St. Louis, MO: W.B. Saunders; 2019. p. 1359–65.e1352.

139. Mitchell MA. Zoonotic diseases associated with reptiles and amphibians: an update. Vet Clin Exot Anim Pract 2011;14(3):439–56.

140. Pasmans F, Blahak S, Martel A, et al. Introducing reptiles into a captive collection: the role of the veterinarian. Vet J 2008;175(1):53–68.

141. Rivera S. 19 - Quarantine. In: Divers SJ, Stahl SJ, editors. Mader's reptile and Amphibian medicine and surgery. 3rd Edition. St. Louis, MO: W.B. Saunders; 2019. p. 142–4.e141.

142. Miller RE. Quarantine protocols and preventive medicine procedures for reptiles, birds and mammals in zoos. Rev Sci Tech 1996;15(1):183–9.

143. Peeler EJ, Reese RA, Thrush MA. Animal disease import risk analysis – a review of current methods and practice. Transbound Emerg Dis 2015;62(5):480–90.

144. Andoh M, Sakata A, Takano A, et al. Detection of rickettsia and Ehrlichia spp. in ticks associated with exotic reptiles and amphibians imported into Japan. PLoS One 2015;10(7):e0133700.

145. Norval G, Robbins RG, Kolonin G, et al. Unintentional transport of ticks into Taiwan on a king cobra (Ophiophagus hannah). Herpetol Notes 2009;2(1):203–6.

146. Wolf D, Vrhovec MG, Failing K, et al. Diagnosis of gastrointestinal parasites in reptiles: comparison of two coprological methods. Acta Vet Scand 2014; 56(1):44.

147. Infectious diseases and immunology. In: Reptile medicine and surgery in clinical practice. Hoboken, NJ: John Wiley & Sons Ltd; 2017. p. 197–216.

148. Forzán MJ, Gunn H, Scott P. Chytridiomycosis in an aquarium collection of frogs: diagnosis, treatment, and control. J Zoo Wildl Med 2008;39(3):406–11.

149. Wallace C, Marinkovich M, Morris PJ, et al. Lessons from a retrospective analysis of a 5-yr period of quarantine at San Diego zoo: a risk-based approach to quarantine isolation and testing may benefit animal welfare. J Zoo Wildl Med 2016;47(1):291–6.

150. Wesson J. Sunshinevirus in Australian snakes: investigating the link with disease. Murdoch, WA, Australia: Murdoch University; 2020.

151. Divers S. Basic reptile husbandry, history taking and clinical examination. In Pract 1996;18(2):51–65.

152. Sergeant E. Epitools epidemiological calculators. In: AusVet animal health Services and Australian biosecurity Cooperative research Centre for emerging infectious disease. Bruce, ACT, Australia: Ausvet; 2009.

153. Nevarez JG. 47 - Euthanasia. In: Divers SJ, Stahl SJ, editors. Mader's reptile and amphibian medicine and surgery. 3rd Edition. St. Louis, MO: Elsevier; 2019. p. 437–40.e431.

154. Leary S, Underwood W, Anthony R, et al. AVMA guidelines for the euthanasia of animals: 2020 edition. Schaumburg, IL, USA: AVMA American Veterinary Medical Association; 2020.

155. AVMA. American Veterinary Medical Association. AVMA guidelines for the euthanasia of animals: 2013 edition. Schaumburg, IL: American Veterinary Medical Association; 2010.

156. Necropsy. In: Reptile medicine and surgery in clinical practice. Hoboken, NJ: John Wiley & Sons Ltd; 2017. p. 409–24.

157. Wellehan JFX, Walden HDS. 32 - Parasitology (Including Hemoparasites). In: Divers SJ, Stahl SJ, editors. Mader's reptile and Amphibian medicine and surgery. 3rd Edition. St. Louis, MO: W.B. Saunders; 2019. p. 281–300.e283.

158. Griffin C. The importance of diagnostic testing and directed therapy in reptiles and amphibians. In: Paper presented at: wild west veterinary conference; 16/10/2009. 2009. Vet Show, Nevada.

159. Wendland LD, Brown MB. 171 - tortoise Mycoplasmosis. In: Divers SJ, Stahl SJ, editors. Mader's reptile and amphibian medicine and surgery. 3rd Edition. St. Louis, MO: W.B. Saunders; 2019. p. 1353–4.e1351.

160. Wellehan JFX, Divers SJ. 31 - Mycology. In: Divers SJ, Stahl SJ, editors. Mader's reptile and amphibian medicine and surgery. 3rd Edition. St. Louis, MO: W.B. Saunders; 2019. p. 270–80.e273.

161. Urbanová D, Halán M. The use of ultrasonography in diagnostic imaging of reptiles. Folia Vet 2016;60(4):51–7.

162. Holmes SP, Divers SJ. 56 - Radiography—Chelonians. In: Divers SJ, Stahl SJ, editors. Mader's reptile and Amphibian medicine and surgery. 3rd Edition. St. Louis, MO: W.B. Saunders; 2019. p. 514–27.e511.

163. Dahlhausen B, Soler-Tovar D, Saggese MD. Diagnosis of mycobacterial infections in the exotic pet patient with emphasis on birds. Vet Clin Exot Anim Pract 2012;15(1):71–83.

164. Marschang RE. 118 - antiviral therapy. In: Divers SJ, Stahl SJ, editors. Mader's reptile and amphibian medicine and surgery. 3rd Edition. St. Louis, MO: W.B. Saunders; 2019. p. 1160–1.e1161.

165. Higbie CT, Nevarez JG, Roy AF, et al. Presence of West Nile Virus RNA in tissues of American Alligators (Alligator mississippiensis) vaccinated with a killed West Nile Virus Vaccine. J Herpetol Med Surg 2017;27(1/2):18–21.

166. Mohan K, Foggin CM, Dziva F, et al. Vaccination to control an outbreak of Mycoplasma crocodyli infection. Onderstepoort J Vet Res 2001;68(2):149–50.

167. Grobler M. The use of an inactivated vaccine in farmed Nile Crocodiles (Crocodylus Niloticus) for the control of Mycoplasma Crocodyli infection. Pretoria, South Africa: University of Pretoria; 2012.

Prevention is Better than Cure

An Overview of Disease Outbreak Management in Herptiles

Shirley Yeo LLizo, VMD

KEYWORDS

- Outbreak • Pathogen • Quarantine • Herptile • Bacterial infection • Viral infection
- Mycotic infection • Parasitic infection

KEY POINTS

- To be able to manage a disease outbreak effectively, there has to be preventative steps in place.
- Prevention includes quarantine or isolation of the specimen, a reliable source where specimen is obtained, and screening processes in place.
- Recognition of the disease in the early stage and rapid diagnosis will allow for more effective control.

INTRODUCTION

This article will focus on the diagnosis and treatment of common diseases affecting reptiles and amphibians (Appendix 1). There will be discussions on the characteristics of each pathogen and treatment strategies based on the differences in pathogens.

As the saying goes, "Prevention is better than cure". The key to successfully manage a disease outbreak is to prevent one, by that, it means to have already in place preventative measures. This will reduce the risk of a disease outbreak.

Preventative measures may include source of specimen, quarantine, types of testing while in quarantine, and treatment protocols based on test results.

SOURCE OF SPECIMEN

A new reptile or amphibian infection may originate from the wild, a zoo or aquarium, a wildlife rehabilitation center, a pet store, or the private sector. This will affect the decision on quarantine length, types of testing indicated, and any necessary treatment. A specimen from the wild is of an unknown status because there is no available

Topeka Zoo & Conservation Center, 635 SW Gage Boulevard, Topeka, KS 66606, USA
E-mail address: sllizo@topekazoo.org

Vet Clin Exot Anim 24 (2021) 647–659
https://doi.org/10.1016/j.cvex.2021.05.002
1094-9194/21/© 2021 Elsevier Inc. All rights reserved.

history, so it runs a higher risk assessment. This is compared to a specimen coming from a zoo or aquarium where it is presumed to have undergone some type of medical examination during its time at that institution so therefore runs a lower risk assessment. Other sources would fall in between these two categories.

QUARANTINE
Length of Stay

When a new animal arrives at an institution, it should first be quarantined. Quarantine length and which events to occur in quarantine may vary, depending on the origin of the specimen. A wild caught specimen may undergo a longer quarantine stay and have more tests performed where applicable because it is of an unknown source. A specimen arriving from another institution may already have undergone a preshipment examination and testing, so a quarantine examination may not be indicated. An average stay duration is usually 30 days, but this can be extended up to 90 days, depending on the test results such as fecal analyses. This is to ensure that each life stage of a parasitic cycle is effectively targeted and disrupted. A new specimen may stop eating after arrival, and quarantine is the period where the specimen is allowed to acclimate, and hopefully start eating regularly again before joining the main collection. They may take an extended time period.

If several animals are expected to arrive into quarantine, they should do so at the same time and then be able to leave at the same time, called "All in-all out". If a specimen arrives later, it should not be added to the existing group, otherwise, the existing group may need to have their length of stay extended.

Housing

Traditionally, a herptile can be housed in the same room as a mammal or bird, making the assumption that a disease will not cross species. If the herptiles come from different sources, it is recommended that they are housed in different rooms, even if they arrive at the same time.

Cleaning Tools

Tools that are used for cleaning the enclosures should not be shared between specimens unless they are originally from the same source and same species to avoid cross-contamination. This includes the water and feeding bowls.

Disinfection

There should be a cleaning schedule in place, and the appropriate disinfectant used for the species and the pathogen in question. Owing to their physiology, amphibians are especially sensitive to the different types of disinfectants and may succumb to toxicity if the appropriate disinfectant and method are not used. Avoid the use of products containing formalin, formaldehydes, phenols, or pine scent. These produce toxic fumes which are detrimental to the reptiles and especially amphibians (Appendix 1 on Disinfectants.).

Staffing

Selected staff should be assigned to only care for the animals in quarantine, and not also work in other animal areas of the same institution. However, if this is not possible, then the animals in quarantine should be serviced last, after the other animals in the main collection are cared for. A change of attire is also recommended between working with the main collection and the quarantined animals. This is to safeguard the existing collection by not introducing a new pathogen to the collection.

Types of Testing

Some of the routine tests are fecal analyses for endoparasites, screening for commonly known diseases in a particular species, for example, by polymerase chain reaction (PCR), weighing the animal to ensure the animal is maintaining its body condition, and obtaining baseline data such as complete blood count (CBC) and chemistry. Additional diagnostics include radiology and ultrasonography. Prophylactic therapies such as anthelmintics may also be indicated. The commonly used ones are ivermectin at 0.2 mg/kg by mouth, subcutaneous (SQ), or intramuscular (IM) or topical in amphibians in the interscapular region, contraindicated in chelonians, and fenbendazole/Panacur at 25 to 50 mg/kg by mouth or per rectum using a feeding tube (Appendix 2).

Observations

During quarantine, observations are made of the animal's behavior, appetite, and excrement, as well as any abnormal clinical signs.

In summary, following these basic steps will reduce the risk of introducing a new pathogen to the collection. In the event of a disease outbreak, steps can be retraced in an attempt to mitigate the risks. This is a form of risk assessment.

Despite incorporating preventative measures, diseases will still occur and may lead to an outbreak. The following sections discuss some of the more common diseases seen in herptiles.

REPTILE DISEASES

They are divided into several broad categories including bacterial, viral, fungal, and parasitic diseases.

Bacterial Infections

Salmonellosis

Over 90% of reptiles and amphibians have *Salmonella* in their gastrointestinal tract which they shed in feces and spread to their skin and environment. Although the bacterium does not usually cause disease in these animals, it is included here because of its zoonotic potential, causing morbidity and mortality in humans.

Clinical signs: rare. Diagnosis: As most herps will harbor this organism, and will shed either intermittently or continuously, a cloacal culture is usually not routinely carried out, and they are assumed positive unless proven otherwise. Other testing methods include PCR and enzyme-linked immunosorbent assay. If necessary, a series of cloacal or fecal culture, at least 5 samples collected over a 30-day period, should be performed to determine the *Salmonella* status of a reptile along with PCR. Of the 3 tests available, the PCR is the most sensitive, and the culture is the most specific.[1]

Treatment: If a herp tested positive but is asymptomatic, then treatment is usually not indicated. However, if treatment is necessary because of the zoonotic potential, then antibiotic selection should be based on culture and sensitivity testing.[1]

Cited case: 1996 Denver Zoo Komodo Dragon (*Varanus komodoensis*) special day, 50 visitors became sick, direct petting of lizard and barriers.[2]

Viral Infections

Inclusion body disease

The most commonly affected snakes with inclusion body disease (IBD) are boas and pythons. IBD was originally thought to be caused by a retrovirus, but more recently the source was confirmed to be a reptarenavirus.[3] The boas are typically the hosts as many are infected and can harbor the virus.

Clinical signs: neurologic signs include slow righting reflex, poor doer, anorexia, and weight loss. Immunosuppression is often involved. Usually, the disease presents more acutely with pythons and more chronic with boas.[3,4]

Diagnosis

Antemortem

1. Clinical pathology: Initially a leukocytosis is seen in the acute phase; as disease progresses, white blood cell counts tend to decline to subnormal levels (**Fig. 1**). Serum chemistry values will differ depending on the snake's hydration status and body condition;
2. PCR (blood sample)[3,4] (The author uses the University of Florida ZooMed Diagnostic Laboratory.);

Postmortem

PCR and histopathology: eosinophilic inclusion bodies found, for example, in the kidney, liver, esophageal tonsils, and stomach.[3,4]

Treatment: no effective treatment, only supportive or palliative; euthanasia.[3,4]

Disease management: In many cases, prognosis is guarded to grave, so it may be more humane to euthanize the animal. If the animal is to be maintained, then isolation should be seriously considered to prevent the spread of the disease.[5]

Ophidian paramyxovirus (Ferlavirus)

It is a highly contagious respiratory disease mostly found in venomous (viperid) snakes but has also been found in nonvenomous snakes and lizards.

Clinical signs: nasal discharge, open-mouth and/or labored breathing, mucoid exudate in oral cavity, occasional neurologic signs such as tremors, and opisthotonus.[6,7]

Diagnosis: serology (Hemagglutination Inhibition test, PCR) (The author uses UF ZooMed Laboratory.), lung biopsy (via endoscopy for histopathology, electron microscopy).[6,7]

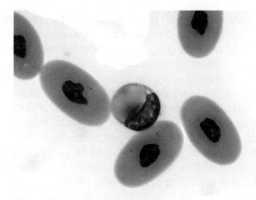

Fig. 1. Photomicrograph of a blood film from a rainbow boa (*Epicrates cenchria*) showing a lymphocyte with a pale basophilic, distinct inclusion of arenavirus (inclusion body disease) pushing the nucleus aside. Several erythrocytes are also present. X100 objective. Wright-Giemsa stain. (Photo courtesy of Nicole Stacy, DVM).

Treatment: no effective treatment, supportive care, or antibiotics for secondary infections; a vaccine is under investigation.[3]

Necropsy: grossly, limited to the lungs and liver.

Disease management: If an animal has a positive titer from the screening test, it should be isolated to prevent the spread of the disease. Strict hygiene should be practiced.

A more recent paramyxovirus but not a ferlavirus is the Sunshine virus in Australian pythons which needs to be considered when a snake presents with a neurorespiratory disease.[8]

Mycotic (Fungal) Infections

There are many classes of fungi affecting reptiles, two of which are Ophidiomyces (commonly known as snake fungal disease) and Nannizziopsis (commonly known as yellow fungus disease). The term Chrysosporium anamorph of *Nannizziopsis vriesii* or CANV has caused some confusion and should not be used.[9] Predisposing factors to mycotic infections may include a concurrent disease, excessive high humidity, low environmental temperature, malnutrition, and inappropriate antibiotic therapy (Normal cutaneous flora inhibit the growth of certain fungi.).

Clinical signs: most commonly cutaneous and respiratory systems affected, respiratory distress leading to death.[9]

Diagnosis: usually requires histologic examination of host response and identification of fungal agents.[9]

Treatment: for localized or superficial lesions, debridement of the lesions followed by antifungal topical applications such as Lugol solution or povidone-iodine, silver sulfadiazine/Silvadene cream 1%; for deep systemic infections, amphotericin B, itraconazole, fluconazole, voriconazole, and terbinafine. Ultraviolet light may also be beneficial.[9]

Disease management: Isolation may be necessary to prevent disease transmission. In severe cases, euthanasia may be indicated.

Cited case: African bush vipers in an North American Zoo.[10]

Parasitic Infections

Ectoparasites

The common one encountered in snakes mostly are the snake mites, *Ophionyssus natricis*, pinpoint black, sometimes red, moving dots on a snake. They feed on the blood of the snake.

Clinical signs: frequent soaks in water bowl, dysecdysis, debilitation in cases of heavy infestation, leading to death due to anemia or other infections.

Diagnosis: identification of mite.

Treatment: permethrin topical, diluted ivermectin topical, and parenteral ivermectin; treat environment concurrently; often requires multiple treatments.

Disease management: identify source of ectoparasite and then eliminate or treat the source. The source may be inanimate, such as the substrate, or animate, such as a conspecific. If infestation is not brought under control, it may have serious consequences.

Cited case: multiple snake and lizard species housed in individual tanks in a large exhibit hall in an North American zoo. (Author)

Cryptosporidiosis

Often called "Crypto", this one-celled microscopic intestinal parasite of the Coccidian subclass causes primarily diarrhea.

Clinical signs: postprandial regurgitation, weight loss, diarrhea, chronic debilitation, palpable swelling in gastric region due to the thickened gastric mucosa.

Diagnosis: acid-fast stains of feces or coating of regurgitated material, contrast radiography, endoscopic examination with biopsy of gastric mucosa.

Treatment: no effective treatment although hyperimmune bovine colostrum has proven to be effective in humans[11]; supportive therapy to prolong life; euthanasia (**Fig. 2** on medicating orally).

Disease management: Euthanasia is often considered because of the debilitative effects of the disease. It has also previously been considered a zoonotic disease, hence another reason for euthanasia, but it is now believed that the species affecting the reptiles are not the same ones affecting mammals.[12]

Cited case: Boelen's pythons at an North American zoo. (Jeff Ettling, Personal communication, 2020)

For a summary of the diseases that commonly affect reptiles, refer to **Table 1**.

AMPHIBIAN DISEASES
Bacterial Infections

A syndrome called "Red Leg" or bacterial dermatosepticemia is sometimes seen in amphibians infected with gram-negative, saprophytic bacteria such as *Aeromonas*, *Citrobacter*, *Proteus*, and *Pseudomonas* spp, with *Aeromonas* being the most common[13].

Clinical signs: ventral skin hyperemic—primarily abdomen and legs, ulcers on nose, skin, toes; hemorrhages on skeletal muscles, tongue, and nictitating membrane; weight loss; lethargy.[14] Bloating from intestinal gas, hydrocoelom, and hydrops can occur, leading up to sudden convulsions and eventually death.[13]

Diagnosis: Histology of affected areas includes inflammatory or necrotic foci in the liver, spleen, and other coelomic organs; blood or coelomic fluid (if present) is obtained for culture.[13,14]

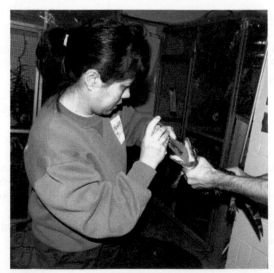

Fig. 2. Medicating a Chinese alligator (*Alligator sinensis*) with metal ball-tipped gavage tube and oral speculum (green block). (Author).

Table 1
Diseases of reptiles

Disease	Clinical Signs	Diagnosis	Treatment
Salmonellosis	Rare	Cloacal culture, series	Supportive treatment, if symptomatic
Inclusion body disease	Neurologic, slow righting reflex, poor doer, anorexia, weight loss	CBC—leukocytosis, acute phase; then leukopenia; PCR; histopathology—inclusion body	Supportive, palliative
Ophidian paramyxovirus	Nasal discharge, open-mouth breathing, oral mucoid exudate, neurologic	Serology—HI, PCR; lung biopsy	Supportive
Ophidiomyces, "snake fungal disease"; Nannizziopsis "yellow fungal disease"	Cutaneous lesions, respiratory distress	Identification of fungal elements	Debridement of lesions, topical antifungals, systemic antifungals, may be UV light
Snake mite Ophionyssus natricis	Frequent soaks in water bowl, dysecdysis, debilitation, death	Identification of mite	Topical permethrins, topical dilute ivermectin, parenteral ivermectin, treat environment
Cryptosporidiosis	Postprandial regurgitation, weight loss, diarrhea, debilitation, palpable swelling in gastric region	Acid-fast stain of feces, regurgitated material; contrast radiography; endoscopy/biopsy stomach	Supportive

Abbreviation: UV, ultraviolet.

Treatment: Before C&S results, start enrofloxacin 5 to 10 mg/kg SID by mouth or IM, oxytetracycline 50 mg/kg by mouth twice a day, or chloramphenicol 50 mg/kg by mouth twice a day; if fungal infection suspected, then itraconazole 0.01% bath (3.5 L of fresh water mixed with 35 mL of itraconazole solution 5 min/d × 8 days).[13,14]

Disease management: In aquatic and semi-aquatic species, spread of infection is often through the environment, that is, the water. Therefore, water quality is key. Separating affected individuals is often necessary to prevent spread to conspecifics sharing the same environment.

Viral Infections

Ranavirus

This virus causes infection in amphibians, reptiles, and fishes. It is transmitted by direct and indirect contact. The virus is able to survive for long periods of time in the aquatic environment without a host. This virus is highly virulent, causing a mortality rate reaching 90% to 100%. As such, the global impact is significant as it has caused the demise of many amphibian species. It is a notifiable disease to the World Organization for Animal Health (OIE).[14]

Clinical signs: acute onset of illness, high mortality rate, over a period of several days; skin hemorrhages near base of hind limbs and vent opening, lethargy, erratic swimming, buoyancy issues, dyspnea, fluid accumulation under the skin of abdomen and hind legs.[14]

Diagnosis: virus isolation in affected tissue; intranuclear inclusions within erythrocyte[13]; postmortem—fluid accumulation in coelom, hemorrhages of epicardial surface, gastric serosae, and hepatic parenchyma. Occasionally, liver or spleen affected, ulcers in skin and palate may be seen; PCR test; viral culture.[14]

Treatment: Currently no treatment or vaccine is available.[14]

Disease management: Prevention is key to control the spread of the disease, so quarantine of the amphibians is essential. Sterilization and disinfection (bleach 1%, chlorhexidine 0.75%) of articles used in the care of the amphibians need to take place. Euthanasia is often the end-result because of the grave prognosis and to prevent the spread due to the highly virulent virus.

Mycotic Infections

Chytridiomycosis

Chytridiomycosis is caused by two fungal species, *Batrachochytrium dendrobatidis* (Bd, affecting frogs) and *B. salamandrivorans* (affecting salamanders). Since 1998, the world has seen the decline of 501 amphibian species (6.5%), 90 presumed extinctions, in the tropics of Australia and Central and South America. This panzootic represents the greatest recorded loss of biodiversity attributable to a disease.[15] The "drink patch," specialized skin located in the ventral pelvic region that absorbs water, and the digits are especially affected. Bd is a OIE notifiable disease.[14]

Clinical signs: abnormal posture, anorexia, lethargy, dehydration, hyperemia, excessive shedding of skin, pupillary miosis, muscle incoordination.

Diagnosis: skin scrape with Wright-Giemsa or Gram stain under light microscope, swabs or pieces of integument for PCR, histopathology (**Fig. 3**).

Treatment:
1. Baths—Itraconazole (0.01% bath for 5 min/d for 10–11 days), maintaining animals well within their normal thermal range; terbinafine (0.01% bath buffered using bicarbonate to a pH of 7.2–7.4 for 5 min/d for 5 days); maintain animals well within their normal thermal range;

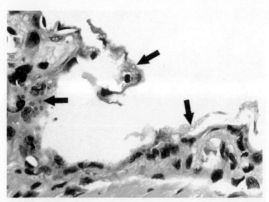

Fig. 3. *Batrachochytrium dendrobatidis* chytridiomycosis in the digital skin of an eastern newt (*Notophthalmus viridescens*). Arrows highlight the fungal organisms within the epidermis and accumulated keratin (hyperkeratosis). 400x magnification, hematoxylin and eosin. (Photo courtesy of Robert Ossiboff, DVM).

2. If appropriate for species, raise environmental temperatures for captive populations to greater than 23°C to help halt the infection;
3. Systemic antifungal drugs appear to be ineffective.

Disease management: with such a devastating disease, prevention in the form of quarantine or isolation is key. Once the animal is infected, the survival rate is poor.

Saprolegniasis
This includes several genera of opportunistic fungi or "water molds" that infect the gills and/or skin of aquatic and larval amphibians.

Clinical signs: whitish cotton-like growth on skin or oral cavity, turns greenish as time passes due to algae, lethargy, anorexia, weight loss, respiratory distress.[13]

Diagnosis: skin scrape—hyphae, thin-walled zoospores.[13]

Treatment:
1. Malachite green dip (67 mg/L for 15 seconds, once daily for 2–3 days);
2. Copper sulfate (500 mg/L for 2 minutes, once daily for 5 days, then once weekly until healed);
3. Treat eggs with Methylene blue.[13]

Disease management: In this case, correcting the poor water quality conditions is important for any chance of survival.

Parasitic Infections

Many of the parasites, protozoans (amebas, ciliates, flagellates) and metazoans (myxozoans, helminths) do not cause diseases in healthy amphibians unless they are debilitated or immunocompromised.

Protozoans

Amoebas
Most amoebas occur in the gastrointestinal tract of stressed amphibians but may also affect the kidney and liver.

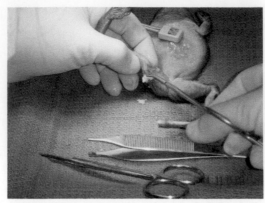

Fig. 4. Extracting encysted parasites in hind limb of White's tree frog (*Litoria caerulea*) (Author).

Clinical signs: anorexia, weight loss, lethargy, diarrhea, hematochezia, dehydration.[13]

Diagnosis: fecal analysis, cloacal wash, histology of affected tissue.[13]

Treatment: supportive therapy, oral or bath treatments with metronidazole.[13]

Ciliates, flagellates

Most of these organisms are also found in the gastrointestinal tract or skin of amphibians and usually are commensal and not pathogenic.

Clinical signs: anorexia, lethargy, pallor, splenomegaly, and splenic necrosis.[13]

Diagnosis: antemortem—skin scrapings, gill clips, feces, cloacal washes, urine, unstained wet mounts of blood (trypanosomes), Wright's Giemsa-stained blood smears; postmortem—impression smears of spleen, histopathology.[13]

Treatment: oral or bath treatments with metronidazole, antimalarial drugs for trypanosomes.[13]

Disease management: For these protozoans, it is needless to say that attention must be given to the environment and the prevention of reinfection are both integral to successful treatment.

Metazoans

Here we will focus on the helminths which are most prevalent.

Helminths

They are also known as flukes or digenes. Amphibians are secondary intermediate or definitive hosts.

Clinical signs: yellowish bumps on the body and legs where the metacercariae have encysted. With high numbers, these cause trauma, compression, or displacement of tissue.[13]

Diagnosis: identification of parasites in the encysted tissue.[13]

Treatment: difficult, multiple doses of praziquantel[13] (**Fig. 4**).

Disease management: Prevention is most effective by removing the snails which are intermediate hosts from the aquariums or closed aquatic systems.

For a summary of the diseases that commonly affect amphibians, refer to **Table 2**.

Table 2
Diseases of amphibians

Disease	Clinical Signs	Diagnosis	Treatment
Dermatosepticemia	Hyperemic ventral skin	Histology of affected areas	Antibiotics, antifungal bath
Red-leg syndrome	Weight loss, lethargy, hemorrhages on skeletal muscles, tongue, nictitating membrane	Culture of blood or coelomic fluid	
Ranavirus	Acute onset, skin hemorrhages at the base of hind limbs & vent opening, lethargy, erratic swimming, buoyancy issues, dyspnea, edema, hydrocoelom	PCR, virus isolation, microscopy	None
Chytridiomycosis "Bd"	Abnormal posture, anorexia, lethargy, dehydration, hyperemia, excessive skin shedding, pupillary miosis, muscle incoordination	Skin scrape with Wright-Giemsa or Gram stain under light microscopy, swabs or pieces of integument for PCR, histopathology	Antifungal baths, raise environmental temperature (appropriate for species)
Saprolegniasis	Whitish cotton-like growth on skin, turns greenish with time, lethargy, anorexia, weight loss, respiratory distress	Skin scrape—hyphae, thin-walled Zoospores	Chemical baths
Amoebas	Anorexia, weight loss, lethargy, diarrhoea, hematochezia, dehydration	Fecal analysis, cloacal wash, histology of affected tissue	Supportive therapy, oral or bath metronidazole
Ciliates, flagellates	Anorexia, lethargy, pallor, splenomegaly	Skin scrapes, gill clips, feces, cloacal washes, urine, unstained wet mounts of blood, Wright-Giemsa stain blood smear; postmortem: impression smears of spleen	Oral or bath metronidazole, antimalarial drugs for trypanosomes
Helminths	Yellowish bumps on body & legs	Identification of parasites in encysted tissue	Difficult, multiple praziquantel

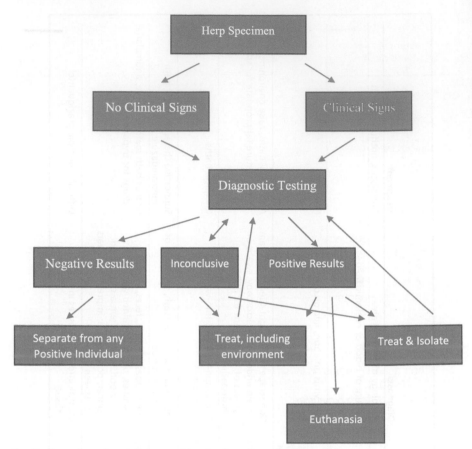

Fig. 5. Flow chart for decision-making in disease outbreak.

SUMMARY

This has been an overview of disease outbreak management, highlighting the more common diseases among herptiles where the potential for a disease outbreak exists if not given the appropriate medical attention. Prevention in the form of quarantine or isolation is key to avoid disease transmission. The source of the infection needs to be identified early to effectively treat the patient. Treatment often consists of not only treating the patient but also its environment as well (**Fig. 5**).

CLINICS CARE POINTS

- It is imperative that when a new specimen arrives, a risk assessment is performed to determine the length of quarantine and which diseases it needs to be screened for.
- Relevant disease testing and the interpretation of the results will help in the decision-making process.
- Prompt testing, diagnosis, and treatment are necessary to mitigate the effects of the disease, whether on one specimen or a group of animals. This will also prevent a disease outbreak from spreading further.

- Protocols need to be in place to offer the best hygiene practices to avoid a disease outbreak.
- The appropriate disinfectant needs to be selected not only to prevent spread of the disease but also to cause no harm to the animals.

DISCLOSURE

The author has nothing to disclose.

SUPPLEMENTARY DATA

Supplementary data to this article can be found online at https://doi.org/10.1016/j.cvex.2021.05.002.

REFERENCES

1. Mitchell MA. Salmonella: Diagnostic Methods for Reptiles. Mader's Reptile Medicine & Surgery, 2nd ed. St. Louis (MO): Saunders, Elsevier; 2006.
2. Collins LM. Denver Zoo Lizard Cause Salmonella Outbreak. AP News 1996.
3. Divers SJ. Viral Diseases of Reptiles. In: Merck Manual, last full review/revision Jun 2020, content last modified Jun 2020. Available at: https://www.merckvetmanual.com/exotic-and-laboratory-animals/reptiles/viral-diseases-of-reptiles.
4. Ritchie B. Inclusion Body Disease. Mader's Reptile Medicine & Surgery, 2nd ed. chp 24 p 404-405
5. Schumacher J. Inclusion Body Disease. Mader's Reptile Medicine & Surgery, 2nd ed. chp 60.
6. Ritchie,B. Paramyxoviridae. Mader's Reptile Medicine & Surgery, 2nd ed. St. Louis (MO): Saunders, Elsevier; 2006. p 401-404.
7. Bronson E, Cranfield M. Paramyxovirus. Mader's Reptile Medicine & Surgery, 2nd ed. chp 63
8. Hyndman TH, Shilton CM, Marschang RE. Paramyxoviruses in reptiles: a review. Vet Microbiol 2013;165(3–4):200–13.
9. Divers SJ. Mycotic Diseases of Reptiles. In: Merck Manual, last full review/revision Jun 2020, content last modified Jun 2020
10. Marrow JC. Diagnosis and Treatment of a *Paranannizziopsis australasiensis* (Onygenales) Outbreak in African Bush Vipers (*Atheris squamigera*). Proc Am Assn Zoo Vets 2020.
11. Steele J, Sponseller J, Schmidt D, et al. Hyperimmune bovine colostrum for treatment of GI infections: A review and update on Clostridium difficile. Hum Vaccin Immnother 2013;9:1565–8.
12. Divers SJ. Parasitic Diseases of Reptiles. In: Merck Manual, last full review/revision Jun 2020, content last modified Jun 2020
13. Wright KA. Overview of Amphibian Medicine. Mader's Reptile Medicine & Surgery, 2nd ed, chp 75, p 956-957.
14. Whitaker, BR. Infectious Diseases of Amphibians. In Merck Manual, last full review/revision Sep 2013, content last modified Sep 2013
15. Scheele BC, Pasmans F, Skerratt LF, et al. Amphibian fungal panzootic causes catastrophic and ongoing loss of biodiversity. Science 2019;363(Issue 6434):1459–63.

Reproduction Management of Herds/Flocks of Exotic Animals

Investigating Breeding Failures in Birds, Reptiles, and Small Mammals

Lorenzo Crosta, DVM, PhD, GP Cert (ExAP), FNOVI (Avian and Zoo Medicine),
DECZM[a],*, Daniele Petrini, DVM, MSc, GPCert (ExAP), SPACS[b],
Shivananden Sawmy, BSc (Hons) Biol, BVM&S (Edinburgh, UK), Cert AVP
Zoological Medicine (UK), MRCVS[c]

KEYWORDS

- Exotic animals • Breeding/reproduction • Flock/herd management
- Flock/herd medicine • Infertility • Breeding failure • Reproductive tract diseases

KEY POINTS

- Breeding exotic species requires a good understanding of the biology of the species.
- Breeding failures are not necessarily caused by a disease.
- Train yourself to consider the herd/flock as a whole organism.
- Deepen your knowledge of diseases that may lead to breeding failure.

FOREWORD

The medical management of a breeding collection of nondomestic pets is challenging, and it is not the typical job for a veterinarian. Even experienced small animal practitioners may find difficult to cope with this multifaceted task, which includes knowledge of biology and especially specific general and reproductive biology of the species being dealt with, and knowledge of nutrition, of behavior, and of environmental enrichment. Doctors must know the physiology and diseases that affect the reproductive systems of different orders of patients. In addition, they also require a deep understanding of the exotic animal breeder community and of their

[a] Sydney School of Veterinary Science, The University of Sydney, Avian, Reptile and Exotic Pet Hospital, 415 Werombi Road, Camden, 2570 NSW, Australia; [b] Medicina e Chirurgia Degli Animali Non Convenzionali, Segretario SIVAE; [c] Avian, Reptile and Exotic Pet Hospital, Sydney School of Veterinary Science, The University of Sydney
* Corresponding author.
E-mail address: lorenzo_birdvet@yahoo.com

Vet Clin Exot Anim 24 (2021) 661–695
https://doi.org/10.1016/j.cvex.2021.06.001
1094-9194/21/© 2021 Elsevier Inc. All rights reserved.
vetexotic.theclinics.com

expectations, which ranges from the canary bird fancier to the curator of a large zoologic collection.

BIRDS (LORENZO CROSTA)
Introduction

This article is tailored to give small animal veterinarians, and also avian practitioners without specific experience in the management of bird collections, some examples and suggestions to be used when evaluating a bird breeding facility, in order to highlight the weak points and help in selecting the best birds to use as breeders.

In most cases, general small animal practitioners find it difficult to work with breeding collections. This difficulty may be caused by a lack of information about breeding animals, and by the very limited number of articles treating the topic, but in the opinion of the author it is mainly caused by the lack of experience in working with a large group of animals (multiple patients). In this respect, the flock is a single, unique organism; therefore, with some exceptions, single birds are of little value, because the clinician is working to exploit and protect the real patient: the bird collection. Hence, medicine, sensu stricto, is only 1 of the tools needed for the sanitary management of the flock, whereas the analysis and evaluation of the flock must be broader and include other aspects. In brief, it is no longer examining a patient, it is examining a group.

Types and Clinical Characteristics of the Flock

As a general rule, there are different kinds of bird collections, but veterinarians mainly face 2 types:

- Collections focused on reproduction and breeding
- Collections more focused on visitors (this applies mostly to zoos)

Depending on the type of collection (purely breeding, or zoo), management uses different techniques, but the focus is still to breed the birds; often, the veterinarian is called to help understand why there is a low breeding performance, or no breeding at all.[1]

One mistake that most practitioners make when approaching a breeding farm or a zoo is to focus on the birds that are obviously unwell, and then start examining and eventually treating them. If the purpose of clinical expertise is to fix breeding problems, that is not the right approach. Instead, the correct course of action is to evaluate the breeding facilities first and then take the breeding stock into consideration.

It is like running a clinical examination, but, instead of examining skin, gastrointestinal system, heart, lungs, and so forth, the plan is to examine several aspects of the collection. The author defines them as the clinical characteristics of the flock, and they are:

- Management, hygiene, and sanitary status of the collection
- Mortality and causes of deaths
- Breeding performance, evaluation of breeding birds, and analysis of breeding failures
- Evaluation of the nursery, and rating of the produced chicks
- Evaluation of new birds to be added to the collection

Management and sanitary status of the collection

When completing this analysis, as if they were working on a single patient, clinicians need to take into consideration different subunits of the same apparatus. The first thing to evaluate are the birds. In detail, clinicians need to understand what bird species are to be bred. This information can make a big difference, because the following things need to be analyzed depending on the bird species. Therefore, clinicians need to know whether birds are kept in pairs, whether they are maintained in colonies, and whether this changes during the different seasons. Also, on a percentage basis, clinicians need to know whether there are single birds, and why.

Look at the aviaries, or the cages, or the paddocks. Observe their design. Are they appropriate for the species? Is there any risk factor, any detail that may disturb or even scare the birds? Is there anything in, or with, the aviary that looks like a good architectural design for the visitors but could be inappropriate for the birds, especially if they are meant to breed? Remember that the final users of the aviary are the birds, and the inner part must be good for them. Multispecies aviaries are seldom used for breeding, but sometimes this can be achieved. In this case, clinicians must make sure the birds are not disturbing each other, or fighting, or even hunting. The enclosure accessories, such as feeding and drinking bowls, perches, and nests, need to be considered. Also, do not forget the flooring, bedding, and the kind of substrate that is used inside the nests. Some species do not need a nest box, and some do not need a substrate.

Nutrition. Nutrition is a weak point in many aviaries. Because there is no gold standard in avian nutrition (and, with almost 10,000 bird species, this is to be expected), there are several opinions about the nutrition of birds in captivity. Exotic animal nutrition, including birds, therefore suffers from so-called nutritional mythology.

On one side, there are breeders that are trying to imitate the birds' natural diet. In the experience of the author, this is almost only possible when breeding birds in their natural area of distribution. In contrast, there are breeders and bird food producers that prefer the use of pelleted, or extruded, diets, which should meet the birds' nutritional requirements in a uniform way. Discussing the best option is beyond the scope of this article, and it depends on the bird species, season, and age.

However, there are some observations, made over many years by breeders, that are supported by science. For example, 1 concept is clear: in addition to providing nutrients for the body, food is a source of enrichment, or, to put it better, the search for food is a source of enrichment, whereas the biochemical composition of food is a source of neuroendocrine stimuli that cause behavioral changes.[2] Excluding poultry and few other commercially raised species, parrots and birds of prey are the most widely studied birds in this respect, but although birds of prey generally are fed a monotypic diet and what is important for their performance is the energy intake, Psittaciformes do use food and its search for several purposes, including to provide energy for the body but also for entertaining with other birds, sexual display, and likely teaching their young.

Therefore, clinicians want to know what is fed to the birds but also how, where, and when the food is provided.

Nutrition: what?. Parrots' diets can now be based largely on extruded foods. The nutritional value of this type of food is not in question, but a possible drawback is the lack of social stimulation offered by a diet based only on monotypic pellets. Therefore, to meet the behavioral needs of parrots, their diet must be enriched with food suitable for the purpose. If the purpose is breeding the birds, then the food must be used as a tool to stimulate breeding, and, to do so, carers want to imitate what happens in nature. Most parrot species do not react to the circannual rhythm as do wild birds that developed in temperate regions. Parrots do not perceive the increasing day length as the start of the breeding season, or, at least, they perceive it in a different way. Most parrot species are stimulated to breed by different factors, such as an increase of fresh food, and/or an increase of rainy days, likely because rain supposedly leads to the presence of a lot of fresh food.

Seen from this perspective, parrot nutrition, with the aim of breeding, should alternate a dry season with a season with free availability of fresh and rich foods. During the dry season, provide a good diet, but it must not stimulate the breeding birds. For example, a diet based only on pellets/extruded foods works well. When the breeding season approaches, it is necessary to imitate what happens in nature: large availability of fresh and rich foods, and an increase of protein and fat. Therefore, apart from the pellets, which always represent a large percentage of the diet, the following items can be used:

- Legumes (beans, peas, lentils, chickpeas) are traditionally served soaked, and sometimes sprouted. The great advantage of sprouted legumes is that they look like a fresh food, like what is available during the rainy season. Furthermore, they are more digestible than dry beans, and legumes increase the protein content of the diet. However, sprouts are dangerous: they represent the perfect medium to grow pathogens. One option is cooking the sprouts and offering them in a limited quantity, to have them consumed rapidly.[3]
- Fruits and vegetables: these are a fresh food, with certain advantages. In addition, they provide vitamins, minerals, and trace elements. All types of long-fiber vegetables are good for entertaining parrots, as well. Although fruit and vegetables can be offered all year round, it is better to avoid them for a short period, when trying to mimic the dry season.
- Nuts and fatty seeds: because of their high fat content, they are unbalanced from the nutritional point of view; however, a small daily number of nuts can stimulate breeding in some species. For example, macaws are known to love having some nuts in their diet, especially during the breeding season. For example, the main dietary item of the Lear's macaw (*Anodorhynchus leari*) in the wild is the licuri palm nut (*Syagrus coronata*). In contrast, some parrot species, such as the Saint Vincent Amazon (*Amazona guildingii*), which developed where the availability of fatty food is very limited, are prone to become obese if offered an unbalanced diet.
- Meat and animal byproducts: some parrot species benefit from a small increase in the protein content of their diet. It seems to stimulate reproduction. In addition, some species offer meaty or bony bites to their partners, as part of the courtship. However, it is important not to exceed certain quantities because kidney damage can be caused by too much protein in the diet.

Nutrition: how and when?. In order to help the physiologic breeding season of Psittaciformes, the way food is provided is also important. In general, it is important to provide adequate food for the physiologic season; avoid offering excess mixed foods, because birds will select the ones they prefer, and they are not necessarily the best ones; prevent perishable foods from being available too long.

Nutrition: where?. Although much of the food is provided in normal feeders, there are techniques that allow food to be used as a form of enrichment, and this may be critical for courtship and other important behaviors that lead to a successful breeding. For example, cracked nuts and similar treats can be scattered on the ground to stimulate the search for them. It important to consider the treats as a part of the diet, in order to have a good nutritional balance.[2]

Summarizing, and independently of the choice of the bird caretaker, or curator, as veterinarians, the important facts to focus on are:

- Kind of feeds and raw material used
- Foodstuff storing room/area
- Appropriateness of foodstuff/diets with the maintained bird species

Hygiene. The rules for the hygiene management of a bird breeding center do not differ from the rules for the management of breeding stocks of any other species:

- Cleaning staff working schedule: birds are messy, especially parrots and birds of prey, and leave a lot of leftovers in the enclosure. Cleaning must be a primary task for the caretakers.
- Observe the presence of fecal material and evaluate how old they are. This point is important because some species produce a large quantity of stools when kept in captivity. For example, some thrush species (Turdidae) may produce in 1 day stools that weight almost as much as the bird itself.[4]
- Watch for the presence of pests, or vermin, and the measures taken to control them.
- Strategy to avoid contact between poison/traps/dead pest and the birds.
- Disinfection plan, and check what kind of detergents and disinfectants are used: some may be irritating for the respiratory tract and some may be toxic.
- In indoor facilities, check the air quality. Some diseases, such as aspergillosis, can be controlled by strict monitoring of the air.[5]

Mortality and causes of deaths

Most aviculturists perceive veterinarians as primary providers of clinical services only, and few maintain a flock health program designed to meet the production goals of the collection. Veterinarians also view themselves in this role.[6] It is common that the veterinarian is called to diagnose the causes of mortality in an avian breeding center.

Most fatalities are caused by long-term incorrect sanitary management. The tired-environment concept is not a myth, and, in most cases, the cure is not easy and seldom gives immediate results. However, the job of veterinarians is to evaluate the breeding center as a whole, and then make the diagnosis.

Several years ago, I coined what seemed to be a joke: Crosta's first axiom. The axiom is that when 1 bird dies it is an accident; when 2 birds die, it is not. I still believe this. Most aviculturist have no idea of what the average mortality is. What is a normal mortality? Are there any published data about it? The answer is no. However, there are some anecdotical indications. In brief, extrapolating from technical discussions with several bird curators and breeders over 30 years, it is thought that the average mortality depends on species, age of the birds, and age of the collection.

In a large collection, older than 10 years, hosting several different psittacine species and managing more than 100 breeding pairs, the yearly mortality of adult birds (>18 months of age) should not exceed 4%.

In contrast, a small bird breeding center, with less than 20 to 30 pairs, managing similar species (for example, only Amazons) and in place for only 5 years, the yearly mortality of adult birds should not exceed 2%.

In addition, if chick mortality is taken into consideration, then the job is far too complicated, because of the many factors that play a role. The analyses should consider: origin of chicks (nest vs artificial incubation); bird species; age of the chicks (first week; first month; 2–6 months, and so forth). Therefore, it is almost impossible to have a clear understanding of what is normal and what is not.

Breeding performance, evaluation of breeding birds, and analysis of breeding failures
At this point, the veterinarian should be able to understand whether the breeding problems of the flock are caused by management or by quality/health of the breeding birds.[1]

In cases of wrong management, it is useless to work with the birds: better to give the best possible advice about how to improve the management and reevaluate the situation later.

If, instead, the problems seem to be related to health, or diseases, then the veterinarian must schedule a complete diagnostic plan on the breeding stock, with the purpose of identifying the birds that are not good for breeding, and helping the owner/curator to plan the future steps, such as the disposal of nonbreeding birds, or acquisition of new birds, if they are needed.

There are many issues related to the health of breeding birds that can cause reproductive problems. Infertility in birds can be defined as the failure to produce fertile eggs. In a wider perspective, the term is erroneously used to define avian pairs that do not produce eggs, or do not seem to have interest in breeding. In addition, the widest definition may include birds that do produce fertile eggs but have a high percentage of embryonic deaths.[7] In a breeding farm, the veterinarian will be asked to solve problems of fertility in the widest meaning of the term.

Specific disease issues

Reproductive apparatus Orchitis, oophoritis, and oviductitis can be primary reasons for a disappointing breeding performance. In addition, in ratites and waterfowl, lesions of the phallus can cause infertility problems.

Musculoskeletal apparatus Arthritis, arthrosis, limb deviation, bumblefoot, missing limbs or toes, kyphosis, and scoliosis are all problems that can have a severe impact on breeding. Missing toes or limbs may limit the ability of birds to mate properly. Apparently, a missing wing is not as bad as a missing leg as a limiting factor to copulation. However, a missing wing may alter the behavior of a bird (display, courtship, and so forth) to the point that the bird does not find a partner or is not be able to copulate properly.[1]

Gastrointestinal system Cloacitis, cloacal paralysis, and cloacal tumors, including papillomas, may all lead to breeding failure.[7] This failure is caused by both the inability to breed and also by the pH and microflora changes caused by chronic cloacal/intestinal inflammation and infection.

Endocrine/metabolic causes Low calcium blood level and pituitary gland deficiency are also medical causes of breeding failure, or breeding-related problems.

Behavior Abnormal behaviors can lead to the inability to find a partner, to build a nest, to copulate, and so forth. In many cases, the wrong behavior is caused by an inappropriate method of rearing the chicks. There are species differences, and some species are more susceptible than others; however, chicks that have been reared alone, with no social contacts, may not be able to behave in an appropriate way.

There are species with peculiar sexual behaviors, and this must always be taken into account. For example, out of the breeding season, captive northern goshawk (*Accipiter gentilis*) females often hunt and eat their males. Hence, the aviary must have a specific design, allowing the birds to watch each other but not have physical contact, until it is the right time.

The eclectus parrot (*Eclectus roratus*) is the only psittacine bird showing polygynandry. Polygynandry is a form of polygamy; in sexually reproducing animals, it is a multimale and multifemale mating system. Polygynandry encapsulates both polygyny (males having multiple female mates) and polyandry (females having multiple male mates) within the same species. Knowing this, eclectuses can be flocked and bred in colonies. Nevertheless, very good results have been achieved keeping them in pairs.

Some male birds can see their neighbors as sexual competitors, and therefore spend much time challenging and trying to fight them. This behavior is the cause of 2 issues: (1) the birds are frustrated; the hierarchy situation remains unresolved, and the fights go on for ages. (2) The contenders spend a lot of time fighting and do not care about breeding.

Toxins Aflatoxins and other mycotoxins can directly or indirectly cause low fertility. Some drugs, such as metronidazole, tetracyclines, and ivermectin, are also thought to produce sterility. This finding may be anecdotal, but it is better to use other drugs during or before the breeding season.

Generalized/chronic diseases There are several diseases that may cause infertility. Chlamydiosis, as with other bacterial diseases, can cause orchitis.[8,9] Many chronic diseases may limit the production or the quality of the eggs. For example, because of the limited production of yolk proteins, hepatitis can cause issues with egg quality. Also, generalized diseases can inhibit mating behavior.[7]

Blindness There are anecdotical reports about blind birds being infertile. Although blindness is a serious disadvantage for animals whose primary sense is sight, and therefore blind birds should not be selected as breeders, the question remains: can a blind bird breed? The personal experience of this author is that there are blind birds that can breed.

In contrast, blindness can also be a strong limitation in recognizing the sexual signals from a possible partner, which is likely to reject the blind bird as a possible partner.

Once it is certain that breeding failures depend more on a medical issue than on management, clinicians can establish a check plan. The diagnostic tests are in 2 main categories:

1. Tests to protect the flock/collection
2. Analysis to evaluate single birds

Tests to protect the flock/collection These are the most widely used analyses. They are conducted to avoid the introduction of pathogens (especially infectious/contagious diseases) in bird collections. There is a continuous revision of how the veterinary community perceives these diseases, and this varies in different parts of the world. Further, there is an intense update about the gold-standard techniques that are best to detect a single disease. However, for psittacine birds, it is recommended to test for Psittacine Circovirus (Psittacine beak and feather disease), Polyomavirus (avian polyoma virus), Pacheco disease (psittacid alphaherpesvirus 1), Adenovirus, Psittacosis, and Bornavirus (avian Bornavirus).

In a flock situation, analyses to evaluate single birds are uncommon, and are generally the last step of a thorough diagnostic process used to screen birds with a high individual value. The clinical examination of a single bird that is apparently not a good breeder does not differ much from that of a normal bird during a standard avian clinical visit, including physical examination, hematology, blood chemistry, microbiology, and parasitology.[1] In contrast, avian flock medicine uses different tools, or gives different importance to the same analytical instruments.

For example, after a thorough clinical examination has been done but no information has been collected for the cause of breeding failure was, a celioscopy is an important tool to evaluate the quality of the reproductive apparatus of both sexes.[10]

To cite some examples, true hermaphroditism is extremely rare in birds,[11] or at least it has been reported very rarely,[12] but some forms of anatomic intersexual features are not as rare; for example, a wrong development of the vas deferens can lead to infertility. Also, abnormalities of the gonads at an early stage can be diagnosed with the use of endoscopy.[10] In addition, some abnormalities of the gonads can be inapparent, even with a celioscopy examination, but biopsy and histopathology can reach a proper diagnosis.[13,14]

Because assisted insemination techniques are becoming more and more popular,[15,16] a semen analysis, also called seminogram or spermiogram, must be used to assess fertility in male birds before the artificial insemination is attempted.[17–19] Clinicians must be aware that although artificial insemination is a widely used technique in commercial poultry, cranes, and birds of prey, and although it is possible in parrots, it is still far from being a routine method in this last family. In the end, artificial insemination is possibly an excellent tool for specific situations, such as recovery programs of endangered avian species, when an increased number of offspring is desired and also mating specific birds is mandatory.[20]

Egg necropsy This topic can be a question of mortality or of breeding failure. In any case, it is of paramount importance to necropsy all the eggs that do not hatch. The primary purpose is to determine whether eggs that are thought to be sterile are really not fecundated, or whether there is a tiny embryo that could not be spotted with candling. This difference is important, because in the first case it is likely that the male is not working properly, or the pair is not a true pair, whereas, in the second case, the male works well but something went wrong during the first stages of incubation.

In older, or end-stage, dead embryos, a good egg necropsy can often lead to a causative diagnosis.

Evaluation of the nursery, determination of sex, and rating of the chicks bred in the facility

Nowadays most institutions and bird breeders are drastically revising their approach to breeding and fewer and fewer bird chicks are hand reared. However, the nursery remains a key point in a bird collection, and its importance is directly related to the species being worked with and the number of chicks the owner wants to hand rear. The first points to verify are whether there are separate areas for incubation and hatching and whether there is a specific room for the hand rearing of chicks. Those 2 facts are most important because they have a great impact on the chick health and physical and mental development: well-managed hand-rearing techniques, done by experienced professionals, may produce healthy chicks, able to have a good and friendly relationship with humans but still able to behave normally for the species and, therefore, become breeding birds; in contrast, rearing techniques that are obsolete and performed by nonprofessional staff lead to the production of young birds that are unable to behave properly, that will develop behavioral problems, and, in the end, will not be able to mate with adequate partners.

Rating of the chicks. Once a first evaluation of the nursing premises has been done, and most of this judgment should be made when evaluating all the breeding farm, the clinician can start evaluating the chicks as single patients. This step takes into consideration several parameters[21]:

- Physical condition and morphology. It is of primary importance to focus on the normal development process of the avian chick. If clinicians do not understand the difference between a normal chick and a chick that is starting to develop problems, their reactions are often too late to be successful. Routine checkups allow clinicians to have a detailed history of every chick and identify any deviation from normality earlier, so that potentially ill birds can be isolated from the other chicks in the nursery as soon as possible.

Sick chicks are generally easier to identify than sick adult birds, because they do not need to hide their symptoms yet. The typical clinical symptoms to be aware of are slow crop emptying, swollen abdomen, generalized edema, dehydration, abnormal feces, and so forth. Growth rate: a simple way to check the general status and condition of a chick, is to analyze its growth and weight gain rates. The generic growing curve of altricial birds always has, more or less, the same shape, so the evaluation of individual growth curves helps to identify chicks with growing problems.

- Routine testing of the chicks is also a useful way to monitor the collection. A random microbiology survey on the chicks, run on a routine basis, even when the chicks are apparently healthy, is a wise way to control outbreaks of bacterial diseases.

Sex of the chicks and sex ratio. The assessment of the sex of the chicks that are produced is also an important part of the job of aviculture veterinarians. In addition, it is better to know in advance what sex the chicks are, in order to avoid the selling of birds that may be useful later on for the collection.

Formation of new pairs. If there is the need to form new pairs, or to replace aging or dead birds, or birds that are no longer breeding, it is better to use birds born in the same collection. This option allows curators to select the best birds as replacements, and without the risk of the introduction of new diseases.[1]

Evaluation and screening of new birds to be added to the collection
As stated earlier, if there is the possibility of making internal replacements, which means to replace aging or nonproductive birds with young, healthy adults from the same farm, that is much better. However, sometimes clients are forced to acquire birds from other institutions, and this exposes the collection to a risk of being exposed to contagious diseases.[22,23]

However, in many avian collections, the selection of the breeding birds is made on the owner's/curator's personal opinion, or birds' sizes and/or colors, on price, and on avicultural mythology. Given this, there is rarely a scientific approach to bird selection, especially when infertility problems arise. However, there are almost no publications or books explaining how to select birds that are more suitable for breeding purposes.[24]

As usual, when a selection of the birds needs to be made, it is not necessary to rate them, and rating will depend on different parameters, such as species, origin, how the bird was reared and weaned, sex, age, physical conditions, and health status.

- Species: the choice of the species depends on the circumstances of the owner, such as financial investment, location, and experience. When giving an expert opinion, always think of the best possible conditions for a given species. This advice implies the analysis of other factors, such as:
  ○ Aviaries (size, hanging vs on the ground, north-south orientation)

- o Environment (indoor/outdoor, need for heating)
- o Temperature (season variations)
- o Food (providers, season variation)
- o Compatible species (in terms of behavior, food, and diseases)
- o Disease testing (may change for the different species)
- Origin: this is also critical. Is it known where the birds come from? Is the source reliable? Depending on the answers to these questions, It may be necessary to test for different diseases. For example, if the bird comes from a well-known breeder, possibly the client, and it is known that there are no diseases circulating in the breeding stock, it is possible to have a different approach compared with when the birds come from an unknown breeding center, maybe located abroad.
- Type of rearing/weaning: depending on what is wanted from a bird, it may also be important to know how it was reared and weaned. It is generally thought that parent-raised birds do better as breeding birds, compared with hand-reared specimens. There are indications that some species cope well with hand rearing and apparently do not have problems in behaving normally when they are adult (for example, Amazons), whereas, for some other species, hand rearing seems to have a greater impact on social behavior later on (for example, cockatoos).[25] Seen from another perspective, this means that hand rearing can be done, but must be done by professionally trained keepers, and the final outcome will also depend on the bird species.

Conclusion

Citing Speer[6] (1994), "Most aviculturists perceive veterinarians as primary providers of clinical services only, and few maintain a flock health program designed to meet the production goals of the collection. Veterinarians also view themselves in this role." Although it is dated, this statement still represents the situation of how aviculture sees veterinarians, and how most veterinarians see themselves with respect to aviculture and bird breeding. Aviculturists are not the easiest clients; they know what they are talking about, they want their problems to be addressed professionally, and, in the end, they want tangible progress. If the veterinarian is not trained to work with aviculturists and to deal with flocks of birds, breeding, and production medicine, the relationship between a possible client and the veterinarian will never start. Or, worse, it will end very soon.

REPTILES (SHIVANANDEN SAWMY)
Reptile Reproductive Biology

A thorough discussion on reptile reproduction and embryology is beyond the scope of this article but a brief review is warranted. In contrast with birds, which are all oviparous, reptiles can either be oviparous (producing shelled eggs that require external incubation to hatch), or viviparous (embryos are retained in the oviduct until fully developed and born live).[26–28] Furthermore, viviparous development varies across taxa; that is, the development of offspring can rely entirely on yolk in the oviduct or a chorioallantoic placenta nourishes the embryos until born. Interestingly, some reptile species are capable of asexual reproduction or parthenogenesis. This phenomenon has been observed in at least 30 species of lizards, the most common being the whiptail lizard (Aspidoscelis [Cnemidophorus] spp) and 1 snake species, the blind snake (Indotyphlops [Rhamphotyphlops] braminus).[28–30] Despite asexual reproduction, females still display courtship behavior and pseudocopulation.[31]

Reproductive Cycles

Reptiles originating from the tropics usually come from habitats experiencing minimal variations in annual temperature or photoperiod. This uniform climate allows most of these species to have a continuous reproductive cycle, which means that they are capable of fertile mating all year round.[28] However, some of these reptiles, such as tropical boids (Boidae) are more inclined to breed in the colder months. In contrast, reptiles from subtropical or temperate zones usually become reproductively active in the spring after a period of brumation (seasonal cooling) and have an associated reproductive cycle.[28,29] Copulation and egg (or fetal) development are stimulated by sex hormone secretion and gonadal development, followed by a final phase of gonadal regression before the next cycle of gonadogenesis. Typically, these reptiles have a long active breeding season and a stable cycle of active and inactive seasons. In addition, some reptiles have a dissociative reproductive cycle; that is, copulation occurs at the start of the active breeding season before gonadogenesis.[28] The male inseminates the female using sperm produced during the previous active season, whereas the females develop ova during the current active season and store the sperm until ovulation.

Management of the Breeding Collection

Record keeping

Detailed record keeping is a crucial part of the management of any captive animal collection in order to help monitor the health and reproductive activity of the colony.[32] Husbandry-related information, such as vivarium temperature, humidity, photoperiod, and cleaning schedule, should be diligently recorded and should be second nature for any reptile enthusiast. Moreover, details regarding the animals in the colony should include their origin, quarantine information, and any tests performed for screening of infectious diseases, identification (microchip or coloration pattern), previous health and medical records, weight, nutrition (diet and frequency of feeding), antiparasitic treatment schedule, appetite, fecal and urate production and frequency (as well as any abnormalities), brumation history, and shedding information.

With regard to breeding management, it is vital to document all reproduction-related activity in the colony, including onset of reproductive behavior, dates when animals are introduced to each other for mating, and confirmed copulation and gestation, as well as previous reproductive history; for example, dystocia. The data should be reviewed before and after the breeding season to help identify whether any issues, such as poor productivity, are related to breeding management (for example, poor incubation technique) or are caused by wider problems involving husbandry, nutrition, and disease. More specifically, these records should help identify and intervene if there are any problems with oviposition or parturition, discern prolific breeders from poor-doers, and remove the latter from the collection.

In addition, egg incubation records should be scrupulously maintained, including type of substrate used, humidity, temperature, previous data on hatchability and fertility, and estimated hatch dates. The date of oviposition or parturition should be recorded. Furthermore, in oviparous species, clutch size and any abnormal eggs, or slugs, should be documented, whereas, in viviparous ones, the number of live young, stillbirths, or mummified fetuses should also be noted.

Husbandry

Hygiene

Strict quarantine protocols should be in place to minimize exposure to and spread of disease within the breeding facility. In addition, high standards of hygiene and biosecurity are required to keep the breeding population healthy. A daily cleaning schedule should be adhered to, and personnel should be extremely careful in mixed species collections because they are at a higher risk of interspecific disease transmission. Routine fecal analysis should reflect the effectiveness of the hygiene protocol based on the level of gastrointestinal parasite burden detected. Regular pest control should also be performed to avoid predation on eggs and neonates as well as adults in some cases.

Housing

The premises where the breeding animals are housed should provide shelter from the elements and protect from unwanted drastic fluctuations in photoperiod, outside temperature and humidity, and potential pests and predators. The facility's design depends on the size of the enterprise, funding, local climate, the species being bred, and whether it is a multispecies breeding collection. A separate building or a well-delineated area should be available for quarantine (for new acquisitions) and isolation (for sick individuals) purposes. Surfaces should be easy to clean and disinfect, with changing facilities and foot baths likely to be required for large breeding facilities. Detailed record keeping and regular checks regarding husbandry-related parameters such as ambient temperature and humidity, ultraviolet (UV) light emission measurement, cleaning, and maintenance of vivaria or other enclosure types are needed. The enclosures should be clearly labeled with the species housed, whether venomous or not, and the number of individuals per housing unit, including their sex and age. Ideally, male and female reptiles should be kept separately outside the breeding season but reunited at the start of the reproductive cycle.

The temperature, humidity, heat lamps and mats, UV lights, and thermometers and thermostats for individual vivaria (terraria) or enclosures (eg, tortoise tables for some terrestrial chelonians) should be regularly checked and defective equipment replaced. Enclosure design should also provide adequate ventilation to reduce the risk of respiratory tract infections. The size of vivaria or other housing units should ideally be based on the latest peer-reviewed international or national published data on captive reptile welfare and housing requirements. The captive environment should allow for a thermal gradient to be created and for the animal to express normal behavior and exercise.[14] The type of substrate used depends on the species concerned. Newspaper is usually a cheap and hygienically excellent substrate to keep most breeding reptiles on, but it is lacking aesthetically and does not provide environmental enrichment. However, it allows the easy monitoring of fecal consistency and the passing of cloacal or seminal plugs. Other types of bedding commonly used include paper mulch or sand or fine wood chips for fossorial species because they require a substrate that allows burrowing.

The provision of a nesting site or nest box (eg, plastic, or cardboard box) with an appropriate medium, such as damp vermiculite, is crucial to encourage oviparous species to lay their eggs. Although viviparous species do not require a nest box to initiate parturition, the provision of a secluded area is beneficial.

Nutrition

The plethora of reptile species kept in captivity means that it is difficult to cover reptile nutrition in great detail here. Therefore, only the basic principles are discussed. In order to support the high energy requirements associated with reproduction, a reptile must have a good plane of nutrition, be in good physical condition, and be free of disease. This requirement is particularly important in females because these factors dictate their ability to reproduce and deliver healthy offspring. For example, in snakes, more than 40% of a female's body mass is allocated to reproduction.[29] Therefore, veterinarians must be familiar with the nutritional requirements of the animals in the breeding colony.[32–34] The diet, mineral and vitamin supplementation, and feeding protocol should be reviewed yearly, ideally outside of the breeding season, so that any adjustments can be made well in advance, thereby allowing time to improve the nutritional status of individuals to be used for breeding. Consequently, both males and females need to be provided with adequate nutrition outside the breeding season, especially in snakes, because they may not consume any food when reproductively active or gestating. Accurate record keeping, such as weight or carapacial length of individuals in the breeding colony, allows veterinarians to determine the suitable weight and size for reproductive maturity and activity.

The breeding colony

The failure to breed reptiles in captivity is largely caused by 3 simple issues:

- Individuals of the same sex (wrongly sexed because of poor sexing technique or inexperience) are housed together.
- Immature individuals are kept as breeding pairs.
- Diseased or geriatric animals are kept in the breeding stock.

In addition, poor nutrition and inadequate husbandry and egg incubation conditions contribute to low breeding success. All newly acquired reptiles should ideally come from a reputable source where they have undergone thorough health screening before shipment. On arrival, all reptiles should undergo a full health check, be tested for infectious diseases, and have ancillary diagnostic tests performed where required. The new acquisitions should be placed in quarantine, up to several months in some cases, and their weight, health status, appetite, and fecal parasite load regularly monitored before joining the breeding stock.

Prebreeding assessment

All animals in the breeding colony should undergo a full clinical examination before the start of the breeding season, with particular attention on cloacal examination to ensure that no abnormalities could affect successful copulation. Further diagnostic tests, such hematology, biochemistry, radiography, ultrasonography, and endoscopic examination of the cloaca, may be required in some cases based on clinical findings.

Stimulation of Reproductive Activity

Timing of reproduction

The onset of sexual maturity in reptiles varies across taxa but largely depends on growth rate and size of the animal, rather than age.[35] In captivity, reptiles housed under ideal environmental conditions may become sexually mature more quickly than their wild counterparts because food availability is not usually a limiting factor.[29] Reptiles that have a distinct breeding season are often regulated by 1 or more environmental cues, with a change in temperature being the most common stimulus.[29] However, reproduction may still be inhibited because of other limiting factors; for example, poor nutrition or disease. Numerous reptile species (snakes in particular) are capital breeders, wherein the energy required for reproduction is derived from fat reserves rather than food consumed.[29,36] As an adaptation to low or unpredictable food availability and poor nutritional status before the breeding season, female reptiles relinquish reproduction because they have to be able to sustain the high energy requirements during this period without consuming any food.[36] In some species, the presence of a male may be an additional cue for the female to mobilize adequate energy reserves for reproduction.[28,29] The significance of the presence of the male reptile in modulating the female reproductive cycle is still unclear and varies between species. For example, completion of the oogenic cycle can occur without a male in green iguanas, whereas, in certain snake species, the presence of the male and copulation may be required for maturation of previtellogenic follicles.[29,37]

Seasonal cooling (brumation)

Many temperate reptile species require a period of cold temperature (also known as brumation), ranging from 10°C to 13°C for 8 to 12 weeks to stimulate reproductive activity.[29,38] In contrast, subtropical and tropical taxa only require daily nighttime temperatures of 20°C to 24°C to initiate reproduction.[28,29] Before brumation, all animals in the breeding colony should undergo a full clinical examination, including fecal analysis and ancillary tests if required.

Brumation is usually timed so that it mirrors natural weather patterns, but this can be modified if necessary. There is still considerable debate about how brumation should be initiated and completed and the required duration to stimulate breeding. Seasonal cooling can range from 4 to 12 weeks, but it depends on the species and the keeper's experience. Some herpetoculturists have historically preferred to induce and terminate brumation by gradually altering the temperature to mimic seasonal transition, but the latest evidence suggests that a drastic change in temperature may be more natural because it reflects changes that the reptile experiences in its microhabitat in the wild.[29]

Photoperiod

In addition to temperature stimulus, induction of reproductive behavior in some temperate species also relies on photoperiod cues. Roughly, a prebrumation period of 6 weeks' duration is needed where 6 to 8 hours of daylight and a corresponding 16 to 18 hours of night are provided, followed by a gradual increase in daylight period postbrumation until reaching a peak of 14 hours.[28] In contrast, tropical reptiles can breed all year round if provided with a photoperiod of 12 hours of daylight.

Copulation

Following the introduction of potential mates, close monitoring is essential because injuries are common during courtship or copulation, especially in lizards and chelonians. The latter tend to cause more serious damage, and males can inflict severe, potentially fatal, bites to females' limbs to prevent them from escaping; for example, Asian box turtles (*Cuora* spp).[28] Trauma to the phallus or hemipenes can also occur during copulation (discussed later in relation to common reproductive disorders).

Determination of gestation and management of gravid female reptiles

Many reptile keepers wrongly use an observed copulation event as the start of gestation, which means that gestation times are often overestimated because the number of matings and duration of copulation in reptiles is species dependent (ranging from a few seconds to more than 24 hours).[29] More importantly, mating does not equate to fertilization, and several factors affect gestational length; for example, season, temperature, food availability, housing, and photoperiod. Early signs of pregnancy vary across species, ranging from behavioral changes, such as increased basking time or anorexia, to coelomic distension, namely in snakes and lizards, which can be palpated to confirm the presence of eggs or fetuses. Radiography and ultrasonography should be used to assess stages of gestation. In addition, ultrasonography can help refine breeding management and reproductive success by measuring ovarian follicles, determining whether ovulation has occurred, and assessing the development of eggs and fetuses. Once confirmed to be gravid, female reptiles can be isolated to be monitored closely for any signs of oviposition or parturition, and ultrasonography can be used in the later stages of gestation to determine the viability of eggs and fetuses and detect any abnormalities.

Oviposition and parturition

Most female reptiles show behavioral changes before oviposition or parturition; for example, gravid females spend more time basking or digging nests in the substrate, especially chelonians and lizards. Another sign of imminent oviposition in gravid snakes is a prelay skin shed, which occurs roughly 7 to 14 days before oviposition in colubrids and 18 to 26 days in pythons.[29] As mentioned earlier, ultrasonography can help determine the viability of eggs and fetuses, whereas radiography can help diagnose obstructive dystocia. These aforementioned behavioral changes should prompt the reptile breeder to provide a nesting site (brood box or ovipositorium) of adequate size and with the appropriate lightly moistened nesting substrate (discussed later). Provision of a nesting site is critical to prevent any potential complications such as dystocia. Brood boxes can be improvised from opaque plastic containers with a small entrance on the side (for lizards) or top (for snakes) and positioned in the vivarium so that the temperature inside is between 28°C and 32°C (82°F–86°F).[29] Lizards may need to have a separate nesting vivarium because they tend to ignore brood boxes, whereas chelonians require deep litter to be able to dig and bury their eggs.

Egg incubation

The use of an incubator helps create a controlled environment where humidity and temperature can be carefully adjusted, and it reduces the risk of damage from adults.[2] Furthermore, 1 incubator can be used for multiple species if separate incubation containers are used to create microenvironments with differing levels of humidity. The relative air humidity should be around 50% to 95% (dependent on species), but a regular supply of fresh air should also be provided; for example, by having set times for opening the incubator door to avoid significant temperature fluctuations.[27]

Commercially available incubators used in the poultry industry can be modified for use in reptiles, but, in general, reptile incubators need to meet the following 3 criteria[39]:

- They need to provide good insulation to prevent loss of heat and humidity.
- Heat should be uniformly distributed throughout the incubator, and there should be no focal hot spots.
- They should be equipped with a fail-safe thermostat as well as a back-up one to control the heat.

Incubation temperatures vary across species but usually range from 26°C to 32°C (80°F–90°F), and although higher temperatures reduce incubation time, they increase the risk of congenital defects, such as anophthalmia, abnormal coloring patterns, or neurologic deficits.[27–39] Eggs may also fail to hatch at excessively low or high temperatures. The duration of incubation also depends on species and is highly variable; for example, 45 to 70 days in most snakes and lizards, but it can be prolonged in chameleons (several months) and chelonians (eg, up to 500 days in the leopard tortoise, *Stigmochelys pardalis*).[27,29,33,40]

Substrate

In general, most reptile species have similar egg incubation requirements, but some are more sensitive than others to disruptions during this period. A wide variety of incubation media have been used, but vermiculite, perlite, sphagnum, and peat mosses remain the most popular substrates, either used on their own or combined. The incubation medium should only be slightly humidified (not soaked) because excessive moisture predisposes to fungal growth, whereas low humidity can lead to excessive water loss and embryonic death in porous eggs. Ideally, only filtered water, aged tap water, or spring water should be used to moisten the substrate because distilled and reverse-osmosis deionized water have been reported to cause hatch-rate problems in leopard geckos.[28] A weight ratio of water to medium of 1:1 to 1:3 is recommended and, in general, a moister substrate is required for species producing leathery eggs and drier media for brittle eggs.[28] A thermometer should be placed into the substrate, level with the bottom of the eggs, and it should be possible to clearly read it from the outside the incubator.[27] Inner chamber incubation temperature should ideally be recorded daily and a graph plotted to monitor any changes and identify any potential issues.

Care of the eggs
When collecting eggs from nesting sites or manipulation during regular inspection, great care should be taken not to rotate them, because this may lead to embryonic death or deformities in numerous reptile species, especially in early to midembryonic development.[27,28,33] Each egg should be carefully inspected, marked on its dorsal surface, weighed, and placed half buried in an appropriate medium (discussed later) in an incubation box before being transferred to an incubator. The eggs should be monitored daily and inspected every 1 to 2 weeks. Although a slight mottling to the surface of the egg may not be significant, pronounced changes in color or the presence of mold usually mean that the egg has died or was infertile.[27] Egg viability can be assessed for the presence of the developing vasculature of the growing embryo by transillumination (candling). An infertile egg has a homogeneous diffuse yellow-white content. Ultrasonography can be used to assess the embryo in noncalcified eggs, and a water-soluble gel should be applied to the egg's surface because ultrasonography gel has been found to interfere with oxygen exchange.[27]

Hatching
The young of most oviparous species possess a caruncle (egg tooth), which they use to pip, or incise, the eggshell at term.[27–29] The neonate may take between 12 and 72 hours to emerge from the egg, during which time the remaining yolk is absorbed.[28,29] Most eggs within a clutch should hatch within 48 hours of each other, and the noise and movement of the hatchlings may stimulate the rest of the clutch to pip.[27,28] In general, the hatching process should be allowed to proceed naturally, and neonates do not require human intervention except in rare cases; for example, a neonate pipping at the bottom of the egg. However, manual pipping is recommended if an unusually prolonged period has elapsed since the pipping times of other eggs in the same clutch. The procedure involves carefully cutting a small triangular window in the eggshell at the top of the egg with either scalpel or sharp scissors using aseptic technique.[27,28] Extreme care is necessary to prevent damage to the egg vessels and shell membranes. If the embryo is fully developed, it should react to gentle stimulation and it may still take several days to leave the egg.[39] If the neonate needs to be extirpated from the egg, then respiratory stimulation and support must be instigated immediately.[27,39] Potential causes of egg death include embryonic diapause, infertile eggs, incorrect incubation temperatures and humidity (high or low), insufficient ventilation, and excessive handling or trauma.[2]

Neonatal care
During the first few days after hatching, neonates can be kept at temperatures similar to incubation and they can be housed singly or in groups, but this depends on the species.[27,38] In those that can be group housed, the enclosure should be large enough to

avoid aggression and competition for food, and feeding should be done under supervision to ensure that all the hatchlings are able to eat without being bullied. In general, neonates derive their nutrition from their yolk during their first few days of life and, in some cases, it can even sustain them through their first brumation. The hatchlings should be visually assessed daily, their appetite monitored once they start eating, and they should be weighed weekly. The diet varies across species groups, and it is impossible to cover neonatal nutrition here.

Common Neonatal Disorders

Neonatal deformities

Most of the medical issues encountered in neonates are either the result of genetic mutations or are caused by developmental abnormalities during embryonic development as a result of inappropriate incubation temperatures.[26–28] These developmental defects tend to occur more frequently in snakes and chelonians, and they are wrongly referred to as fetal monsters; for example, double-headed snakes. If a high number of neonatal deformities are recorded at a breeding facility, the incubation records should be thoroughly examined before embarking on genetic analysis and other ancillary tests.

Retained yolk sac and omphalitis

In most neonates, the yolk sac is absorbed into the coelomic cavity before hatching.[26–28,39] However, in some cases, the yolk sac is still attached to the animal after hatching and this is often the result of the reptile owner overhandling the eggs during later stages of incubation, leading to the emergence of premature neonates. Affected hatchlings should be placed on clean, moist paper towels until the yolk gets absorbed, usually within 24 to 96 hours.[27,28] If this does not happen, then the yolk sack can be cleaned with dilute iodine or chlorhexidine solutions to minimize the risk of infection or it can be excised following ligation of the proximal umbilical stalk, especially if the yolk sac is discolored (which suggests infection).[27] Once resected, the umbilical stump can be disinfected as mentioned earlier.

In contrast, despite having a closed umbilicus, some hatchlings present with a firm, palpable intracoelomic mass in the umbilical area, which suggests an omphalitis or infected yolk sac and requires urgent intervention because the neonate is usually septic by the time of presentation. The patient should be stabilized with fluids and started on empiric systemic antibiotics and anesthetized for an omphalectomy.[28] A detailed account of the procedure can be found in Wright and Raiti[28] (2019). The coelomic cavity should be thoroughly flushed after excision and a sample can be taken of the infected material for culture and sensitivity. Postoperatively, fluid therapy, antimicrobials, and nutritional support should be continued.

Common Reproductive Disorders in Adult Reptiles

Dystocia

Dystocia is the most common reproductive disorder in female reptiles, with a higher prevalence in oviparous species, snakes in particular.[27,29,32,39,41,42] The condition is usually multifactorial in origin; for example, inappropriate nesting sites, malnutrition, or salpingitis.[29,42] The clinical signs can be nonspecific and vary across species, ranging from lethargy to anorexia or coelomic distension. In lizards and terrestrial chelonians, the animal may be restless and dig frantically in the nesting area but with no eggs passed. In snakes, the gravid female may not pass any eggs past the due date or only a part of the eggs or neonates. A cloacal prolapse may also develop as a consequence. Dystocia can be readily diagnosed based on clinical history and diagnostic imaging modalities such as radiography or ultrasonography. Before treatment, a full blood count and biochemistry are recommended to try get a more accurate clinical picture. The treatment of dystocia depends on whether the condition is obstructive or nonobstructive, the clinical status of the animal, and the duration of the condition. Medical management can usually be attempted in nonobstructive cases and often involves supplementation of calcium, fluid therapy, and oxytocin administration. Egg manipulation and ovocentesis can also be attempted under general anesthesia in certain cases. Surgery is usually recommended if the aforementioned procedures fail and is usually the treatment of choice in obstructive cases. The medical and surgical management of dystocia is beyond the scope of this article and readers are referred to the specialist reptile literature.

Cloacal prolapse

As mentioned earlier, cloacal prolapse, usually involving eversion of the oviduct or shell gland, occurs mostly secondary to dystocia but can also happen during normal oviposition or parturition.[32,39,41–43] This condition represents a surgical emergency and the prolapsed tissue should be kept clean and lubricated while investigating the underlying cause through radiography, ultrasonography, and blood biochemistry. Celiotomy is often required to remove any retained eggs or neonates from the oviduct before the prolapsed tissue is reduced back into the coelom, and cloacopexy is required in some cases. Purse-string sutures are contraindicated because they can lead to more straining and mask reeversion of prolapsed tissue.[29] In cases where severe damaged has occurred to the oviduct, then surgical removal is recommended, which will affect future breeding, so this should be discussed with the owner before surgery.

Egg-yolk coelomitis

Egg-yolk coelomitis is commonly encountered across the various reptilian taxa and is either caused by the rupture and leakage of contents from vitellogenic ovarian follicles or the rupture of an oviduct and spillage of its contents, secondary to dystocia (and owners trying to manually correct the dystocia).[29,32] The diagnosis is similar to the aforementioned conditions, and treatment involves medical stabilization followed by surgical repair of the damaged oviduct. If severe, it may affect breeding in the future (ie, recurrence of dystocia), so the animal may have to be retired from breeding.

Hemipenile and penile trauma

Trauma to the male copulatory organ occurs as a result of aggressive copulation or high number of matings leading to swelling of the damaged tissue and potentially subsequent infection.[3,7,17] Therefore, it is important to monitor reptiles during courtship and copulation to minimize the risks of injuries. The reptile should be removed from the breeding colony for the remainder of the season. In some cases, the trauma and swelling to the penis or hemipenis is so severe that a prolapse or paraphimosis results and retraction back through the cloaca is impossible. The engorged tissue may bleed extensively if further traumatized. If the organ is still viable, it can be cleaned, debrided, and replaced under general anesthesia and a stay suture temporarily applied. However, if the tissue is necrotic and not amenable to reduction, then amputation can be performed under general anesthetic because the male reproductive organ does not have any urinary function. Because squamates possess 2 hemipenes, they are still capable of breeding with the intact hemipenis if 1 is amputated. However, chelonians and crocodilians possess a single phallus or penis, which means that amputation of the copulatory organ usually means the end of the breeding life.

SMALL MAMMALS (DANIELE PETRINI)
Introduction

The Rabbit
The domestic rabbit (*Oryctolagus cuniculus*) is a small mammal belonging to the order of Lagomorpha, in the family Leporidae and genus *Oryctolagus*. It is commonly thought that the original site of domestication was the Iberian Peninsula. However, southwest France is recently reported to be the site of domestication because of archaeological and historical evidence.[44] The first recorded rabbit husbandry was in early Roman times, when rabbits were captured in the wild and introduced in leporaria, sort of enclosed walled gardens. By 1700, 7 distinct colors and patterns had been selected: nonagouti solid color, brown, albino, dilute (blue), yellow, silver, and Dutch spotting. By 1850, 2 new colors and the Angora-type hair had been developed. Between 1850 and the present, the remaining colors and fur types have been developed and selected. Nowadays, more than 300 breeds of rabbits that differ in size, coat color, length of ears, and type of fur are reported to be recognized worldwide,[45] and several hybrid lines for meat production have been created.[46] The British Rabbit Council held the breed standards of more than 70 breeds, divided in fancy, lop, standard fur, and rex breed sections.[47] Rabbits are now bred for various reasons: as a source of meat, wool, and fur; as animal models in scientific research; and for pets and exhibition animals.

Breeding and reproduction in rabbits
Adult females are known as does and have 2 cervices that are separate from each other and lead to each uterine horn. There is no uterine body. Puberty is generally reached earlier in smaller breeds, whereas larger breeds mature later. Rabbits do not have a definite estrous cycle and, as in the cat and ferret, ovulation is induced by the copula. Does vary in their sexual receptivity: approximately 7 to 10 days, followed by a short period of 1 to 2 days during which they are not receptive to the male. The time of ovulation after copulation is shorter than in ferret and cats, usually 10 hours in does and 30 hours in cats and ferrets. To be sure of successful ovulation, a single dose of 100 IU of hCG (human chorionic gonadotropin) can be administered to the doe after mating. Rabbits are prolific and can become pregnant monthly because of a fertile postpartum estrus within 24 hours of kindling.[48]

In adult males, known as bucks, the inguinal ring remains open after the testicles descend and so the testicles can move between the scrotum and the abdominal cavity. The breeding period is usually 5 to 6 years in bucks and 3 to 4 years in does.

In wild rabbits, the mating season is from January to September and the ovarian activity decreases in autumn. However, if rabbits are kept in conditions of food availability and artificial light, they can mate all year round. Furthermore, ovarian activity, reflecting hypothalamic changes, is diminished as days shorten. The use of a 16:8 or 14:10 hour light/ dark cycle, adequate caloric intake, and a slightly increased environmental temperature may prevent or reduce this suppressive seasonal and environmental effect.[49]

Husbandry, housing, and breeding programs in rabbits
Rabbits should be housed in areas that are suitable for the animal's use, size, and weight and in accordance with current guidelines.

The room temperature should be maintained within a range of 16°C to 22°C (61°F–72°F) with a humidity level between 30% and 70%. Rabbits are quite resistant to cooler temperature, but they can quickly develop hyperthermia at higher temperature.[50] Hence, they are very susceptible to heat stress, because they have few functional sweat glands and have difficulty in eliminating excess body heat when the environmental temperature is high. In these conditions, conception rate, embryonic development, litter size, litter weight, and milk production decrease. In males, testosterone concentration, spermatogenesis, temporary sterility, sexual desire, ejaculate volume, motility, sperm concentration, and total number of spermatozoa in an ejaculate decrease, and sperm abnormalities and dead sperm increase by exposure to the same factors.[51]

Adequate ventilation is also a key point and there must be around 10 to 15 air changes per hour.

Rabbits tend to be social and, when possible, should be housed in groups, or in pairs. However, housing rabbits in a group, in a pair, or individually is still debated. The best solution seems to be 4 to 5 rabbits (maximum a litter) per cage or pen, but not exceeding the density of 15 to 17 rabbits/m^2.[52]

Environmental enrichment is also highly recommended: gnawing sticks of soft wood with 3-cm diameters decreases aggressiveness.[52] Toys such as balls, plastic chain, wooden blocks, polyvinyl chloride tubing, huts, and other commercial items designed for use with laboratory animals may be provided. Interactions with items that the rabbit directly manipulates decrease with time, and they should be swapped frequently to keep up the rabbit's interest. Rabbits tend to chew these items, which, therefore, must be safe and nontoxic. In addition, they must be easily disinfected and replaced once damaged.[53,54]

Most rabbit breeders house does and bucks in separate cages and put them together only for breeding. The doe is usually brought to the buck's cage and, if she is receptive, the copulation occurs. In this way, a buck can be used with multiple does and breeding usually takes place on the same day so as to have foster mothers if needed at the time of the birth of the kits.[55]

In breeding programs that use postpartum estrus, the females have a greater dietary demand to cover the nutritional needs of pregnancy and lactation, especially calcium, proteins, and vitamins. It is common in these cases to notice a delay in the implantation of the embryo and therefore a pregnancy of longer duration.[55]

Reproductive Disorders

Reduced fertility

Factors that may contribute to infertility or reduced fertility in rabbits are:

- Age (immaturity or senescence of the buck or doe)
- Heat stress
- Systemic illness
- Nitrate contamination of food or water
- Caloric or other nutritional imbalances, such as low-protein diets; hypovitaminosis A, D, or E; or hypervitaminosis A
- A decrease in daylight
- Overcrowding
- Overuse of the bucks for breeding
- Autumnal breeding depression
- Uterine neoplasia (eg, uterine carcinoma)
- Metritis/uterine infection: *Pasteurella multocida*, *Staphylococcus aureus*, *Listeria* spp, *Chlamydia* spp, *Moraxella* spp, *Brucella* spp, *Salmonella* spp
- Uterine venous aneurysm
- Excessive noise
- Retained placentas

- Orchitis and epididymitis
- Venereal spirochetosis[49,56,57]

Abortion and resorption

A critical moment of pregnancy in rabbits is around the 21st day, when, because of the size of the uterus and fetuses, there is a reduced blood supply to the organ. Fetal death before the 21st day of pregnancy results in fetal resorption, whereas fetal death after the 21st day results in abortion. Causes of abortion and resorption are many and include:

- Stress
- Trauma
- Dietary imbalances (deficiencies of vitamin E, vitamin A, and protein)
- Infections, in particular with *Listeria monocytogenes*, affect animals in advanced pregnancy because the uterus and placenta present the most favorable environment for growth of the organism; clinically, the abortion is seen in late term pregnancy[49,58,59]

A herpesvirus infection affecting mini rex and crossbred meat rabbits was identified in a rabbitry in Alaska. The disease affected rabbits of all breeds and occurred over approximately a 2-month period. Clinical signs included conjunctivitis and periocular swelling, ulcerative dermatitis, progressive weakness, anorexia, respiratory distress, and abortion.[60,61]

In cases of unwanted mating, the pregnancy can be interrupted by administering aglepristone at 10 mg/kg once daily on days 15 and 16 after mating.[61]

Mastitis

Disorders of the mammary gland can interfere with normal nursing and survival of both the doe and the kits.[55] Acute inflammation of the mammary gland is most often encountered during lactation, when milk provides an excellent substrate for bacterial growth, the glands are pendulous and easily injured, and the young traumatize the teats. Mastitis is established when bacteria enter the gland via the bloodstream, through a cutaneous lesion, or via the teat canal. This condition usually occurs in lactating or pseudopregnant does, and predisposing factors that can worsen the onset of the disease are:

- Abrasive bedding
- Inappropriate caging
- Unsanitary environment
- Biting young
- Mammary impaction after early weaning or death of neonates

Rabbit mastitis may be diffuse or focal and suppurative. Clinical signs are depression and lethargy, pyrexia, anorexia, polydipsia, septicemia, rejection of kits, or death of doe or the young. The mammary glands are hot, swollen, firm, painful, and erythematous, and the skin is discolored red to dark blue. When the mastitis is diffuse, the lesion is known as blue breast. The bacteria most often isolated in mammary glands affected by mastitis are *S aureus*, *Pasteurella* spp, and *Streptococcus* spp.[62]

A presumptive diagnosis is usually made on clinical signs, and milk samples should be submitted for culture and sensitivity test. Treatment consists of administration of antibiotics based on sensitivity, nonsteroidal antiinflammatory drugs (NSAIDs) and opioids as painkillers, gentle massage of the mammary tissue to promote drainage, hot packing, fluid therapy, assisted feeding if necessary, and supportive care. In severe cases, mastectomy may be required. Early weaning of the young is required in lactating does; the use of a foster doe is not recommended to avoid transmission of the infection, and the kits should be hand raised.

Venereal spirochetosis

Venereal spirochetosis, also known as rabbit syphilis, is caused by *Treponema paraluiscuniculi*, a gram-negative, spiral rod.

The disease is transmitted by direct contact, especially during mating, but occasionally by extragenital routes as well. Exchange of the bucks among breeders promotes dissemination of the organism. Breeding animals are at higher risk than individual pets or laboratory animals, in which the disease is uncommon.

Clinical signs begin with vesicular swelling and reddening, followed by dry scaliness of the swollen prepuce and vulva. As the disease progresses, macules, papules, erosions, ulcers, and crusts on the external genitalia, perineal areas, nose, lips, and eyelids may appear. If the prepuce is affected severely, apparent and transient infertility may result. Females can develop metritis, retained placentas, and abortions, possibly unnoticed, which occur at 12 to 22 days of pregnancy. The herd may have a history of low conception rates and a high incidence of nest box fatalities in young less than 9 days of age.[63]

The diagnosis is based on clinical signs, and the condition must be differentiated from sarcoptic mange, ear mites, bacterial dermatitis, dermatophytosis, myxomatosis, and urine scald. Available laboratory test are a polymerase chain reaction test and an antibody test. It is important to remember that, because antibody levels are slow to increase, false-negatives are possible, and suspect animals may have to be tested multiple times over several weeks to verify a negative status. A single positive test result in a clinically healthy rabbit has no clinical relevance because many rabbits harbor the organism within their nasal cavities without ever becoming infected or having previously been exposed. Rabbits younger than 2 months may still have maternal antibodies, and positive results must be interpreted carefully.

Large rabbitries can benefit from a serologic survey with the microhemagglutination test to screen and verify infected animals because asymptomatic infections are common in infected colonies.

Treatment consists in the use of penicillin G procaine at 40.000 U/kg intramuscularly (IM) every 24 hours for 5 to 7 days.[64]

Infected animals should not be bred, and it may be possible to eliminate the infection from small herds by treating all animals simultaneously. Maintaining a closed breeding herd prevents introduction of venereal spirochetosis. If new animals must be introduced, they should be clinically and serologically free of the disease. It is advisable to quarantine all newly introduced animals in the breeding center.

Pseudopregnancy

Pseudopregnancy frequency was reported to be as high as 23% in a commercial rabbit breeding facility where does were group housed.[53] Pseudopregnancy in rabbits can result from a sterile or unsuccessful mating, an injection of luteinizing hormone, or from the stimulation caused when 1 doe mounts another,[47] given that rabbits are induced ovulators. Pseudopregnancy usually lasts 16 to 18 days after breeding, and the continuous secretion of progesterone causes physical and behavioral changes mimicking a normal pregnancy.[47] Under this hormonal influence, the uterus and mammary glands start to enlarge in preparation for gestation and lactation. The pseudopregnant doe frequently engages in maternal behaviors and often pulls hair from her body to build a nest.[47,49] In general, pseudopregnancy resolves spontaneously but can also evolve to hydrometra or pyometra.

Pseudopregnancy depresses fertility, and its cause is still unknown.[65] In particular, pseudopregnancy does not seem to affect the receptivity of nulliparous does; however, their fertility is highly reduced (37.55 vs 96.1%), leading to low productivity at birth (3.0 vs 7.4 born alive/artificial insemination). In primiparous does, pseudopregnancy affects receptivity (60.0% vs 81.3%), fertility (24.0% vs 82.5%) and as a consequence productivity at birth (2.1 vs 8.3 born alive/artificial insemination). In multiparous does, pseudopregnancy depresses fertility (53.8% vs 86.2%) and to a lower degree productivity (6.1 vs 8.6 born alive).[66] Pseudopregnancy is thus liable to strongly depress reproduction performances. Ovariohysterectomy is the treatment of choice.

Uterine infection

Endometritis, metritis, and pyometra may all be seen in breeding and nonbreeding does. History often includes recent breeding or birth, infertility, inability to rebreed, or pseudopregnancy. Does with endometritis can breed successfully or have fetal resorptions and stillbirths. The infection can start with mating, although infection in nonbreeding does may occur by the hematogenous route. A retrograde infection can develop secondary to vaginitis.[67] In a recent study, 7 out of 13 does treated once or twice with a slow-release deslorelin implant to suppress ovarian function developed endometritis.[68]

Clinical features may consist of mucopurulent vaginal discharge, anorexia, abdominal distension, and reduced fertility.

Diagnosis is based on reproductive history, and gentle palpation of the abdomen may reveal an enlarged uterus; it is essential to be careful during palpation to avoid rupture of the uterine wall. Laboratory findings may include leukocytosis and heterophilia, but these findings are not always present. Serum biochemistry may show prerenal azotemia because of dehydration, or because the chronic inflammation may lead to renal amyloid deposition.[69] Radiology may aid in the diagnosis, but only ultrasonography can confirm the disease.

The 2 commonly isolated organisms are *Pasteurella multocida* and *S aureus*[62,70]; however, other bacteria, such as *Chlamydia*, *L monocytogenes*, *Moraxella bovis*, *Actinomyces pyogenes*, *Brucella melitensis*, and *Salmonella* spp, have also been isolated from animals with pyometra.[58,71–73]

The treatment of choice is ovariohysterectomy, but, if the affected doe is a breeding rabbit with mild disease, treatment with broad-spectrum antibiotics, fluid therapy, NSAIDs, and supportive care may be attempted.

Dystocia

Dystocia is less common in rabbits than in guinea pigs and small rodents. Signs of dystocia may include a bloody or greenish-brown vaginal discharge or contractions without passage of kits.[74] The cause of dystocia should be investigated before therapy is decided, and if the kits are oversized or malpositioned, a cesarean section is indicated. In animals where obstruction is not suspected, 1 to 2 mL/kg 10% calcium gluconate can be administered by injection or orally, 30 minutes before administering oxytocin at 0.1 to 0.3 IU/kg subcutaneously (SC) or IM. Nonobstructive dystocia can be managed through medical treatment, assisted vaginal delivery, or both.[75]

It is important to review the husbandry of the rabbitry, looking for stressors that could inhibit parturition, as well as dietary problems (eg, vitamins, calcium) that could lead to uterine inertia.

A radiographic study is mandatory to evaluate abnormalities in the fetuses or in the width of the pelvic canal, and ultrasonography of the abdomen is useful to assess the viability of fetuses.

Dystocia can result from maternal and fetal causes[75,76]:

- Age: doe bred too young (3–4 months) or too old (>3 years)
- Narrow pelvic canal
- Obesity
- Uterine torsion
- Pregnancy toxemia
- Uterine inertia
- Stress during parturition
- High temperature
- Oversized kits
- Mispositioned kits
- Congenital birth defects (eg hydrocephalus, anasarca)

Agalactia/hypogalactia

The normal lactating behavior of the doe is to nurse the kits once or twice a day for a few minutes and staying away from the nest. Kits drink the milk rapidly, taking up to 20% of their body weight during these quick nursing sessions. To assess whether kits are receiving enough milk, is useful to weight them daily and to add supplemental feeding if they are not gaining weight.

Lack of milk is common in very young or aged animals, and this can be responsible for losses in the herd.

Causes of agalactia include genetics, poor nutrition, and environmental stressors. Analysis of the herd environment and diet can reveal problems that can be corrected, such as overcrowding, insufficient or poor-quality food, and stress. Administration of oxytocin to facilitate milk letdown has been described, at a dose of 0.2 to 3.0 IU/kg administered IM, SC, or intranasally.[73–76]

Other, less common female genital tract diseases

- Ovarian disease
- Uterine torsion
- Endometrial aneurism
- Ectopic pregnancy
- Pregnancy toxemia
- Mammary tumors

Male Genital Tract Disease

Orchitis and epididymitis

Orchitis and epididymitis can occur in breeding and pet bucks. Causes include *P multocida* and other bacteria, myxomatosis, and trauma.

Clinical signs include pyrexia, swollen testes and scrotum, anorexia, depression, weight loss, and reproductive failure. The diagnosis is based on clinical signs, and treatment of the specific cause is advisable (eg, antibiotic therapy); in most cases the therapy is castration.

THE GUINEA PIG
Introduction

The domestic guinea pig (*Cavia porcellus*) is a small mammal native to the Andean regions of South America and was domesticated approximately 4500 years ago. Different phylogenetic and morphologic studies indicated that South American and European ancient and modern strains of domestic guinea pig originate from a single domestication of wild montane guinea pig (*Cavia tschudii*) from the Peruvian highlands.[77] Systematically, the domestic guinea pig, *C porcellus*, belongs to the order Rodentia. Guinea pigs are further classified in the suborder Hystricomorpha and family Caviidae, which includes tailless South American rodents with a single pair of mammary glands.

Breeding and Reproduction in Guinea Pigs

Guinea pigs are prolific animals, and their growth and reproduction may be achieved under a wide range of climates and diets. Mature male guinea pigs are usually called boars, whereas mature females are called sows. In 2018, Sánchez-Macías and colleagues[77] reported that, assuming sufficient diet and thermally neutral ambient conditions, photoperiod does not affect reproduction or growth in guinea pigs. However, the investigators reported that a short-photoperiod condition (8 hours of lights on) may retard puberty in boars. The age at which sexual maturity is achieved varies with sex differentiation, environment conditions, and genetic background. Sexual maturity in boars is reached between 70 and 130 days of age.[78] Sows do not usually show their first heat until after 30 days of age, and the first occurrence of this physiologic event can take placed between 33 and 135 days of age.[78] Mills and Reed[79], in 1971, reported that the body weight at puberty is a more constant parameter than age; the breeding onset occurs when sows attain an approximately body weight of 450 g (range, 400–500 g) and boars reached 650 g. Under farming conditions, domestic guinea pigs are polyestrous nonseasonal breeders, even if slight seasonal variations in reproductive performance have been reported.[78] The duration of the estrous cycle is between 15 and 17 days, and estrus lasts 24 to 48 hours.[78] During estrus, the intact vaginal closure membrane perforates, and ovulation occurs spontaneously approximately 10 hours after the onset of estrus. During estrus, sows tend to show lordosis and mount other sows. The female accepts the boar for 6 to 11 hours. Most sows present a postpartum estrus, which usually occurs 2 to 15 hours after delivery, and, if mated, approximately 70% of the sows become pregnant. A standard method of estrus synchronization that respects animal welfare in guinea pigs has been determined by Grégoire and colleagues.[80] This method consists of a 15-day treatment of 0.1 mL of oral progestogen (Altrenogest) by mouth once daily, and this induces ovulation within 4 to 5 days. The estrus synchronization represents an improvement in the breeding techniques from a zootechnical point of view because it allows the use of artificial insemination and the consecutive improvement of both production and sanitary control in breeding farms. However, a complete and easily practicable technique for large-scale artificial inseminations has not yet been described. Electroejaculation and intraperitoneal insemination techniques have been reported.[81,82]

Mating in guinea pigs can be detected by the presence of a vaginal plug that fills the vagina from cervix to vulva. A few hours after mating, the plug falls out of the vagina and can sometimes be observed as a waxy mass on the cage floor. The guinea pig has a long gestation period, and its duration is reported to be inversely related to the number of fetuses carried.[78] The gestation length ranges from 59 to 72 days, with an average length of 68 days.

Reproductive Disorders

Ovarian cysts

The most common reproductive disorder in guinea pigs is ovarian cysts; in a study on 1000 animals, the disorder was mainly found in older specimens. The overall prevalence of ovarian cysts was 21.9%; however, in middle-aged guinea pigs, the prevalence was 42.9%. Cystic endometrial hyperplasia was diagnosed in 11 cases and was always associated with ovarian cystic disease.[83]

In general, up to 76% of female guinea pigs develop ovarian cysts during their lives (1.5–4 years of age); they may occur in 1 or both ovaries, but they are usually bilateral.[84]

Guinea pigs may develop 2 different types of ovarian cysts: serous cysts (nonfunctional cysts deriving from the rete ovarii) and hormone-producing follicular cysts. No significant correlation has been identified between reproductive history and the prevalence of cysts.[85]

Clinical signs vary according to whether the cysts are hormone producing or not, and include infertility, bilateral symmetry, nonpruritic alopecia, abdominal swelling, enteritis (secondary ileus), and pain-induced anorexia. Common sequelae include mucometra, cystic endometrial hyperplasia, and fibroleiomyomas.

A suspected diagnosis arises from the clinical signs. Abdominal palpation can help, but care must be taken because the cysts can easily be broken. The best technique to confirm the diagnosis is ultrasonography. Ovariectomy is the best way to prevent ovarian cyst, and ovariohysterectomy is curative.

Therapy for serous cysts consist of percutaneous ultrasonography-guided drainage of the cysts, but this is often palliative because they usually grow back in a few days. Unlike follicular cysts, serous cysts do not respond to hormone treatment. Follicular cysts are derived from preovulatory follicles that fail to ovulate[86] and may respond to gonadotropin-releasing hormone (GnRH) and hCG by inducing a surge of luteinizing hormone, resulting in luteinization of cysts. These drugs are an option when a medical treatment is desired. Gonadorelin is a short-acting GnRH agonist and can be used in guinea pigs at 25 μg/animal every 14 days for 2 injections; no adverse effects from the use of GnRH in guinea pigs have been reported. hCG can also be used, but its choice should be secondary to short-term GnRH agonists because after the second or third administration the formation of antibodies that make the molecule no longer effective is common and this potentially can trigger an allergic reaction on long-term use.[87] Long-term GnRH agonists (eg, deslorelin implant) have not been shown to be effective for the treatment of follicular cysts; furthermore, guinea pigs treated with deslorelin can have an intermittent and prolonged vaginal opening, potentially a risk factor for vaginal infections.[88]

Pregnancy toxemia

Toxemia of pregnancy is commonly seen in breeding guinea pigs and it is most common in the last 2 weeks of gestation and in the first 1 to 2 weeks postpartum. The prognosis is often poor, and it is advisable to know the factors that can predispose to the disease, such as obesity, lack of exercise, large fetal loads, change in diet and/or environment, heat stress, and primiparity.[73,89]

Pregnancy toxemia can be caused by a metabolic disorder mainly affecting obese sows, or by hemodynamic problems and uteroplacental ischemia. It can be caused by a negative energy requirement of the sows resulting from the heavy requirement of the fetuses. Another cause is when the uterus in an advanced stage of pregnancy weighs on its own vascularity and that of the kidneys and gastrointestinal tract, resulting in lack of blood supply, ischemia, hypertension, DIC, and death.

Clinical signs include anorexia, depression, lethargy, uncoordinated movements, and dyspnea, and the breath may smell of ketones, which is attributable to ketonemia.

Laboratory findings may include alterations in urine panel, such as proteinuria, ketonuria, and urine pH of 5 to 6 (normal pH is 9). On blood panel, hypoglycemia, acidosis, hyperlipemia, and hyperkaliemia are usually present.

Treatment is often not effective, so prevention is the key: stress, obesity, and changes in diet or environment in late pregnancy should be avoided. It can be advisable not to breed during the postpartum estrus, which is very fertile. Some breeders suggest offering supplements to the regular diet that are high in carbohydrates in the last 2 weeks of gestation, as well as calcium supplementation and close observation. The treatment includes intravenous warm fluids, glucose, and assisted feeding with a diet containing available carbohydrates[90]; in cases of limited uterus blood supply and presence of hypertension, a cesarean section is indicated after stabilization of the sow.

THE CHINCHILLA
Introduction

The chinchilla, like its closer relatives, the guinea pigs and degus, is a small rodent native to South America. It belongs to the order of Rodentia, family Chinchillidae, and genus *Chinchilla*. Two species belong to this genus: *Chinchilla lanigera* and *Chinchilla chinchilla* (formerly known as *Chinchilla brevicaudata*). In the wild, chinchillas live in colonies in extensive burrow systems or rock crevices. Their distribution areas can be found in the cold, semiarid, rocky slopes of the Andes of northern Chile at elevations of about 3000 to 5000 m above sea level. Environmental conditions of these areas are typical of tropical desert, with climatic variations showing drastic temperature changes during daytime and between the seasons (from 30°C to −22°C) and low rainfall. The domestic chinchillas are known to descend from 13 individuals belonging to the species *C lanigera*, brought to California by Matthew Chapman.[91] *C chinchilla* was also reported to be domesticated in Chile at the beginning of the twentieth century. The specific information given here refers only to *C lanigera*.

Chinchillas were initially domesticated for the use of their fine and extremely esteemed coat in fur industries, and nowadays they are better known as popular pets. Selective breeding has produced a large number of color mutations.

Breeding and Reproduction in Chinchillas

Wild female chinchillas are seasonally polyestrous.[91] However, in captivity, births may occur throughout the year, with 2 annual activity peaks in spring and summer,[92] and similar results have also been reported on some farms in South America. Males are generally thought to remain fertile throughout the year. Busso and colleagues[92] (2012), investigating testicular activity in animals exposed to a natural photoperiod, observed seasonal changes in sperm concentration and testicular endocrine activity during the year. Higher mean values were observed during winter for both examined parameters.

The length of the estrus cycle varies according to different investigators and the rearing conditions of the studied animals; Busso and colleagues[92] reported the length of estrus cycle to range between 15 and 50 days, with an average length of 21 to 35 days. Estrus mainly lasts 24 hours up to 4 days, and the ovulation occurs spontaneously.[91] Chinchilla females present, like guinea pigs, a postpartum estrus, which can be used to minimized litter intervals. The vagina presents a closure membrane that covers the vaginal orifice at all times, except at parturition and during estrus. Sexual maturity is achieved earlier in females than in males (4–6 and months and 8–9 months respectively).[91] Gestation is long compared with other rodents. The average length is 111 days, and 1 to 6 kits can be produced per litter.

Chinchilla Nutrition

Proper diet is important in chinchilla breeding programs and herd management. Busso and colleagues[92] reported that low nutrition and/or high caloric restriction can delay puberty, suppress ovulation, and reduce performance during lactation in captive chinchillas.

Chinchillas are herbivores and in their natural environment they eat any available wild grasses and leafy plants, usually during early morning and evening. A good captive diet should be based on a high fiber content. Fresh, good-quality hay must be fed ad libitum. Grass hay (eg, timothy hay) should be given to adult chinchillas, and pregnant and lactating females and growing kits may be fed with alfalfa hay.[93] A measured amount of commercial specific pelleted feed is usually administered. The diet can be supplemented with small amounts of fresh vegetables and fruits. The use of nuts, seeds, and other treats must be limited. Commercial pellets should contain between 16% and 20% crude protein, 2% to 5% crude fat, and at least 18% crude fiber.[94] The author observed lower reproductive performances with commercial pellets containing 14% crude protein. However, further studies are needed to determine the nutritional requirements in the different physiologic phases of chinchillas to maximize performance.

Reproductive Disorders

Lethal factor in chinchillas

The existence of a lethal factor is well known among chinchilla breeders, even if it is rarely reported in the literature. When planning mating in a chinchilla herd, it is important to remember that mating certain phenotypes is not recommended. Some genes do not allow the fetus to survive in a condition of homozygosity (lethal factor). The lethal coat color genes involved in chinchilla are white and touch of velvet (TOV). If there is a homozygous condition for the white + white or TOV + TOV, there is a 25% chance that the embryo will be reabsorbed; sometimes there are stillbirths, or lifeless kits that die a few hours after birth. Sometimes kits are aborted, but not expelled, causing a uterine infection and impairment of the fertility of the chinchilla. It is possible to pair a TOV and a white.

Fur ring in male chinchillas

Fur rings are common in male chinchillas and are characterized by a ring of fur in the prepuce encircling the penis. This condition can predispose to balanoposthitis and paraphimosis, leading to constriction of the penis.

Clinical signs can be represented by stranguria, excessive grooming of the preputial area, lethargy, and decreased appetite. Chinchillas with fur ring may have problems in mating.

The therapy consists of applying a lubricant and unrolling the hair ring to the tip of the penis to be removed. Care must be taken not to traumatize the penis; in the most serious cases, the administration of analgesics, fluid therapy, and antibiotics is recommended.

Reproductive Disorders Common in Guinea Pigs and Chinchillas

Pyometra and metritis in guinea pigs and chinchillas

Pyometra and metritis can occur in breeding and nonbreeding sows and chinchillas.

In guinea pigs, the most commonly isolated organisms are *Bordetella bronchiseptica* and hemolytic *Streptococcus* spp. The most common sources of infection are mating, contaminated or irritating bedding material, and hematogenous spread. Certain types of bedding may predispose sows to vaginitis: these include wood chips, sawdust, or other types that can become impacted into the vaginal area. Other possible pathogens include *Salmonella enterica*, *Escherichia coli*, *Corynebacterium pyogenes*, and *Staphylococcus* spp.[73]

Diagnosis can be made by palpating the enlarged uterus, and by the presence of bloody or purulent vaginal discharge (if the vulva is open), depression, anorexia, and pyrexia. The uterus can be visualized on radiographs, and abdominal ultrasonography confirms the fluid-filled uterus. In chinchillas, some mucoid vaginal discharge is normal during estrus and should not be confused with pathologic vaginal discharge. Cytology may aid in this differentiation. The predominant cells during estrus are partially to completely cornified superficial epithelial cells. Neutrophils are absent during estrus but common during proestrus and metestrus.[91]

Ovariohysterectomy is the treatment of choice, whereas long-term antibiotic therapy may be used in breeding sows if fertility needs to be maintained.

The author has treated pyometras in chinchillas by administering aglepristone, a competitive progesterone antagonist, 15 mg/kg SC on days 1, 2, and 8, along with enrofloxacin 10 mg/kg by mouth every 12 hours and supportive care; in breeding sows, the same treatment can be administered.[95,96]

Dystocia in guinea pigs and chinchillas

Dystocia is rare in chinchillas, whereas is quite common in guinea pigs. Causes may include oversized kits; narrow pelvic canal; nutritional deficiencies; uterine inertia; and, in guinea pigs, also the inability of the pubic symphysis to separate, hypovitaminosis C, and uterine torsion.

In guinea pigs, most dystocia cases occur in sows that are first bred after 8 to 12 months of age. However, no evidence was found of ossification of pubic symphysis in either nonbreeding or breeding female guinea pigs.[97] Continuous straining for 20 minutes or unproductive contractions for more than 2 hours is abnormal. Bloody or green-brown vaginal discharge can be found in severe cases without giving birth to pups.

The fibrocartilaginous pubic symphysis under the influence of relaxin begins to separate during the second half of gestation, and continues parting until a palpable gap of around 15 mm is present, which happens 48 hours prepartum. At parturition, this opening may reach 2.5 cm or more in diameter.[65] Palpating the vaginal canal may reveal a pup that must be manually removed or assisted in delivering. It is important to point out that, if the dystocia is caused by failure to separate the pubic symphysis, the use of oxytocin is absolutely contraindicated; in this case, cesarean section is the therapy of choice.

If uterine inertia is suspected, then the treatment consists of diluted calcium gluconate. Doses are 25 to 50 mg/kg SC in chinchillas[87] and 50 to 100 mg/kg SC, or orally in guinea pigs.[71] If there is no response, treatment with oxytocin 0.2 to 0.3 up to 1 IU/kg SC is indicated.

Surgical intervention is imperative if the labor lasts more than 3 to 4 hours and the kits are not delivered; chinchillas respond well to cesarean section, and a survival rate of 67% has been reported.[98]

Mastitis in guinea pigs and chinchillas

Mastitis is more common in guinea pigs than in chinchillas because they are more pot-bellied and touch the ground with their mammary glands. Kits may cause damage to the mother's nipples, which is followed by an infection. The main bacteria involved are E coli, Pasteurella, Klebsiella, Staphylococcus, Streptococcus, and Pseudomonas spp. The mammary gland appears red, edematous, swollen, hard, and painful; in some cases, there is also a mucopurulent discharge with or without blood in the milk. If not properly treated, these lesions can progress to abscess or necrosis of the tissue. Therapy is supportive with the administration of antibiotics based on culture, NSAIDs, opioids, and hot compresses. In severe cases, mastectomy is indicated.

In chinchillas, mastitis is usually caused by trauma from kits. The young are born with well-developed and sharp incisors; in large litters, or in cases of hypogalactia or agalactia, the kits can fight and cause damage to the teats. In the author's experience, excellent results may be achieved by carrying out shifts and leaving 1 or 2 kits with the mother at a time, trying to identify the most aggressive kits. The time spent with the mother varies according to the age of the newborns and according to the weight; in principle, for the first days of life the shifts will be short, lasting about 3 to 4 hours, taking care to keep the kits warm. With increasing age, shifts of longer than 6 to 8 hours occur. If the kits do not grow up or the mother dies, another chinchilla can try to adopt them because they are normally good nurses and accept the young of other females.

CLINICS CARE POINTS

- Diet and dietary changes can be used as a tool to stimulate breeding in some bird species.
- Every specimen that dies can be useful to understand the causes of mortality within a collection.
- Apply scientifically sound evidence to the selection of animals for breeding purposes.
- Diseases not related to the reproductive tract can also be the cause of breeding failures.
- Behavioral abnormalities often contribute to breeding failures.
- There are many different bird and reptile species: each has different reproductive biology and different requirements for breeding.
- There is not a hygiene for birds, a hygiene for reptiles, and one for small mammals: there is hygiene, and clinicians must be strict with it.
- Brumation can be an important part of a reptile breeding program.
- Most neonatal issues in birds and reptiles depend on the quality of incubation.
- Abortion in rabbits can depend on stress, trauma, dietary imbalances, and infections.
- Deslorelin can cause endometritis in rabbits and ascending infections in guinea pigs.
- Ovarian cysts in small mammals may be ruptured by abdominal palpation: use ultrasonography.
- Dystocia is less common in rabbits than it is in guinea pigs and chinchillas.

DISCLOSURE

The authors have nothing to disclose.

REFERENCES

1. Crosta L. Medical management & selection of breeding birds. In: Annual conference proceedings Adelaide South Australia, 26. Journal of the association of avian veterinarians Australasian Committee Ltd, NSW, Australia; 2018. p. 34–7.
2. Crosta L. Enriquecimiento Ambiental en Criaderos: una cuestión de bienestar. In: Proc. Practical veteducando course. Mexico City: Chapultepec Zoo; 2013. p. 1–116.

3. Wolff PL. Husbandry practices employed by private aviculturists, bird markets and zoo collections, which may be conducive to fostering infectious diseases. Rev Sci Tech 1996;15(1):55–71.

4. Melillo A, Carubbi G, Crosta L, et al. A study on the microbial population of the cloaca of some Turdidae species, both in free ranging and captive birds. In: Proc. of the 5th conference of the European committee of the association of avian veterinarians. 1999. p. 96–7. Pisa, Italy.

5. Crosta L, Timossi L, Burkle M. Management of zoo and park birds. In: Harrison GJ, Lightfoot TL, editors. Clinical avian medicine. Palm Beach, FL, USA: Spix Publishing, Inc; 2011. p. 991–1004.

6. Speer BL. The pathogen vs. the pathogenesis: a different view of avicultural medicine. In: Proc Assoc Avian Vets, Reno, NV. 1994. p. 373–7.

7. Crosta L, Schnitzer P. Infertility. In: Graham JE, editor. Blackwell's five-minute veterinary consult: Avian. Elsevier; 2016. p. 150–2.

8. Gerlach H. Chlamydia. In: Ritchie BW, Harrison GJ, Harrison LR, editors. Avian medicine: principles and practice. Lake Worth, FL: Wingers Publishing, Inc; 1994. p. 984–96.

9. Monleon R, Martin MP, Barnes JH. Bacterial orchitis and epididymo-orchitis in broiler breeders. Avian Pathol 2008;37(6):613–7.

10. Crosta L. Endoscopia em Aves. In: Cubas ZS, Ramos da Silva JC, Catão-Dias JL, editors. Tratado de Medicina veterinária de Animais selvagens. 2rd edition. São Paulo, Brazil: Editora Roca Ltda; 2014. p. 1751–67.

11. Contar Adolfi M, Nakajima RT, Nóbrega RH, et al. Intersex, hermaphroditism, and gonadal plasticity in vertebrates: evolution of the Müllerian Duct and Amh/Amhr2 signaling. Annu Rev Anim Biosci 2019;7(1):149–72.

12. Mikulas JE, Brooks DM. A case of hermaphroditism in a wood duck (Aix sponsa). Bull Tex Ornith Soc 2013;46(1–2):63–5.

13. Crosta L, Gerlach H, Bürkle M, et al. Endoscopic testicular biopsy technique in Psittaciformes. J Avian Med Surg 2002;16(2):106–10.

14. Crosta L, Schnitzer P, Timossi L. Testicular biopsy. In: Samour J, editor. Avian medicine and surgery. 3rd edition. Elsevier; 2016. p. 535–6.

15. Gee GF, Mirande CM. Artificial insemination. In: Ellis DH, Gee GF, Mirande CM, editors. Cranes, their biology, husbandry, and conservation. Hancock House Publishers; 1996. p. 205–18.

16. Lierz M, Ortiz OA, Samour J. Reproduction. In: Speer BL, editor. Current therapy in avian medicine and surgery. Elsevier; 2016. p. 433–60.

17. Stelzer G, Crosta L, Bürkle M, et al. Attempted semen collection using the massage technique and semen analysis in various psittacine species. J Avian Med Surg 2005;19(1):7–13.

18. Samour J. Semen collection. In: Samour J, editor. Avian medicine and surgery. 3rd edition. Elsevier; 2016. p. 525–34.

19. Dogliero A, Rota A, von Degerfeld MM, Quaranta G. Use of computer-assisted semen analysis for evaluation of Rosy-faced lovebird (Agapornis roseicollis) semen collected in different periods of the year. Theriogenology 2015;83(1):103–6.

20. Lierz M, Reinschmidt M, Müller H, et al. A novel method for semen collection and artificial insemination in large parrots (Psittaciformes). Sci Rep 2013;3:2066.

21. Schubot RM, Clubb KJ, Clubb SL. Psittacine aviculture: perspectives, techniques and research. Avicultural Breeding and Research Center; 1992.

22. Speer BL. Avicultural medical management: an introduction to basic principles of flock medicine and the closed aviary concept. Vet Clin North Am Small Anim Pract 1991;21(6):1393–404.

23. Wallace C, Marinkovich M, Morris PJ, et al. Lessons from a retrospective analysis of a 5-yr period of quarantine at San Diego zoo: a risk-based approach to quarantine isolation and testing may benefit animal welfare. J Zoo Wildl Med 2016; 47(1):291–6.

24. Crosta L. Avian neonatology and pediatrics. In: Proceed. 11° FSAPAI & 18° WSAVA CE conference Mumbai - India. 2019. p. 184–7.

25. van Zeeland YRA, Friedman SG, Bergman L. Behavior. In: Speer BL, editor. Current therapy in avian medicine and surgery. Elsevier; 2016. p. 177–251.

26. Frye FL. Biomedical and surgical aspects of captive reptile husbandry. 2nd edition. Malabar, FL: Krieger Publishing; 1991. p. 345–92.

27. Mader DR. Perinatology. In: Mader DR, editor. Reptile medicine and surgery. Philadelphia: WB Saunders; 2005. p. 365–75.

28. Wright K, Raiti P. Breeding and neonatal care. In: Girling SJ, Raiti P, editors. BSAVA manual of reptiles. 3rd edition. Cheltenham: BSAVA Manual of Reptiles; 2019. p. 70–88.

29. DeNardo D. Reproductive biology. In: Mader DR, editor. Reptile medicine and surgery. 2nd edition. Philadelphia: WB Saunders; 2005. p. 376–89.

30. Crews D, Moore MC. Psychobiology of reproduction of unisexual whiptail lizards. In: Wright JW, Vitt LJ, editors. Biology of whiptail lizards (Genus Cnemidophorus). Oklahoma: University of Oklahoma Press; 1993. p. 257–82.

31. Schuett GW, Fernandez PJ, Gergits WF, et al. Production of offspring in the absence of males: evidence for facultative parthenogenesis in bisexual snakes. Herp Nat His 1997;5:1–10.

32. Stahl SJ. Veterinary management of snake reproduction. Vet Clin Exot Anim 2002; 5:615–36.

33. Frye FL. A practical guide for feeding captive reptiles. Malabar, FL: Krieger; 1991.

34. Stahl SJ, Donoghue S. Feeding reptiles. In: Hand MS, Thatcher CD, Remillard RL, et al, editors. Small animal clinical nutrition. 4th edition. Topeka, KS: Mark Morris Institute; 2000. p. 961–78.

35. Porter KR. Herpetology. Philadelphia: WB Saunders; 1972.

36. Bonnet X, Naulleau G, Shine R, et al. Short-term versus long-term effects of food intake on reproductive output in a viviparous snake Vipera aspis. Oikos 2001;92: 297–308.

37. DeNardo DF, Autumn K. The effect of male presence on reproductive activity in captive female blood pythons, Python curtus. Copeia 2001;2001(4):1138–41.

38. Seigal RA, Ford NB. Reproductive ecology. In: Seigal RA, Collins JT, Novak SS, editors. Snakes: ecology and evolutionary biology. New York: McGraw Hill; 1987.

39. Ross RA, Marzec G. The reproductive husbandry of pythons and boas. Stanford, CA: Institute for Herpetological Research; 1990.

40. Fife RJ. Observations on incubation, diet, and sex determination in hatchling tortoises. In: Proc int herpetol symp captive propagation husbandry. 1992. p. 16.

41. Denardo D. Dystocias. In: Mader DR, editor. Reptile medicine and surgery. 2nd edition. Philadelphia: WB Saunders; 2005. p. 787–92.

42. Lock BA. Reproductive surgery in reptiles. Vet Clin North Am Exot Anim Prac 2000;3:733–52.

43. Bennett RA. Cloacal prolapse. In: Mader DR, editor. Reptile medicine and surgery. 2nd edition. Philadelphia: WB Saunders; 2005. p. 751–5.

44. Donnelly TM, Vella D. Basic anatomy, physiology, and husbandry of rabbits. In: Quesenberry KE, Orcutt CJ, Mans C, et al, editors. Ferrets, rabbits, and rodents: clinical medicine and surgery. 4th, edition. St. Louis (MO): Saunders; 2021. p. 133.
45. Dorożyńska K, Maj D. Rabbits–their domestication and molecular genetics of hair coat development and quality. Anim Genet 2021;52(1):10–20.
46. Available at: https://hypharm.fr/lignees-reproducteurs-cunicoles/. Accessed December 2020.
47. Available at: https://thebritishrabbitcouncil.org/FINAL%20Mono%20Breed%20Standards%20Book%20AUGUST%202019.pdf. Accessed December 2020.
48. O'Malley B. Rabbits. In: Clinical anatomy and physiology of exotic species. London, UK: Elsevier; 2005. p. 191.
49. Harkness J, Wagner J. The biology and medicine of rabbits and rodents. 5th edition. Ames, Iowa: Wiley-Blackwell; 2010. p. 31, 204-206; 321-322.
50. Colby LA, Nowland MH, Kennedy LH. Rabbits. In: Clinical laboratory animal medicine: an introduction. Hoboken: Wiley Blackwell; 2020. p. 295.
51. Marai IF, Habeeb AA, Gad AE. Rabbits' productive, reproductive and physiological performance traits as affected by heat stress: a review. Livestock Prod Sci 2002;78(2):71–90.
52. Szendrő Z, Dalle Zotte A. Effect of housing conditions on production and behaviour of growing meat rabbits: a review. Livestock Sci 2011;137(1–3):296–303.
53. Johnson CA, Pallozzi WA, Geiger L, et al. The effect of an environmental enrichment device on individually caged rabbits in a safety assessment facility. J Am Assoc Lab Anim Sci 2003;42(5):27–30.
54. Shomer NH, Peikert S, Terwilliger G. Enrichment-toy trauma in a New Zealand White rabbit. J Am Assoc Lab Anim Sci 2001;40(1):31–2.
55. Cynthia R, Bishop CR, Burgess ME. Reproductive physiology, normal neonatology, and neonatal disorders of rabbits. In: Lopate C, editor. Management of pregnant and neonatal dogs, cats and exotic pets. Aims; 2012. p. 218–23.
56. Di Giacomo RF, Deeb BJ, Anderson RJ. Hypervitaminosis A and reproductive disorders in rabbits. Lab Anim Sci 1992;42(3):250–4.
57. St Claire MB, Kennett MJ, Besch-Williford CL. Vitamin A toxicity and vitamin E deficiency in a rabbit colony. J Am Assoc Lab Anim Sci 2004;43(4):26–30.
58. Watson GL, Evans MG. Listeriosis in a rabbit. Vet Pathol 1985;22(2):191–3.
59. Gray ML, Singh C, Thorp F Jr. Abortion, stillbirth, early death of young in rabbits by Listeria monocytogenes. I. Ocular instillation. Proc Soc Exp Biol Med 1955; 89(1):163–9.
60. Jin L, Valentine BA, Baker RJ, et al. An outbreak of fatal herpesvirus infection in domestic rabbits in Alaska. Vet Pathol 2008;45(3):369–74.
61. Özalp GR, Temizel EM, Özocak-Batmaz E. Clinical, ultrasonography and haematology of aglepristone-induced mid-gestation pregnancy terminations in rabbits. J South Afr Vet Assoc 2013;84(1):e1–4.
62. Segura P, Martinez J, Peris B, et al. Staphylococcal infections in rabbit does on two industrial farms. Vet Rec 2007;160(25):869–72.
63. Di Giacomo RF, Talburt CD, Lukehart SA, et al. Treponema paraluis-cuniculi infection in a commercial rabbitry: epidemiology and serodiagnosis. Lab Anim Sci 1983;33(6):562–6.
64. Fish RE, Besch-Williford C. Reproductive disorders in the rabbit and guinea pig. In: Current veterinary XI. WB Saunders; 1992. p. 1175–9.
65. Theau-Clément M. Preparation of the rabbit doe to insemination: a review. World Rabbit Sci 2007;15(2):61–80.

66. Carter CL, Adams JK, Czarra JA, et al. An incidence of pseudopregnancy associated with the social enrichment of rabbits (Oryctolagus cuniculi). J Am Assoc Lab Anim Sci 2016;55(1):98–9.
67. DeLong D, Manning PJ. Bacterial diseases. In: Manning PJ, Ringler DH, Newcomer CE, editors. The biology of the laboratory rabbit. New York: Academic Press; 1994. p. 131–70.
68. Geyer A, Poth T, Otzdorff C, et al. Histopathologic examination of the genital tract in rabbits treated once or twice with a slow-release deslorelin implant for reversible suppression of ovarian function. Theriogenology 2016;86:2281–9.
69. Hofmann JR, Hixson CJ. Amyloid A protein deposits in a rabbit with pyometra. J Am Vet Med Assoc 1986;189:1155–6.
70. Tirpude RJ, Jain R, Tuteja U, et al. Isolation, identification and characterization of Staphylococcus aureus from systemic infection in New Zealand white rabbits. Indian J Anim Sci 2007;77:207–10.
71. Bishop C. Emergency medicine and surgery of rabbits and rodents. Toronto: Ontario Veterinary Medical Association; 1999.
72. Soave OA, Dominguez J, Doak RL. Moraxella bovis-induced metritis and septicemia in a rabbit. J Am Vet Med Assoc 1977;171:972–3.
73. Bishop CR. Reproductive medicine of rabbits and rodents. Vet Clin North Am Exot Anim Pract 2002;5(3):507–35.
74. Paré JA, Paul-Murphy JR . Disorders of the reproductive and urinary systems. In: Ferrets, rabbits and rodents: clinical medicine and surgery. Elsevier Inc; 2003. p. 183–93.
75. Gleeson MD, Sanchez-Migallon Guzman D, Paul-Murphy JR. Clinical and pathological findings for rabbits with dystocia: 10 cases (1996–2016). J Am Vet Med Assoc 2019;254(8):953–9.
76. Bishop CR, Burgess ME. Reproductive physiology, normal neonatology, and neonatal disorders of rabbits. In: Lopate C, editor. Management of pregnant and neonatal dogs, cats and exotic pets. Aims; 2012. p. 217–38.
77. Sánchez-Macías D, Barba-Maggi L, Morales-delaNuez A, et al. Guinea pig for meat production: a systematic review of factors affecting the production, carcass and meat quality. Meat Sci 2018;143:165–76.
78. Sisk DB. Physiology. In: Wagner JE, Manning PJ, editors. The biology of the Guinea pig. London: Academic Press; 1976. p. 79–91.
79. Mills PG, Reed M. The onset of first oestrus in the guinea-pig and the effects of gonadotrophins and oestradiol in the immature animal. J Endocrinol 1971; 50(2):329–37.
80. Grégoire A, Allard A, Huamán E, et al. Control of the estrous cycle in guinea-pig (Cavia porcellus). Theriogenology 2012;78(4):842–7.
81. Hoar RM. Biomethodology. In: Wagner JE, Manning PJ, editors. The biology of the Guinea pig. London: Academic Press; 1976. p. 17.
82. Ueda H, Kosaka T, Takahashi KW. Intraperitoneal insemination of the guinea pig with synchronized estrus induced by progesterone implant. Exp Anim 1998; 47(4):271–5.
83. Minarikova A, Hauptman K, Jeklova E, et al. Diseases in pet guinea pigs: a retrospective study in 1000 animals. Vet Rec 2015;177(8):200.
84. Bishop CR. The Guinea Pig Patient: emerging infectious diseases, genetic predisposition and surgical hints. Proc ExoticsCon 2018. p. 673-685.
85. Nielsen TD, Holt S, Ruelokke ML, et al. Ovarian cysts in guinea pigs: influence of age and reproductive status on prevalence and size. J Small Anim Pract 2003;44: 257–60.

86. Shi F, Petroff BK, Herath CB, et al. Serous cysts are a benign component of the cyclic ovary in the guinea pig with an incidence dependent upon inhibin bioactivity. J Vet Med Sci 2002;64:129–35.
87. Pignon C, Mayer J. Guinea pigs. In: Quesenberry KE, Orcutt CJ, Mans C, et al, editors. Ferrets, rabbits, and rodents: clinical medicine and surgery. 4th Edition. Saunders: St. Louis; 2020. p. 274.
88. Kohutova S, Jekl V, Knotek Z, et al. The effect of deslorelin acetate on the oestrous cycle of female guinea pigs. Vet Med 2015;60:155–60.
89. Harkness JE, Turner PV, vnde Woude S, et al. Harkness and Wagner's biology and medicine of rabbits and rodents. Ames: Wiley-Blackwell; 2010.
90. Kondert L, Mayer J. Reproductive medicine in guinea pigs, chinchillas and degus. Vet Clin Exot Anim Pract 2017;20(2):609–28.
91. Mans C, Donnely TM. Chinchillas. In: Quesenberry KE, Orcutt CJ, Mans C, et al, editors. Ferrets, rabbits, and rodents: clinical medicine and surgery. 4th Edition. Saunders: St. Louis; 2020. p. 298–322.
92. Busso JM, Ponzio MF, De Cuneo MF, et al. Reproduction in chinchilla (Chinchilla lanigera): current status of environmental control of gonadal activity and advances in reproductive techniques. Theriogenology 2012;78(1):1.
93. Colby LA, Nowland MH, Kennedy LH. Chinchillas. In: Clinical laboratory animal medicine: an introduction. Hoboken (NJ): Wiley-Blackwell; 2020. p. 243–63.
94. Burgess ME, Bishop CR. Reproductive physiology, normal neonatology, and neonatal disorders of chinchillas. In: Lopate C, editor. Management of pregnant and neonatal dogs, cats and exotic pets. Aims; 2012. p. 295–307.
95. Baron von Engelhardt A. Behandlung des Endometritis/Pyometrakomplexes eines Meerschweinchens mit Aglepristone-ein Fallbericht. Prakt Tierarzt 2006; 3(1):14–6.
96. Pisu MC, Andolfatto A, Veronesi MC. Pyometra in a six-month-old nulliparous golden hamster (Mesocricetus auratus) treated with aglepristone. Vet Q 2012; 32:3–4, 179-181.
97. Hugon H, Bruyas J. Suivi de l'évolution du tissu fibro-cartilagineux de la symphyse pubienne par tomodensitométrie chez des cobayes femelles précocément primipares ou non mises a la reproduction au cours de la premiere année de vie. Doctoral thesis, veterinary medicine. Université de Nantes; 2015.
98. Tomaskovic A, Cergolj M, Makek Z, et al. Einfluss des Kaiser-schnitts auf die Fruchtbarkeit der Südamerikanischen Chinchillas. Tieraerztl Umschau 2002; 57:40–2.

Recommended Health Care and Disease-Prevention Programs for Herds/Flocks of Exotic Animals

Michelle Sutherland, BVM&S, BSc (Hons), MANZCVS (Avian Health), CertAVP
(ZooMed), DiplABVP (Avian Practice)[a],*,
Hamish Baron, BVSc (Hons), FANZCVS (Avian Medicine & Surgery)[a],
Joshua Llinas, BVSc (Hons), MVS, BSc (Hons)[b]

KEYWORDS

- Disease prevention • Exotic pets • Health care • Herd health

KEY POINTS

- Preventative health care is a key component of exotic pet ownership and begins primarily with client education.
- Providing clients with up-to-date, detailed information regarding the nutrition and husbandry requirements of their animals is paramount to ensuring the welfare needs of both individual and collections of exotic pet species.
- Prevention of infectious diseases entering a collection via isolation of new animals, quarantine, and testing for diseases of concern during a quarantine period is easier and more cost-effective than managing disease outbreaks.
- Vaccines are available for some species and in some locations and should be administered on the basis of risk and impact of contracting the diseases of concern.

INTRODUCTION

Preventative medicine is an essential part of veterinary medicine and exotic pet ownership, and it primarily begins with client education. Despite the advances made in the ever-growing field of exotic pet medicine, much of the advice given to new pet owners is often outdated or incorrect, leading to many disease states that may have been preventable. Exotic pet owners should be provided with an understanding of the general environmental and husbandry needs of their animal, including information regarding nutritional requirements, safe and adequate enclosures,

[a] The Unusual Pet Vets, 210 Karingal Drive, Frankston, VIC 3199, Australia; [b] The Unusual Pet Vets, 62 Looranah Street, Jindalee, QLD 4074, Australia
* Corresponding author.
E-mail address: michelle@unusualpetvets.com.au

Vet Clin Exot Anim 24 (2021) 697–737
https://doi.org/10.1016/j.cvex.2021.05.003
1094-9194/21/© 2021 Elsevier Inc. All rights reserved.

potential environmental hazards, necessary hygiene and sanitation measures, and normal behavior. For many exotic animals, inadequacies in any or all of these can lead to disease states than can significantly shorten both their quality of life and their lifespan. Existing and potential owners should also be aware of the risk factors that lead to the introduction of an infectious disease, or the acquisition of an animal that is already unwell. Educating clients about potential health issues in exotic pet species is best achieved before the purchase of an animal and ideally works best if veterinarians, breeders, and pet store owners work together to educate themselves, ensure that animals are healthy before purchase/sale, and provide accurate information to new pet owners. Exotic pet veterinarians should seek to further their own knowledge via continuing education, as well as to perform outreach by speaking to local hobby groups and contributing to industry publications to help educate existing and future exotic pet owners.[1]

Preventative health care is often overlooked in exotic species, particularly in those in which annual or semiannual vaccinations are not routinely required. Routine health checks provide veterinarians with the opportunity to engage with pet owners and discuss animal health and husbandry, as well as the potential to detect any underlying health issues that have not been identified by the owner. Preventative health care strategies ensure maximal welfare as well as eliminating the need to treat avoidable disease states. Correct nutrition and appropriate husbandry are essential cornerstones to preventative health care in exotic species; the reader is advised to consult articles elsewhere in this issue for further information on these topics. This article aims to provide veterinarians with guidelines on recommended preventative medicine for companion and aviary psittacine birds and poultry, rabbits, ferrets and other small mammals, reptiles, and amphibians. Although the information provided here is accurate at the time of publication, veterinarians are advised to consult their local veterinary bodies and pharmaceutical companies for up-to-date guidelines and legislation relevant to their country of practice, particularly in relation to vaccinations.

HEALTH PLANS

A health care plan may take many forms, from general advice to collection-, flock-, or individual animal-specific advice. Particularly for groups of animals, by considering and formulating a preventative health care plan, owners will become more aware of the needs of their pets. The development of tailored health care plans is an ideal opportunity for veterinarians to offer clients good-quality advice and will enhance the client-veterinarian bond.[2] A health care plan should consider housing, including outdoor ranges where appropriate, food and water provision, flock or herd behavior, procedures for introducing new animals, hygiene practices, external disease risks, and the identification of disease issues.[2] Once these factors have been evaluated, appropriate measures can be recommended. A target date should be set for the review of health care plans; this will be variable depending on the needs of the collection or flock, but 6-monthly reviews accompanied by routine health examinations or site visits may be appropriate in many cases. Such a review schedule will also allow veterinarians to ensure that the flock or collection can be legitimately regarded as under their care, a key component of responsible prescribing practice.[2]

HEALTH SCREENING FOR AVICULTURAL/BREEDING PSITTACINE COLLECTIONS

The role of veterinarians in avicultural collections takes many forms. The most common involvement is during health screening of incoming birds or an outbreak of disease in a collection. Biosecurity is crucial for the successful management of an avian collection; appropriate biosecurity requires a vigilant owner and an engaged and informed veterinarian.

Any new bird that presents as outwardly healthy may harbor subclinical infections that can be transmitted to the collection. It is with these diseases where the informed avian veterinarian can make significant contributions to the health and disease status of an avicultural collection. Knowledge of the diseases that are present in the country of origin as well as the diseases of concern for the collection will allow appropriate quarantine duration and disease screening to occur. A comprehensive table of diseases in psittacine aviculture and the recommendations for screening is found in **Table 1**.

Depending on the location and the risk factors associated with incoming bird or birds, individual assessment and analysis should be carried out to determine which of the pathogens in **Table 2** are relevant to the collection. Quarantine is always recommended; a common quarantine period of 30 to 45 days is applied in many situations (**Fig. 1**). Specific details of the diagnostic procedures implemented depend on the species, diseases of concern, and the implications of those diseases on the collection. Before any bird is introduced to a new collection or when a new collection is to be managed by a veterinarian, the suggested protocol for introduction is as follows.

INTRODUCTION OF NEW BIRDS

The collection should undergo a thorough review of its biosecurity framework, including quarantine protocols and the current disease status of the collection. The new aviary should have a document composed of an overarching summary, flock production records, aviary structural and traffic flow maps, financial information, and finally, the individual diagnoses obtained from the aviary's birds themselves. The source of the new birds should be thoroughly explored, and different options should be sought so as to best align with the goals and biosecurity framework of the collection. Preference should be given to collections or flocks where thorough records and diagnostic testing have been undertaken so as to ensure the healthiest possible specimens and to reduce risk.

METHODS
Hazard Identification

Hazard identification should be carried out; **Table 2** may act as a framework from which these hazards are identified and considered.

Risk Assessment

The likelihood of infection, country of origin, age, sex, and known disease status of the collection should all be considered. These considerations will help to build information for a risk assessment that should be carried out for each likely or possible hazard. The risk assessment should include information about the epidemiology, host susceptibility, and modes of transmission, incubation period, persistence in the environment, distribution and prevalence, status of the collection, pathogenesis, clinical signs, and the available diagnostic testing. The last point is specifically important given that, in many countries, testing modalities are not available for all identified hazards.

Risk Management

Following the assessment of these risks, the collection managers, in conjunction with their veterinarian, should then undertake a risk-management plan, establishing the most appropriate quarantine, treatment, and testing regimen for their collection.

Table 1
Infectious disease hazards to psittacine avicultural collections

Hazard	Hazard Affects and/or Spread by Psittacine Birds	Hazard Capable of Producing Disease	Recommendation for Screening	Incubation Period	Recommended Samples
Avian adenoviruses affecting psittacine birds	Yes	May occur during stress or immunosuppression[1]	PCR	N/A	N/A
Avian influenza viruses	Yes	Yes	Virus isolation or real-time PCR, HI	World Organisation for Animal Health defines the maximum incubation period for regulatory purposes as 21 d[2]	Oropharyngeal and cloacal swabs or serum
Avian orthoavulavirus 1	Yes	Yes	Virus isolation, HI, HA, PCR	Incubation period is 2–28 d	Blood
Avian paraavulavirus 3	Yes	Yes	HI, PCR	Incubation period ~2 d	Both tracheal or oropharyngeal swabs and cloacal swabs
Avian metaavulavirus 5	Yes	Yes	Virus isolation via egg inoculation and HI testing or serology	Likely averages 5–6 d[3]	Droppings, tracheal, cloacal, and fecal swabs
Avian polyomavirus	Yes	Yes	Virus isolation or PCR	Incubation period 10–14 d	Blood, blood feather
Avian pox viruses (other than Psittacine pox virus)	Yes	Yes	Virus isolation or PCR	Incubation period 4–10 d	Skin lesions
Mycoplasma gallisepticum	Yes	Yes	Isolation on mycoplasma medium, PCR	Incubation period 6–10 d	Choanal, tracheal, and nasal swabs

Organism			Diagnostic tests	Incubation period	Sample
Mycoplasma synoviae	Yes	Yes	Bacterial isolation, serologic assays, and PCR	Incubation period 11–21 d	Choanal, tracheal, or joint fluid swabs
Parrot bornavirus	Yes	Yes	Quantitative PCR for specific PaBVs or PCR with degenerate primers but these tests are problematic due to the genetic variability of PaBVs	Highly variable, some birds never develop disease; others have an incubation period of weeks to years	Pooled samples of urofeces over consecutive days
Psittacine circovirus	Yes	Yes	PCR, HI, HA	Incubation period variable, from 21 d to years	Blood or blood feather
Psittacid alphaherpesvirus 1 and psittacid herpesvirus 2 (PsHV-1/PsHV-2)	Yes	Yes	PCR	Incubation period 5–14 d	Combined oral mucosal and cloacal swabs (Tomaszewski, Wigle, & Phalen 2006)
Psittacine pox virus	Yes	Yes	Virus isolation	Unknown	Skin or oral plaque lesions
Respiratory herpesviruses including Amazon tracheitis virus and psittacine herpesvirus 3 (PsHV-3)	Yes	Yes	Virus isolation, PCR	Unknown	Lung or tracheal tissue
Salmonella spp[a]	Yes	Yes	Culture, PCR	Incubation period 12–72 h	Feces
Sarcocystis falculata	Yes	Yes	Histopathology, PCR	Incubation period in the intermediate host 11–12 d	Formalin-fixed tissues
Spironucleus	Yes	Yes	Fecal wet preparation, PCR	Incubation period approximately 7 d	Feces

(continued on next page)

Table 1
(continued)

Hazard	Hazard Affects and/or Spread by Psittacine Birds	Hazard Capable of Producing Disease	Recommendation for Screening	Incubation Period	Recommended Samples
West Nile virus	Yes	Yes	Virus isolation, PCR, serology, immunofluorescent staining, immuno-histochemistry	Incubation period highly variable, can develop disease from 3 to 15 d	Infected tissues, blood within the first day after infection
Y pseudotuberculosis	Yes	Yes	PCR	Incubation period between 5 and 10 d	Feces
Avibacterium paragallinarum	Yes	Generally considered to be a poultry pathogen	Not required	N/A	N/A

Abbreviations: N/A: Not applicable; HI: Hemagglutination inhibition; HA: Hemagglutination; PaBVs, Parrot bornavirus.
[a] *Salmonella* spp includes *S arizonae, S enteritidis, S gallinarum, S pullorum,* and *S typhimurium* (antibiotic-resistant strains).
Adapted from Australian Government, Department of Agriculture, Water and Environment[37]

Table 2
Summary of diagnostic testing that may be used as part of a health screen on a new psittacine bird

Diagnostic Test	Pathogens to be Identified	Benefits	Limitations
Complete blood count	Nonspecific, evaluates inflammation, infection, or the patient's response to stress; hemoparasites	One of the most sensitive tests to detect illness in avian patients. Cheap and easy to perform, can be performed in-house with only a small amount of blood	Biological variability, variability associated with chronic, stable conditions, subclinical disease, iatrogenic effects, laboratory variability, and interclinician or intraclinician variability. For a more thorough review, see Ref.[38]
Biochemical analysis	Organ damage or dysfunction	Readily available in laboratories across the globe. One of the most common tools used in the evaluation of avian patients with likely access to normal ranges for the species in question	Poor sensitivity and specificity for assessment of kidney and liver dysfunction[39]
Fecal examination (wet mount, floatation)	Intestinal parasites, *Macrorhabdus ornithogaster*, motile protozoa (*Spironucleus* spp or *Histomonas* spp)	Cheap and easy to perform with limited equipment, does not require invasive sample collection, rapid and specific results when carried out by a trained and skilled operator	Poor sensitivity in some sensitivity
Crop fluid cytology	Motile protozoa (*Trichomonas* spp), spiral bacteria	Cheap and easy to perform with limited equipment, does not require invasive sample collection, rapid and specific results when carried out by a trained and skilled operator	Poor sensitivity

(continued on next page)

Table 2
(continued)

Diagnostic Test	Pathogens to be Identified	Benefits	Limitations
Screening radiographs	Nonspecific pathologic changes	Available in most general practices, immediate results	Requires anesthesia and interpretation by a skilled clinician or radiologist required to increase sensitivity
Serology	Detects antibodies to specific pathogenic organisms	Good specificity and some point-of-care analysers are available	Poor sensitivity in some cases, requires blood collection, turnaround time variable
PCR	Detects DNA/RNA of target organisms (eg, C psittaci salmonella, psittacine beak and feather disease virus, polyomavirus, psittacid herpesviruses, avian bornavirus and mycoplasma/mycobacterium)	Good sensitivity and specificity when carried out by an accredited laboratory and sample submissions are appropriate	Turnaround time variable. Can become costly when sampling a large number of birds

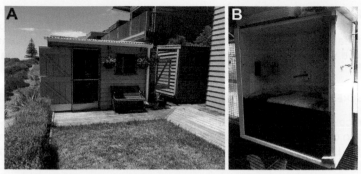

Fig. 1. (*A*) A classic small backyard aviary setup. The shed on the left houses the internal and external flights as well as a wall of breeding cabinets. The shed on the right is the quarantine aviary where any new birds are housed for 3 months before introduction to the main flock. (*B*) Avian hospital cage with a heat source and thermostat, located next to the quarantine aviary and used for the management of sick birds while in quarantine. This prevents the need to move birds from the quarantine aviary while undergoing medical treatment. Image credit: H. Baron, The Unusual Pet Vets.

Information provided should include the duration of quarantine, evaluation of control or management possibilities, including vaccination or prophylactic treatment, and diagnostic testing and disease screening.

Conclusion of Risk Management

A conclusion should be reached, evaluating the risks, mitigating factors, and the management options for the collection to limit the risk of exposure or introduction of diseased individuals into the collection. If these factors and diagnostic modalities are considered appropriate and the level of risk is deemed suitable, both by the attending veterinarian and by the collection management, then a protocol should be put in place to allow the acquisition of the new birds and samples collected for disease screening before or during quarantine.

Surveillance programs and routine screening for diseases such as *Chlamydia psittacid*, because of its zoonotic (and sometimes notifiable) potential, especially in zoologic parks, should be carried out annually in at-risk species. This screening can be in conjunction with vaccination programs that will depend on the region and species being managed. Vaccination against avian influenza (AI) infections caused by viruses of the H5 and H7 subtypes has been used on several occasions in recent years. Vaccination strategies implemented for AI depend on the eco-epidemiological status of the collection in question. Techniques used include routine vaccination performed in endemic areas; emergency vaccination in the face of an epidemic; and preventative vaccination carried out in high-risk or high-value collections whenever a severe risk of viral incursion is identified. It is essential that AI vaccination programs are adapted to local conditions and according to the strain involved, to guarantee efficacy and sustainability. Vaccination should only be used as part of a comprehensive control strategy that also includes biosecurity, quarantine, surveillance, education, and elimination of infected and at-risk poultry or migratory bird species. Despite a wide variety of vaccines that have undergone testing under experimental conditions, only inactivated whole AI virus vaccines and recombinant H5-AI vaccines have been licensed and widely used around the world.[3] Vaccines are also available for West Nile virus, eastern equine encephalitis virus, and although not registered in Aves, make up part of disease-prevention programs for susceptible species in many parts of the United States.[4] Experimental vaccinations have demonstrated efficacy against psittacine beak and feather disease virus, psittacid herpesvirus-1, and psittacine bornavirus-1-5, but these vaccines are not commercially available or registered for use in avian species.[4]

HEALTH SCREENING FOR INDIVIDUAL/HOUSEHOLD/SMALLER AVIAN COLLECTIONS

In smaller collections or in households with only a small number of birds, a different approach to quarantine and disease screening may be taken. This approach focuses more on the bird as an individual entity and affords greater scope for evaluation of organ function and individual bird health rather than a flock-medicine approach. Recommendations for health and disease screening of individual birds are based mostly on experience and clinician preference, rather than peer-reviewed literature. **Table 2** summarizes diagnostic testing that may be assessed as part of a health screen on a new bird.

The clinician must undertake a modified, but active approach in applied preventative medicine in cases of smaller collections or individual bird health examinations. The goal is to identify common pathogens that can be identified and excluded from the smaller collections, even if, in many cases, the complete disease status of the collection is unknown. This situation is commonly encountered by veterinarians working with backyard hobbyists who keep or breed birds in smaller numbers. The application of reasoned decision-making and cost-effective, but diagnostically valuable, testing is a fine line and requires extensive knowledge of the region, the disease prevalence, and the species in question. Disease screening may be carried out annually or more commonly on an as-required basis during outbreaks of mortality or poor breeding successes.

Individual birds, or birds housed as companion pets, can be treated differently also. Annual health checks are often recommended for these birds, despite their intermittent and uncommon contact with pathogens. These annual examinations are useful for early identification of disease processes, and especially useful for establishing "normal" ranges for the individual birds while healthy. Such information can prove enormously valuable when evaluating complete blood counts or biochemical analysis during times of disease or stress and can provide an internal control that would otherwise be unavailable. Because of the lack of sensitivity and specificity in biochemistry and hematology in avian patients, there is little evidence to support annual blood work (biochemistry and hematology) or routine diagnostic testing for infectious diseases (eg, C psittaci) unless there is evidence of exposure to a likely infected source, or for disease screening reasons (ie, quarantine, before the bird going into boarding, or after exposure to birds from outside the collection).[5] The use of an internal control (ie, blood collection from an individual when healthy) and evaluation of trends may help to mitigate some of these difficulties in interpretation of the diagnostic tests, but as a snapshot of patient health, the clinical value in biochemical analysis and hematology in an otherwise outwardly healthy patient is limited.[5,6]

HEALTH SCREENING AND PREVENTATIVE HEALTH CARE FOR BACKYARD POULTRY FLOCKS

Similar to avicultural collections, veterinarians are frequently called on to be involved in the health screening of newly acquired poultry and the management of disease outbreaks in backyard flocks, although with the increase in popularity of poultry as pets, owners are also more commonly requesting routine health examinations to be performed. The principles of preventative health care for backyard poultry flocks are similar to that discussed above relating to avicultural collections; biosecurity and quarantine are critical and preventing diseases from entering a flock is generally simpler and more cost-effective compared to treatment. Veterinarians attending to backyard poultry should have a sound knowledge of the common diseases affecting poultry on a local and national scale, especially those that are considered notifiable.

It should be noted that many backyard poultry are acquired from professional poultry breeding operations or are ex-laying hens, and as such, may have been vaccinated in ovo or as very young chicks, which may limit the interpretation of some diagnostic tests for infectious diseases because of the presence of antibodies. As such, testing for common bacterial and viral diseases as part of a health care assessment may have limited value. In addition to animal welfare implications, because of human health concerns relating to the consumption of eggs from backyard poultry, tests for blood lead levels, *C psittacid*, and endoparasitic and ectoparasitic diseases are suggested as part of an initial health examination for backyard poultry flocks (**Table 3**).

Vaccination of Poultry

The financial losses incurred from morbidity and mortality associated with infectious diseases can be significant in commercial poultry flocks; hence, vaccination for several diseases is considered routine in many countries. In commercial poultry operations, the costs associated with vaccination programs are minimal in comparison to production losses associated with disease. In smaller flocks, vaccination is relatively rare because of cost, availability, and lack of planning. In addition, many small flocks contain birds from a variety of sources, which may be of different vaccination status.[2] Vaccination of small flocks should be based on a risk-benefit analysis, taking into consideration the likelihood of a disease event occurring, the severity of such an event, and any potential adverse vaccination reactions. There may be some circumstances in which the vaccination of poultry may be prohibited or mandated (eg, in the case of a national disease outbreak), thus overriding an individual flock risk-benefit analysis.[2]

Table 3
Diagnostic tests recommended as part of flock health assessments in backyard poultry

Diagnostic Test	Pathogens/Disease Process to Be Identified
Fecal examination (wet mount, floatation)	Intestinal worms (eg, *Capillaria* spp, *Ascaridia* spp, *Heterakis* spp, cestodes) Coccidian parasites (eg, *Eimeria* spp) Motile protozoa (*Spironucleus* spp, *Giardia* spp, or *Histomonas* spp)
Crop fluid cytology	Motile protozoa (*Trichomonas* spp), spiral bacteria, *Candida* spp yeasts
Feather microscopy	Ectoparasites Feather lice (eg, *Menopon* spp, *Lipeurus* spp) Mites (*Ornithonyssus gallinae*) (NB: *Dermanyssus gallinae* is unlikely to be identified by feather microscopy, but birds should be examined clinical for evidence of these mites)
C psittaci PCR/enzyme-linked immunosorbent assay (ELISA)	*C psittaci* (zoonotic potential)
Blood lead levels	Blood lead level (toxic effects in humans via egg consumption)

Another consideration is that many vaccines are only sold in multidose packages (typically a minimum of 500 doses) to administer to large numbers of birds, and these vaccines usually need to be administered immediately after opening. This may make administration uneconomical for small flocks. Although in some instances breed associations may organize sharing of a vaccine package between several owners, attention must be paid to correct prescribing procedures and biosecurity in such circumstances.[2] The poultry vaccinations currently available have been developed for commercial birds, and hence, the age at administration and duration of immunity are targeted toward birds with a relatively short productive lifespan. Backyard poultry flocks often contain birds that live to an older age than those in commercial flocks, so vaccine producers should be contacted in order to determine immunity data for older birds and give advice regarding administration of vaccines to older birds.[2] **Table 4** summarizes the vaccinations that are available for poultry.

DISEASE SCREENING AND PREVENTATIVE HEALTH CARE FOR RABBITS, FERRETS, GUINEA PIGS, CHINCHILLAS, RATS, MICE, GERBILS, HAMSTERS, HEDGEHOGS AND SUGAR GLIDERS

Preventative medicine for collections of rabbits, ferrets, guinea pigs, other rodents, hedgehogs, and marsupials is similar in many ways to the management of any other herd health management. Effective quarantine of incoming animals and careful and accurate implementation of appropriate husbandry, especially dietary management, are essential for the maintenance of a healthy captive population. It is less common for these species to be kept in large breeding collections, and as such, the authors focus on disease-prevention programs with the individual animal as the core of their management. **Tables 5 and 6** outline the different species and their disease-prevention recommendations alongside species-specific considerations. New animals being added to an existing collection should be quarantined to prevent the introduction of potential pathogens, even if (in the case of rabbits and ferrets) they are vaccinated.

Vaccinations are considered routine for rabbits and ferrets, but not for other species of small mammals. For rabbits, vaccination is recommended against 2 main viral pathogens of concern: rabbit hemorrhagic disease virus (RHDV) and myxomatosis. Recently, RHDV-2 has replaced the circulating RHDV and RHDVa strains in most European countries, Australia, and North America.[7–9] Because there are several vaccines available, and current recommendations in endemic countries are to vaccinate against RHDVa and RHDV-2, it is important for clinicians to be familiar with the specifics of each vaccine (see **Table 5**).[8,9] A general vaccination schedule for RHDV includes an initial vaccination aged 8 to 12 weeks, and then subsequently every 6 to 12 months depending on risk; however, manufacturers' guidelines should be followed.[8–11] In Europe, vaccinations to protect against myxomatosis are available, but these are not available in Australia, Asia, or North America because of government legislation preventing their use and import (see **Table 5**).[12] An initial vaccination at 8 to 12 weeks followed by a booster 1 month later and then annually is recommended. A combined RHDV and myxomatosis vaccination is also available in Europe (see **Table 5**), with a recommended vaccination schedule as for RHDV above.[11–13]

REPTILES

Although reptiles are commonly kept exotic pets,[14] evidence suggests many animals die shortly after acquisition,[15] with estimates of mortalities in certain species sold in pet stores reaching levels of 23% within the first year of ownership.[16] It is reasonable

Table 4
Summary of vaccines available for use in poultry in Australia, the United States, and the United Kingdom

Disease	Target Birds	Typical Age	Route of Administration	Duration of Immunity	Available in Combination Vaccine	Minimum No. Doses	Country Available
Avian encephalomyelitis	Breeder hen progeny	Before lay	In water	12 mo in progeny	No	1000	UK, US, Australia
Avian infectious laryngotracheitis (GaHV-1)	Pre-lay chickens	Growers	Eye drop	One laying period	No	1000	UK, US, Australia
Avian influenza	Chickens, ducks, some other species	Growers	IM or SC	12 mo	No	1000	UK
Avian pneumovirus	Breeder, broiler, and pre-lay chickens	Young chicks, then before lay	In water, eye drop, or spray	3 wk, or as a primer	Yes	1000	UK
Avian poxvirus	Chickens	Twice, before lay	SC	12 mo, annual boosters recommended	Yes	1000	US, Australia
Avian rhinotracheitis virus	Broiler and future layer and breeding chickens	Day old and/or growers	Eye drop, nasal drop, spray, or IM	16 wk or 1 laying period	Yes	250	UK
Chicken anemia virus	Broiler breeder hen progeny	Growers then before lay	IM or SC	At least 10 wk	No	500	UK
Escherichia coli	Broiler breeder hen progeny	Growers then before lay	IM or SC	First 7 wk in progeny	No	500	UK, US, Australia
Eimeria spp	Chickens	Young chicks	In feed, water, or spray	40 d to 36 wk	No	500	UK, US, Australia
Erysipelas	Turkeys	Twice as growers	SC	23 wk	No	500	UK

(continued on next page)

Table 4
(continued)

Disease	Target Birds	Typical Age	Route of Administration	Duration of Immunity	Available in Combination Vaccine	Minimum No. Doses	Country Available
Egg drop syndrome (adenovirus)	Future laying and breeding hens	Before lay	IM	One laying period	Yes	1000	UK, Australia
Infectious bursal disease virus	Chickens	Eggs, day old, and young growers	SC, in ovo, spray or in water	At least 42 d	Yes	500	UK, US, Australia
Infectious bronchitis virus	Chickens	Day old onwards	Spray, eye drop, nose drop, or in water	6 wk	Yes	500	UK, US, Australia
Marek disease virus (GaHV-2)	Chickens	Egg, day-old up to point of lay	IM, SC, or in ovo	At least 4 wk Antibodies persist for 2 y	Yes	1000	UK, US, Australia
M gallisepticum	Future laying chickens	Growers	Spray	24 wk	No	500	UK, US, Australia
M synoviae	Laying chickens	Growers	Spray	44 wk	No	500	UK, Australia
Newcastle disease virus (PMV-1)	Broiler, broiler breeding, and future laying chickens; turkeys	Day old and young chicks	Spray, eye drop, or PO	4-6 wk	Yes	1000	UK, US, Australia
Ornithobacterium rhinotracheale	Broiler-breeder progeny	Growers then before lay	IM or SC	43 wk or lay to give 14 d in progeny	No	1000	UK, Australia

P multocida (fowl cholera)	Future layer and breeder hens, ducks and turkeys	Twice as growers	SC	6–16 wk	No	1000	UK, US, Australia
Reovirus	Adult birds and their progeny	Growers	IM or SC	Susceptible period in progeny	Yes	1000	UK, US
Salmonella spp	Breeding and laying chickens and their progeny	Young chicks and growers then before lay	IM or PO	40 wk; 14 d in progeny	Yes	500	UK, US, Australia
Tenosynovitis (viral arthritis)	Chickens	Young chicks	SC	3 wk	No	1000	US, Australia
Turkey rhinotracheitis virus	Turkeys and chickens	Young chicks then as growers	IM, spray or eye drop	6–9 wk or laying period with booster	Yes	500	UK

Abbreviations: Administration route: IM, intramuscular; PO, orally; SC, subcutaneous.
Adapted from Poland,[1] Porter Jr.[2]

Table 5
Summary of preventative health care recommendations for ferrets and rabbits

Species	Vaccination	Quarantine Screening	Sterilization Recommendations	Parasite Prevention	Health Examination Recommendations	Species-Specific Recommendations
Ferrets	*Distemper:* Administered at 6–8 wk and 10–12 wk as an initial course. Unvaccinated adults should receive 2 vaccines, 1 mo apart. Annual boosters thereafter *Rabies:* Some US states require annual rabies booster. Only required in endemic areas	Ectoparasites: Fleas (*Ctenocephalides* sp), ear mites (*Otodectes cynotis*), and sarcoptes mites (*Sarcoptes scabiei*) Internal parasites (fecal floatation and direct wet smear): Coccidia, giardia, and cryptosporidium	Surgical sterilization is recommended after 6 mo old where possible (uncommon in the United States where all ferrets are sold sterilized) Medical sterilization using deslorelin acetate provides efficacy for 301–1249 d in male ferrets and 637–872 d in female ferrets Sterilization (or mating with a vasectomized hob) is essential for female ferrets to prevent hyperestrogenism and accompanying fatal anemia/thrombocytopenia	*D immitis* Ferrets typically carry a low worm burden, but echocardiography is useful for detecting mature worms in the hearts of infected ferrets In endemic areas, ferrets should be administered a monthly preventive beginning at 12–16 wk of age. Year-round administration of the preventive is recommended. Ferrets who have lapsed or have not been treated should receive an ELISA antigen test before starting prophylaxis Treatment of other ectoparasites/ endoparasites is based on risk factors or presence of disease	All ferrets should receive a physical examination and vaccines at least annually At 4 y of age and older, an in-house measurement of blood glucose (to assess for early pancreatic disease; ferrets are prone to insulinomas) is recommended with each examination In geriatric animals (older than 6-y-old), a plasma chemistry panel, complete blood count ± abdominal ultrasound are recommended on an annual basis to assess for common problems, for example, adrenal disease, insulinoma, & lymphoma	Ferrets, particularly those fed soft foods, have a high incidence of periodontal disease. Tartar, gingivitis, periodontitis, and tooth loss may be seen. Affected ferrets may exhibit halitosis, dysphagia, ptyalism, or anorexia. It is highly recommended that owners brush their ferrets' teeth several times weekly if possible Young ferrets are highly prone to gastric foreign bodies. Advise clients to provide ferret-safe toys and ensure no small objects are left on the floor

| Rabbits | Rabbit hemorrhagic disease virus (RHDV) Current recommendations in endemic countries are to vaccinate for RHDVa and RHDV-2, so it is important to be familiar with the specifics of each vaccine[11,13] Europe - Nobivac Myxo RHD (MSD Animal Health) - Combined RHDV and myxoma vaccination - No cross-protection against RHDV-2 - Eravac (Hipra Ltd) - RHDV-2 - Filavac VHD K C + V (CEVA Animal Health) - RHDVa and RHDV-2 Australia - Cylap RCD (Zoetis) - RHDVa - Unclear if provides cross-protection for RHDV-2 | Ectoparasites: Rabbit flea (Spillopsylla cuniculi) important vector for myxomatosis Cediopsylla simplex & Odontopsyllus multispinosus in US Ctenocephalides felis can also affect rabbits Fur mites Cheyletiella parasitivorax - 5-wk lifecycle on host but can survive in environment - Zoonotic Listrophorus gibbus not pathogenic or zoonotic Demodex cuniculi rare Lice Haemodipsus ventricosis Myiasis (fly strike) May be primary or secondary Fly control recommended for outdoor rabbits + environmental hygiene; treat underlying causes Prevention with cyromazine (Europe) | Surgical sterilization is recommended from 4 mo old for males, and 6 month old for females Uterine adenocarcinoma is common in older does (incidence up to 80%). Progressive uterine changes from hyperplasia to adenocarcinoma; rapidly metastasizes locally and to lungs[41–43] | Routine treatment not generally required; treatment is based on risk factors or presence of disease Worming rabbits is not considered routine | All rabbits should receive a physical examination and vaccines at least annually where available Particular attention should be paid to reviewing diet and husbandry, examining for dental disease and otitis externa | Weight should be carefully monitored; consistent weight loss without other clinical signs can be an early indicator of renal disease in rabbits |

(continued on next page)

Table 5
(continued)

Species	Vaccination	Quarantine Screening	Sterilization Recommendations	Parasite Prevention	Health Examination Recommendations	Species-Specific Recommendations
	New Zealand Cylap RCD Filavac North America/Asia RHDV vaccination not routine but recommended in case of an outbreak Vaccination schedules - Maternal antibodies affect vaccination success if performed early - General recommendations: - Initial vaccination aged 8–12 wk - Booster performed after 1 mo - Boosters recommended every 6 mo in high- risk areas or every 12 mo in low-risk areas - Manufacturer's guidelines for specific vaccines should be consulted	Avoid fipronil spray for ectoparasite control, adverse reactions re- ported Ear mites *Psoroptes cuniculi* 3-wk lifecycle on host Treat with ivermectin/ moxidectin Endoparasites Pinworm *Passalurus ambiguus* Usually nonpathogenic even with heavy burden *Coccidiosis* *Eimeria* spp; *Eimeria stie- dae* (hepatic coccidiosis) Can cause high morbidity/ mortality in young rabbits[40]				

Myxomatosis

Vaccination with live attenuated strains of MYXV (eg, Dervaximyo SG33, Merial, Lyons, France) or the heterologous rabbit fibroma virus (RFV) (Nobivac Myxo, MSD-Animal Health; Hoddeston, Herts, UK) is used to protect against myxomatosis in Europe

The homologous vaccinations appear to provide longer-lasting protection than vaccination with RFV but some have been associated with immunosuppression in young rabbits

This has led to recommendations to vaccinate initially with RFV followed by a boost with attenuated MYXV[14]

The Australian federal government does not permit commercial use of myxomatosis vaccines in domestic rabbits in Australia

(continued on next page)

Table 5
(*continued*)

Species	Vaccination	Quarantine Screening	Sterilization Recommendations	Parasite Prevention	Health Examination Recommendations	Species-Specific Recommendations
	Neither type of vaccination provides 100% protection against high-dose challenge, and protection may be short-lived (3–12 mo) Vaccinated rabbits can become infected on challenge and shed virus Myxomatosis vaccinations are not available in North America or Asia					

Table 6
Disease-prevention recommendations and considerations for health screening in rodents and small pet marsupials

Species	Vaccination	Quarantine Screening	Sterilization Recommendations	Parasite Prevention	Health Examination Recommendations	Species-Specific Recommendations
Guinea pigs	Not required	*Dermatophytosis:* Most commonly caused by *Trichophyton mentagrophytes*, diagnosis is based on clinical signs, but fungal culture is required for definitive diagnosis *Ectoparasites:* mites (*Trixacarus caviae*, *Chirodiscoides caviae*), lice (*Gliricola porcelli*, *Gyropus ovalis*), or fleas (*C felis*) *Internal parasites:* (fecal floatation and direct wet smear): coccidia, giardia, and cryptosporidium	Surgical sterilization will prevent unwanted pregnancy, cystic ovarian disease, uterine neoplasia, pyometra, and metritis In males, sterilization will prevent testicular neoplasia and scrotal plug formation and the resultant dermatitis and urinary/fecal obstructions Routine sterilization is not widely accepted but is recommended by some exotic mammal clinicians	Treatment of ectoparasites/ endoparasites is based on risk factors or presence of disease	Annual health examinations with specific attention paid to the molars and premolars.	Dental disease is one of the most common veterinary presentations of guinea pigs. Diets deficient in fiber or vitamin C, infection, and trauma are thought to be common reasons for malocclusion in guinea pigs; genetic predisposition, while not proven, is also strongly suspected Guinea pigs are incapable of endogenous synthesis of vitamin C. Lack of dietary vitamin C results in clinical signs that include a rough hair coat, anorexia, or difficulty prehending food, diarrhea, teeth grinding, vocalizing, lameness, and swollen joints. Guinea pigs require 10–

(continued on next page)

Table 6
(continued)

Species	Vaccination	Quarantine Screening	Sterilization Recommendations	Parasite Prevention	Health Examination Recommendations	Species-Specific Recommendations
						25 mg/kg per day of vitamin C added to their diet; pregnant animals require 30 mg/kg per day.
Rats, mice, hamsters, and gerbils	Not required	Ectoparasitic infestation is more common in rats than in mice. Occasionally the fur mite *Radfordia ensifera* is seen and usually produces few ill effects. However, heavy infestation may lead to self-trauma and ulcerative dermatitis
The tropical rat mite *Ornithonyssus bacoti* is an opportunistic ectoparasite often found on pet rats, mice, gerbils, and hamsters. It spends a relatively short time on a host and penetrates the skin for feeding only. Severe infestations	Routine sterilization of rats is uncommon in clinical practice. There are benefits to sterilization, which include decreased aggression in male rats and decreasing the frequency of mammary tumors in ovariectomised vs sexually intact rats. Neutering sexually mature females often reduces incidence of tumor recurrence in cases where mammary neoplasia has already developed. The placement of GnRH agonists (Deslorelin acetate) can reduce the need to surgically	Treatment of ectoparasites/ endoparasites is based on risk factors or presence of disease	Bi-annual health examinations – no vaccinations are undertaken but routine treatment with the avermectins, although not approved for use in any rodent species, allows routine treatment for pet rodents for pinworms, mites and lice.	Prevention of disease in rodents is far more successful than treatment. Disease prevention is based on the application of appropriate husbandry. Clients should be advised that they should purchase healthy, genetically sound animals; supply appropriate food with balanced protein and caloric content; avoid obesity through exercise and nutrition; provide clean fresh water; preventing the accumulation of excess feces and

	can cause anemia, debilitation, and death in rodents	sterilize female rats following mammary mass removal but was recently found to have no effect on the risk of either developing subsequent mammary tumors or with an increased survival Recommendation: Spay or castrate if necessary			urine; isolating sick animals; and protecting vulnerable animals from more aggressive members of their group (eg, young animals from older animals and male hamsters from female hamsters).
Chinchillas	Not required	Ectoparasites: Fleas (Ctenocephalides sp), ear mites (O cynotis)	Housing is commonly in single-sex groups, and sterilization is not routine. Females tend to be aggressive toward the much smaller males Recommendation: Spay or castrate only if necessary	Treatment of ectoparasites/ endoparasites is based on risk factors or presence of disease Dust baths essential for coat maintenance	Annual health examinations with thorough dental examination assessing signs of early dental changes. Appropriate information regarding diet and husbandry is essential during the initial health examination to ensure a long and healthy life.	Dental disease similar to that described for ferrets is common in pet hedgehogs. Calculus, gingivitis, gingival recession, tooth fractures, and periodontal abscesses may be present. Clinical symptoms are ptyalism, pawing at the mouth, decreased food intake, and bad breath. Clinical signs of dental disease are often missed by owners because of the chinchilla's thick fur coat

(continued on next page)

Table 6
(continued)

Species	Vaccination	Quarantine Screening	Sterilization Recommendations	Parasite Prevention	Health Examination Recommendations	Species-Specific Recommendations
Hedgehogs	Not required	Ectoparasites: mites (*Caparinia tripilis*), (*Chorioptes* sp) are common. Internal parasites: Hedgehogs are susceptible to nematodes, cestodes, and protozoa. *Isospora* and *Eimeria* species coccidia can cause diarrhea. *Cryptosporidium* and *Giardia* infections have been documented. Lungworms infection (*Capillaria* or *Crenosoma* species) will result in bronchopneumonia	Not routinely performed; however, hedgehogs are prone to uterine hyperplasia and neoplasia. The uterus and ovaries are arranged like those of a cow, with the uterine horns coiled caudally and ovaries situated within the coil. Surgical ovariohysterectomy is performed via ventral midline approach. Recommendation: Spay or castrate only if necessary	Treatment of ectoparasites/endoparasites is based on risk factors or presence of disease	A complete physical examination is recommended at the time of purchase, then annually. Review the diet and husbandry. Fecal floatation and direct smear to screen for intestinal parasites. Skin scrapings and ear swabs frequently reveal mites. As with other species, baseline radiographs, urinalysis, and CBC/Chemistry can provide the clinician with a "normal" range for this individual. Identification with a microchip will allow identification even if the patient is rolled up.	Hedgehogs are prone to obesity and dental disease in captivity and should be managed with an appropriate diet, exercise, and dental examination carried out annually to ensure early detection
Sugar gliders	Not required	Internal parasites: *Parastrongyloides* and *Paraustrostrongylus* and a liver trematode	Reproductive disease is fairly uncommon in sugar gliders. A few cases of mammary tumors are reported	Treatment of ectoparasites/endoparasites is based on risk factors or	Annual physical examinations after the initial post-purchase examination. Fecal	

float and direct smear and nail clipping form the baseline for the wellness examination.

presence of disease

and presumably could be prevented by spaying. In males, prolapse of the penis is the most common reproductive disorder. Castration of males will help to decrease scent and staining. Intact males kept with other males often fight; intact males kept with females will often breed This is the most common reason for surgical alteration. The reproductive tract of female marsupials is complicated and closely associated with the ureters. In addition, the pouch and its associated blood supply sits in the middle of the surgical field for a midline surgical approach. The procedure in males is brief and relatively safe.
Recommendation: Castrate if necessary

of the genus Athesmia. Wild sugar glider nests generally contain a range of host-specific mites and fleas, but ectoparasites are uncommon in captivity to think that morbidity levels are significantly higher than this considering the increased rates of stress related to transit, environmental instability, and poor husbandry practices. Because of the variation of reptile species found in captivity, this section aims to give guidelines for the veterinarian to discuss with clients while supplying a framework to make sound recommendations to identify infectious disease most relevant for the specific patient.

HEALTH CARE PROTOCOL FOR REPTILES PRESENTING FOR ROUTINE HEALTH CHECKS
General Recommendations

Any newly acquired reptile or amphibian should be isolated and placed into quarantine. The quarantine period should be based on the disease profile for the species in question. For most infectious diseases, a quarantine period of 3 months has been recommended.[17] Reptiles with certain viruses may take months or even years to show signs of illness,[18,19] and therefore, quarantining for these diseases may not be practical. Polymerase chain reaction tests (PCR) can be used to screen for individual carriers of these diseases.[20]

Quarantine

Similar to that outlined for avian species above, the concepts of quarantine should be discussed with the owner, as proper quarantine is difficult to achieve, requires advanced planning, and may not be feasible for the general hobbyist. In these cases, the real risk of introduction of disease into a collection needs to be discussed. Suggested quarantine lengths for many infectious diseases have been listed in **Table 7**.

General Health Examination

A full health assessment should be performed with any new acquisition. This visit should consist of a full history, including correct species identification, where the animal has originated, assessment of the owners current knowledge and experience with the species in question, other animals in collection, enclosure size and design, plans for enclosure changes as the animal matures, proposed environmental enrichment, stress avoidance, a complete physical examination, dietary plan, and recommended screening tests appropriate for the species in question (**Table 8**).[21] Routine health examinations should also include a yearly health care management plan.

The reader is advised to consult other articles in this issue for a detailed guide to husbandry and diet for captive reptiles. Appropriate provision for the species in question, including enclosure size and designs, lighting, heating, substrate, enrichment, and safety, should be evaluated, and recommendations for improvements should be provided in writing to the owner.

Diagnostic testing is essential for evaluating the overall health of reptile and amphibians because of their ability to mask disease. As many conditions are secondary to immunosuppression caused by poor husbandry, diet, and stress, the presence of an infectious agent on a screening test does not necessarily mean it is the primary cause of the disease; many potential pathogens are commensal under ideal keeping conditions and when the immune system is working efficiently. Careful consideration must be taken when interpreting the significance of a parasite and subsequent recommendations for management, as treating may alter the delicate symbiotic balance. Diagnostic tests should be selected based on consideration of the patient or collection of animals, the prevalence of the disease in question, the pathogenicity of the organism, and the specificity/sensitivity of the test. Screening tests should be performed as part of an intake examination and at subsequent health examinations with the purpose

Table 7
Summary of infectious diseases of reptiles commonly seen in practice and preventative health care recommendations

Pathogen	Organs Systems Affected	Commonly Affected Groups of Reptiles and Amphibians	Common Affected Species Seen in Practice	Recommended Minimum Quarantine Period with Testing	Recommendation for Screening	Recommended Sampling from Live Patient
Viral						
Adenovirus	Gastrointestinal tract Liver Pulmonary Neurologic	Lizards, snakes, chelonians, crocodiles	*Pogona* spp	3 mo	Intake examination 1–3 mo into quarantine (does not 10% reliably detect all carriers)	PCR on cloacal swab
Arenavirus	Neurologic Pulmonary Gastrointestinal tract Integument Hepatic Hematological	Snakes (inclusion body disease)	Boids Pythons	6 mo	Intake examination If negative results retest after: - 3 mo & - 6 mo	PCR on esophageal swab and whole blood Visualization of inclusion bodies on blood smear using immunohisto chemistry
Bornavirus	Neurologic Upper gastrointestinal tract	Snakes	Pythons in Australia	6 mo	Intake examination If negative result retest after 1 mo	PCR combined oral/tracheal/esophageal/cloacal swab
Herpesvirus	Upper gastrointestinal tract Upper respiratory tract Integument	Lizards Snakes Chelonians Crocodiles	Terrestrial tortoises	6 mo	Intake examination, at 6 wk and again several months into quarantine	PCR on oral swabs and lesions in clinical patients Antibody titers in asymptomatic patients

(continued on next page)

Table 7
(continued)

Pathogen	Organs Systems Affected	Commonly Affected Groups of Reptiles and Amphibians	Common Affected Species Seen in Practice	Recommended Minimum Quarantine Period with Testing	Recommendation for Screening	Recommended Sampling from Live Patient
	or shell Hepatic Neurologic					
Nidovirus	Upper and lower respiratory tracts	Lizards Snakes	*Tiliqua* spp *Morelia* spp	3–6 mo	Intake examination Up to weekly for 12 wk as intermittent shedders	PCR on oral cloacal swab or pulmonary wash
Sunshine virus	Neurologic Lower respiratory tract Upper gastrointestinal tract Integument Hematological	Snakes	Morelia species (in Australia	6 mo	Intake examination 1 mo	PCR combined oral/ tracheal/esophageal/ cloacal swab
West Nile virus	Hematological Integument	Crocodiles		3 mo	Intake examination Before leaving quarantine	
Bacterial						
Mycoplasma spp	Respiratory tract Carrier state possible Zoonotic potential (rare)	Tortoises Crocodiles Snakes	Recorded in numerous species *Testudo* spp Pythons	3 mo?	Not recommended unless clinical disease present due to inadequate understanding of carrier state	Culture, PCR, or ELISA of nasal lavage, oral/ choanal swab

Organism	Body systems affected	Species	Notes	Screening interval	Screening recommendation	Detection
Chlamydia spp	Respiratory tract Hepatic Conjunctiva Carrier state possible Zoonotic potential (rare)	Chelonians Crocodiles Snakes Lizards	Recorded in numerous species[52] Crocodiles high prevalence	N/A	Not recommended unless screening for public health reasons	Detection by PCR, immunofluorescence, ELISA, or cell culture from oral swabs, tracheal wash, and from direct lesion sampling
Salmonella spp	Gastrointestinal tract Skin Carrier state Zoonotic potential	High prevalence in all reptile species with lizards and chelonians being natural reservoirs	All reptiles should be considered potential carriers with zoonotic potential[52]	N/A	Not recommended unless screening for public health reasons	Detection by culture from cloacal swab, serial fecal sampling ± pooling
Mycobacterium spp	Systemic; multiple organ systems affected (ie, lung, hepatic, spleen, kidney, heart reproductive tract, nervous system, and articular spaces) Carrier state Zoonotic potential	Snakes Lizards Chelonians Crocodiles	Reptiles appear to be resistant	N/A	Not recommended unless clinical disease present due to inadequate understanding of carrier states	PCR ± acid-fast staining on feces or organs (necropsy) Presence in feces without clinical sign or lesions may not be significant
Protozoan						
Choleoeimeria	Liver Biliary tract	Snakes Lizards Chelonians Crocodiles	Central bearded dragon (*P vitticeps*)	3 mo	Intake examination New patients monthly for 3 mo Before leaving quarantine Then 6–12 monthly	Fecal floatation ± wet mount

(continued on next page)

Table 7
(continued)

Pathogen	Organs Systems Affected	Commonly Affected Groups of Reptiles and Amphibians	Common Affected Species Seen in Practice	Recommended Minimum Quarantine Period with Testing	Recommendation for Screening	Recommended Sampling from Live Patient
Coccidia (*Isospora* spp)	Gastrointestinal tract	Snakes Lizards Chelonians Crocodiles	Central bearded dragon (*P vitticeps*) Blue tongued skinks (*Tiliqua* spp) Chameleons Iguanids	3 mo	Intake examination New animals monthly for 3 mo Before leaving quarantine Then 6–12 monthly	Fecal floatation ± wet smear
Cryptosporidium	Gastrointestinal tract	Snakes Lizards	Reported in multiple snake species Leopard geckos (*Eublepharis macularius*)	3 mo	Intake examination Before leaving quarantine	Repeated cloacal swabs acid-fast stain, PCR with sequencing, microscopy, ELISA of fresh feces, gastric lavage or brushing (snakes), slime from surface of regurgitated food items

Entamoeba invadens	Gastrointestinal tract Liver Kidney	Snakes Lizards Chelonians Crocodiles	High morbidity in snakes and lizards Chelonians and crocodiles are frequent reservoirs	3 mo	Intake examination Before leaving quarantine	Fecal microscopy using iodine staining
Hexamita parva	Kidney Gastrointestinal tract	Snakes Lizards Chelonians Crocodiles	Potentially fatal infection in chelonians	3 mo	Intake examination 6–12 monthly	Wet mount cytology of feces and urine
Intranuclear coccidiosis	Liver spleen Respiratory tract Gastrointestinal tract	Chelonians	Tortoises	3 mo	Intake examination Before leaving quarantine	PCR on nasal lavage, oral/cloacal swab

Table 8
Disease screening and preventative health care testing recommended for reptiles and amphibians

Diagnostic Test	Pathogens/Disease Process to Be Identified	Frequency of Testing	Benefits	Limitations

Dermal examination	Ectoparasites
	- Acariasis
	  ○ Hard- and soft-bodied ticks
	  ○ Mites (*Ophionyssus natricis*)
	- Myasis o Bufolucilia (toads)
	- Leeches
	  ○ Hirudineans: aquatic turtles and amphibians
		At first visit
		Annually thereafter
			Easy to perform
			Many external parasites are also potentially zoonotic[44]
				Specific attention to areas of raised skin, skin folds, the periocular region, groin or inguinal areas, and ear openings reduces the risk of a missed diagnosis

Fecal examination (wet mount, floatation, stains (Wright-Giemsa, iodine solution, Acid-fast)
Collected in clinic opportunistically or using cloacal flush, cloacal stimulation, or colonic massage techniques
Alternatively, samples can be collected at home and refrigerated in a sealed container or zip-lock bag for testing within 24 h of collection, although can reduce the sensitivity for certain parasites (motile parasites)
	Endoparasites
	Protozoan
	- Amoebas
	- *E invadens*,
	  Acanthamoeba
	- Opalinids: Zelleriella
	- Flagellates: Hexamita,
	  Chilomastixis,
	  Tritrichomonas,
	  Trichomonas, Giardia
	- Ciliates: Balantidium,
	  Nyctotherus
	- Apicomplexa: Isospora,
	  Eimeria, Sarcocystis,
	  Toxoplasma,
	  Cryptosporidium
	Nematodes
	- Rhabdias (lungworm)
		Captive-bred reptiles and amphibians
		Fecal assessment on first visit, and either annually or biannually depending on environmental conditions, stocking densities, and general health. Additional sampling before brumation (species dependent), after brumation (species dependent, persistent abnormalities in fecal quality, or quantity. The presence of a compromised immune system or comorbidities should be considered (ie, *Pogona vitticeps* with concurrent
			Cheap and easy to perform with limited equipment, does not require invasive sample collection, rapid and specific results when carried out by a trained and skilled operator	Complicated by intermittent shedding of many organisms requiring multiple tests and preparations (ie, cryptosporidium)
				Fresh samples required for motile parasites to increase sensitivity
				Samples must be collected and processed in such a way to ensure accuracy of the diagnosis[23]
				Small volumes of feces may limit sensitivity. Serial testing required for some pathogens (eg, cryptosporidium)[46]

- *Kalicephalus* spp and Oswaldocruzia (Hookworms) - Oxyurids - Capillaria (Trichurid) - Ascarids - Spiurids Cestodes - Tapeworms Trematodes - Flukes Acanthocephalans (thorny headed worms) Pentastomes	agamid adenovirus-1, *Tiliqua* species with nidovirus) as lower burdens of endoparasites may contribute to increased morbidity and mortality Wild caught, as for captive-bred individuals but with additional screening monthly for first 3 mo and then 6 monthly.[45]			May not be feasible for the smallest patients
Packed cell volume and total solids	Nonspecific Evaluated for red blood cell percentage assessed for anemia and hydration status, buffy coat, and serum color/clarity Total solids assess for inflammation, nutritional status, hydration, inflammation	Intake 6-12 monthly Options to check before and after brumation/hibernation or around stressful events	Cheap and easy to perform with limited equipment, minimally invasive sample collection Small volume of blood required	
Blood smear (stained) - Complete blood count - Hemoparasitic examination Wet mount	Nonspecific, evaluates inflammation, infection, or the patient's response to stress Hemoparasites Hemogregarines, Hemoproteus, Leishmania, Plasmodium, Lankesterella, Trypanosomes, microfilaria,	Intake 6-12 monthly Options to check before and after brumation/hibernation or around stressful events	Sensitive tests to detect illness in reptile and amphibian patients. Cheap and easy to perform, can be performed in-house with only a small amount of blood	Biological variability, variability associated with; chronic, stable conditions, subclinical disease, iatrogenic effects, laboratory variability, and interclinician or intraclinician variability. For

(continued on next page)

Table 8
(continued)

Diagnostic Test	Pathogens/Disease Process to Be Identified	Frequency of Testing	Benefits	Limitations
	flukes, Pirhemocyton Intracytoplasmic inclusion bodies Reptarenavirus, especially boids.[47] Intraerythrocytic iridovirus (*Pogona* spp)[48]			a more thorough review, see Ref.[49] and Ref.[50]
Plasma/serum biochemistry	Organ damage or dysfunction (glucose, protein, uric acid, urea, AST, LDH, ALP, Ca_2^+, and phosphorus minimum database) Reproductive status	Intake 6–12 monthly Options to check before and after brumation/hibernation or around stressful events	Readily available in commercial laboratories as well as in house analysers One of the most common tools used in the evaluation of reptile patients with likely access to normal ranges for many commonly kept species Because of variation between and within species, obtaining baseline blood levels and at least annual monitoring can help to establish normal ranges for an individual	Poor sensitivity for organ function and disease state Seasonal variations in many species Larger volume of blood required, which may not be feasible for many species >9000 species of reptiles alone with many normal reference ranges unknown For a more thorough review, see Ref.[51]
Water testing (aquatic species) Ammonia, nitrite, nitrate, phosphate, general hardness, KH, pH, and salinity	Assesses water quality and life support system function	Each visit	Readily available in house testing Newer automated inhouse testing available	Often subjective assessment of results with variation in interpretation by different readers Water parameters may change rapidly during transport if not handled correctly

of detecting diseases in individuals not yet showing clinical signs of illness. **Tables 7 and 8** provide outlines of potential pathogens of concern for reptiles and recommended disease screening protocols.

Fecal Testing

Direct fecal smear is best used for ciliates, amoeboids, and flagellates, as the high osmolarity of fecal float solutions reduces their motility.[22–25] Direct smears will also assist in detection of nematode larvae, tapeworm eggs, trematode eggs, and some nematode eggs, as these structures are heavy and float poorly. The sensitivity of direct smear for many of the parasitic ovum is poor, and fecal floatation techniques are recommended.[26]

Fecal flotation has the added benefit of concentrating different stages of the parasite and removing debris, allowing better visualization. Most endoparasites being screened for in captive reptiles and amphibians are more readily detectable by standard fecal float techniques.[25–27] Zinc chloride/sodium chloride solutions are superior for detecting nematode eggs and coccidian oocysts, whereas heavier structures, such as large ciliates, certain nematode, and most trematode eggs have higher specific gravities and require sedimentation techniques (ie, Sodium acetate-acetic acid-formulation [SAF] technique) to increase the sensitivity for the heavier organisms.[26] A list of commonly encountered endoparasites and recommended testing regimen can be found in **Table 8**.

Water Testing for Aquatic Species

Water testing for aquatic reptiles and amphibians should be performed at each visit regardless of physical health, as most ailments are related to environmental, and specifically, water-quality issues. It is not possible to effectively treat aquatic reptiles and amphibians without understanding the water quality in their home environment. Parameters that are typically assessed are ammonia, nitrite, nitrate, phosphate, general hardness, carbonate hardness (KH), pH, and salinity (see **Table 8**).

Ultrasound

Ultrasound is a noninvasive tool that can be used to supplement the general health examination for reptiles and amphibians. With the advent of handheld portable machines and probes, these procedures can often be performed with the owner present, increasing both the information gained and the overall value of the consultation. Additional information regarding a healthy squamates body condition (fat bodies), liver, kidneys, gall bladder, urolithiasis in those animals containing bladders, gastrointestinal tract, and confirms gender and gains insights into the current and past reproductive status.[24,25,28] Although more limited, ultrasound examinations can be used for chelonians to evaluate the female reproductive tract. Where possible, ultrasound should be performed at the initial general health examination, before and after breeding periods, and before and after brumation.

Bacterial Infections Encountered in Captive Reptiles and Amphibians

Bacterial infections are generally secondary to reduced immune function. Routine testing for bacteria is not generally recommended, and the presence of bacterial infections needs to be interpreted in light of history and other clinical findings. Screening for the purpose of identifying zoonotic potential may be considered for the organisms outlined in **Table 7**.

Viral Infections Encountered in Captive Reptiles and Amphibians

It is important for the clinician to be aware of the commonly seen viruses within their region as well as those that may be present because of the wide legal and illegal movement of reptiles. It is also necessary to discuss the sensitivity and specificity of the test in asymptomatic patients with your laboratory when performing these screening tests so appropriate recommendations for quarantine and collection management can be made. In many cases, there is still limited information available, making these recommendations difficult.

Further complicating recommendations are the current limited understanding of the impact of many viral infections on reptile. Koch's postulates have only been fulfilled for a limited number of reptilian viruses, so further investigation is required before general recommendations can be made.

The viruses that have been most commonly detected in reptiles include herpesviruses, especially in chelonians, adenoviruses, especially in lizards and snakes, reoviruses, especially in lizards and snakes, paramyxoviruses, especially in snakes, picornaviruses in tortoises, and iridoviruses, with ranaviruses detected predominantly in chelonians, and invertebrate iridoviruses detected in lizards.[19,29] Many summaries of viruses affecting reptiles, the clinical and pathologic presentations, and the diagnostic methods used have been published and are frequently being revised.[19,20,30] It is recommended that the clinician should stay up-to-date on the current and evolving field of reptile virology. Viruses commonly encountered in general practice and recommended screening protocols are listed in **Table 7**. Testing occurs using molecular diagnostic techniques from samples obtained from the commonly affected organ systems (**Fig. 2**).

Fungal Diseases Commonly Detected in Captive Reptiles

Little is known about the normal mycoflora of reptiles and amphibians. As most are considered opportunistic, currently, there may not be benefit to screening for these organisms unless there is a high suspicion based on physical examination and clinical signs. Several studies investigating the "normal" flora of specific reptiles and amphibians are coming to light,[31–33] but wide variation in species and their habitats makes it difficult to extrapolate. Some specific fungi that may be of interest and the diagnostic test that can be performed are listed below:

Chamaeleomyces granulomatous-: culture, cytology, PCR: oral cloacal swabs, liver biopsy
Nannizziopsis spp: cytology, culture, PCR: skin scrapings, skin biopsy
Ophidiomyces: cytology, culture, PCR: skin scrapings, skin biopsy
Microsporidium: histopathology, fecal PCR, blood PCR
Yeast (Candida spp) culture, cloacal swabs, and feces
Chytridiomycosis: cytology (wet mounts of shedding skin), PCR (skin or mouthparts of tadpoles), histopathology.[33]

PROTOZOA

This group of common parasites includes amebas, flagellates, coccidia, plasmodia, cryptosporidium, ciliates, and Opalinida. Most have a direct lifecycle and are capable of reaching high levels in a short period of time. Low levels of some of these parasites in healthy individuals with an intact immune system are often commensal. Pathogenicity occurs when numbers increase and when the immune system is compromised. Reptiles and amphibians may be asymptomatic carriers, and newly acquired

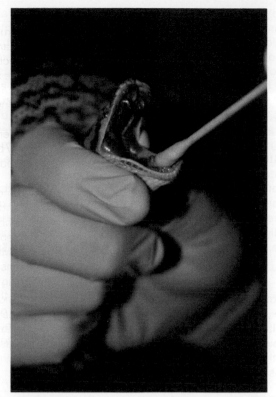

Fig. 2. A swab of the oropharyngeal conjunctiva is taken from a Murray Darling Carpet Python (*Morelia spilota*) for viral PCR screening (Photo credit, M. Sutherland, The Unusual Pet Vets).

individuals should be appropriately quarantined. A list of commonly encountered protozoa can be found in **Tables 7 and 8**

Emerging Diseases

It is important for the clinician to be aware that newly discovered infectious diseases occur frequently. Updates are periodically published with recent information on emerging conditions in squamates and chelonians available.[30,34,35] Care and attention must be given to peer-reviewed literature so as to be able to offer the best advice to owners when it comes to the safe introduction of new reptiles or amphibians to a collection.

PEST CONTROL

Pest species encountered in relation to backyard poultry, aviary birds, and small mammals housed outdoors include rodents, wild birds, and insects. Effective pest control reduces morbidity and mortality through transmitted diseases, food spoilage and losses, and damage to housing. For birds, rodents may be a source of *Yersinia pseudo-tuberculosis*, *Pasteurella multocida*, AI, *Campylobacter jejuni*, *Salmonella* spp, and infectious bronchitis virus.[2] To reduce the incidence of rodent incursions, feed should be stored in a cool, secure, dry place to prevent rodent entry. Sheds and hutches sited on a concrete plinth are more resistant to rodents tunneling underneath them.[2] Any spilled food should be regularly cleaned up to prevent accumulation. Any rodent population control should be carefully considered from an ethical perspective, as well as a risk assessment of the potential effect on nontarget species, such as livestock, pets, and wildlife. Wild birds can also be an important disease reservoir and may cause a significant loss of feed. Wild birds are commonly implicated as sources of *Trichomonas* spp parasites, as well as being reservoir hosts of infectious viral diseases, such as AI and several viral encephalitis viruses.[36–38] The primary control mechanism for wild birds should be good husbandry practices and enclosure design to minimise exposure, such as netting or reduction in overhanging vegetation.[2] Care should be taken to minimise the fecal contamination of water supplies.

Transmission of the viral diseases RHDV myxomatosis to rabbits involves insect vectors; hence, pet rabbits should be prevented from coming into contact with wild rabbits, and screening of cages/buildings to prevent transmission is recommended (see **Table 5**). Similarly, in ferrets, the heartworm *Dirofilaria immitis* is mosquito-borne, and hence, outdoor housing should be insect-proofed (see **Table 5**).

SUMMARY

As in other fields of veterinary medicine, efforts should be made to move from reactive health care for exotic pet species to preventative health care strategies. Adopting a preventative health care approach ensures maximal animal welfare in addition to saving time and expense associated with treating preventable diseases. Correct husbandry and nutrition are the cornerstones to all preventative health care plans and should be discussed in detail with all exotic pet owners.

CLINICS CARE POINTS

- Isolation and quarantine of new animals entering a collection is essential to prevent infectious disease transmission.
- Health care plans should be established with agreement between veterinarians and caregivers and regularly reviewed to ensure they encompass the main husbandry, mental and physical health issues, and infectious diseases of concern for the flock or herd at the individual level.
- Companion and aviary birds should, at a minimum, be tested for gastrointestinal parasites, *Chlamydia psittaci*, and gastrointestinal bacteria and yeast populations before entering a new flock. Testing for other viral diseases may be appropriate depending on individual circumstances. Poultry should in particular be evaluated for respiratory diseases of concern and vaccination status before entering a new flock.
- Reptiles and amphibians should be examined and assessed for the presence of gastrointestinal parasites and some ectoparasites and potential viral pathogens as relevant to the species and geographic area. Water testing is an essential part of maintenance health care for all aquatic species. Ultrasound should be performed to assess the coelomic organs where possible, with particular attention to the reproductive organs and their status.
- Small mammals are prone to respiratory diseases as well as endoparasites and ectoparasites. Individuals should be assessed for these during the initial quarantine and isolation period. Vaccination is recommended for rabbits and ferrets according to the infectious disease risk factors and vaccine availability in the relevant geographic location.

DISCLOSURE

The authors declare no conflicts of interest.

REFERENCES

1. Phalen D. Preventive medicine and screening. In: Harrison G, Lightfoot T, editors. Clinical avian medicine. Palm Beach, FL: Spix Publishing; 2006. p. 573–87.
2. Poland G. Preventative healthcare. In: Poland G, Rafterty A, editors. BSAVA manual of backyard poultry. Quedegley, Glos: BSAVA; 2019. p. 51–8.
3. Marangon S, Cecchinato M, Capua I. Use of vaccination in avian influenza control and eradication. Zoonoses Public Health 2008;55(1):65–72.
4. Heatley JJ, Payne S, Tizard I. Avian vaccination: current options and strategies. Vet Clin North Am Exot Anim Pract 2018;21:379–97.
5. Beaufrère H, Ammersbach M. Advances in clinical pathology and diagnostic medicine: variability and limitations in clinical avian hematology. In: Speer BL, editor. Current advances in avian medicine and surgery. St Louis, Missouri: Elsevier; 2016. p. 461–530.
6. Vergneau-Grosset C, Beaufrère H, Ammersbach M. Advances in clinical pathology and diagnostic medicine: clinical biochemistry. In: Speer BL, editor. Current advances in avian medicine and surgery. St Louis, Missouri: Elsevier; 2016. p. 461–530.
7. Hall RN, Peacock DE, Kovaliski J, et al. Detection of RHDV2 in European brown hares (Lepus europaeus) in Australia. Vet Rec 2017;180:121.
8. Mahar JE, Hall RN, Peacock D, et al. Rabbit hemorrhagic disease virus 2 (RHDV2; GI.2) is replacing endemic strains of RHDV in the Australian landscape within 18 months of its arrival. J Virol 2018;92(2). e01374-17.
9. Rouco C, Aguayi-Adan JA, Santoro S, et al. Worldwide rapid spread of the novel rabbit haemorrhagic disease virus (GI.2/RHDV2/b). Transbound Emerg Dis 2019; 66:1762–4.
10. Saunders R. Vaccinating rabbits against RVHD-2. Vet Rec 2016;178:100–1.
11. Woodland D. A vaccine against rabbit hemorrhagic disease virus. Viral Immunol 2016;29:535.
12. Kerr P, Donnelly TM. Viral infections of rabbits. Vet Clin North Am Exot Anim Pract 2013;16:437–68.
13. Gleeson M, Petritz OA. Emerging infectious diseases of rabbits. Vet Clin North Am Exot Anim Pract 2020;23:249–61.
14. Auliya M. Hot Trade in Cool Creatures -A review of the live reptile trade in the European Union in the 1990s with a focus on Germany. Brussels, Belgium: Traffic Europe; 2003.
15. Robinson JE, St John FAV, Griffiths RA, et al. Captive reptile mortality rates in the home and implications for the wildlife trade. PLoS One 2015;10:e0141460.
16. Lawrence K. Mortality in imported tortoises (Testudo graeca and T. hermanni) in the United Kingdom. Br Vet J 1988;144:187–95.
17. Jacobson ER, Morris P, Norton TM. Quarantine. J Herpetological Med Surg 2001; 11:24–30.
18. Kubiak M. Detection of agamid adenovirus-1 in clinically healthy bearded dragons (Pogona vitticeps) in the UK. Vet Rec 2013;172:75.
19. Marschang RE. Viruses infecting reptiles. Viruses 2011;3:2087–126.

20. Marschang RE. Reptile virology: understanding the methods and their interpretation. In: ExoticsCon Proc Session 142. 2015. p. 583–7. Association of Reptile Veterinarians, San Antonio Texas.

21. Wilkinson SL. Reptile wellness management. Vet Clin North Am Exot Anim Pract 2015;18:281–304.

22. Rataj AV, Lindtner-Knific R, Vlahovic K, et al. Parasites in pet reptiles. Acta Vet Scand 2011;53:33.

23. Raś-Noryńska M, Sokół R. Internal parasites of reptiles. Ann Parasitol 2015;61: 115–7.

24. Holland MF, Hernandez-Divers S, Frank PM. Ultrasonographic appearance of the coelomic cavity in healthy green iguanas. J Am Vet Med Assoc 2008;233:590–6.

25. Bucy DS, Guzman DS-M, Zwingenberger AL. Ultrasonographic anatomy of bearded dragons (Pogona vitticeps). J Am Vet Med Assoc 2015;246:868–76.

26. Wolf D, Globokar Vrhovec M, Failing K, et al. Diagnosis of gastrointestinal parasites in reptiles: comparison of two coprological methods. Acta Vet Scand 2014; 56:44.

27. Rom B, Kornaś S, Basiaga M. Endoparasites of pet reptiles based on coprosopic methods. Ann Parasitol 2018;64:115–20.

28. Banzato T, Russo E, Finotti L, et al. Ultrasonographic anatomy of the coelomic organs of boid snakes (Boa constrictor imperator, Python regius, Python molurus molurus, and Python curtus). Am J Vet Res 2012;73:634–45.

29. Ariel E. Viruses in reptiles. Vet Res 2011;42:100.

30. Latney LV, Wellehan JFX. Selected emerging infectious diseases of squamata: an update. Vet Clin North Am Exot Anim Pract 2020;23:353–71.

31. Barbosa LN, Seabra Ferrerira R Jr, Mello PL, et al. Molecular identification and phylogenetic analysis of Bothrops insularis bacterial and fungal microbiota. J Toxicol Environ Health A 2018;81:142–53.

32. Ross AA, Rodrigues Hoffmann A, Neufeld JD. The skin microbiome of vertebrates. Microbiome 2019;7:79.

33. Chai N, Whitaker BR. Amphibian chytridiomycosis. In: Stahl SJ, Divers S, editors. Mader's reptile and amphibian medicine and surgery. Third Edition. St. Louis, MO: W.B. Saunders; 2019. p. 1292–3.

34. Schmidt V. Fungal infections in reptiles—an emerging problem. J Exot Pet Med 2015;24:267–75.

35. Adamovicz L, Allender MC, Gibbons PM. Emerging infectious diseases of chelonians: an update. Vet Clin North Am Exot Anim Pract 2020;23:263–83.

36. Pello S, Olsen GH. Emerging and reemerging diseases of avian wildlife. Vet Clin North Am Exot Anim Pract 2013;16:357–81.

37. Lumeij J. Infectious diseases: usutu virus. In: Speer BL, editor. Current advances in avian medicine and Surgery. St Louis, Missouri: Elsevier; 2016. p. 98–106.

38. Calistri P, Giovannini A, Hubálek Z, et al. Epidemiology of West Nile in Europe and in the Mediterranean Basin. Open Viral J 2010;4:29–37.

39. Australian Government Department of Agriculture, Water and Environment. Import risk review for psittacine birds from all countries: Draft report. 2020. Available from: https://www.agriculture.gov.au/sites/default/files/documents/draft-psittacine-review-for-public-comment.pdf. Accessed December 15, 2020.

40. Porter RE Jr. Vaccination of poultry. In: Greenacre CB, Morishita TY, editors. Backyard poultry medicine and surgery: a guide for veterinary practitioners. Ames, Iowa: Wiley & Sons; 2015. p. 1181–204.

41. Mancinelli E, Lord B. Urogenital system and reproductive disorders. In: Meredith A, Lord B, editors. BSAVA manual of rabbit medicine. Quedgeley, Glos: BSAVA; 2014. p. 191–204.

42. Saito K, Nakanishi M, Hasegawa A. Uterine disorders diagnosed by ventrotomy in 47 rabbits. J Vet Med Sci 2002;64:495–7.

43. Heatley J, Smith A. Spontaneous neoplasms of lagomorphs. Vet Clin North Am Exot Anim Pract 2004;7:561–77.

44. Mendoza J, Modry D, Otranto D. Zoonotic parasites of reptiles: a crawling threat. Trends Parasitol 2020;36:677–87.

45. Stahl SJ. Mader's reptile and amphibian medicine and surgery. St Louis (MO): Elsevier Saunders; 2019. p. 124–30.

46. Graczyk TK, Cranfield MR. Cryptosporidium serpentis oocysts and microsporidian spores in feces of captive snakes. J Parasitol 2000;86:413–4.

47. Chang L-W, Jacobson ER. Inclusion body disease, a worldwide infectious disease of boid snakes: a review. J Exot Pet Med 2010;19:216–25.

48. Grosset C, Wellehan JFX, Owens SD, et al. Intraerythrocytic iridovirus in central bearded dragons (Pogona vitticeps). J Vet Diagn Invest 2014;26:354–64.

49. Stacy N, Alleman A, Sayler K. Diagnostic hematology of reptiles. Clin Lab Med 2011;31:87–108.

50. Arikan H, Çiçek K. Hematology of amphibians and reptiles: a review. North West J Zool 2014;10:190–209.

51. Thrall MA. Veterinary hematology and clinical chemistry. Ames (IA): Wiley-Blackwell; 2012.

52. Ebani VV. Domestic reptiles as source of zoonotic bacteria: a mini review. Asian Pac J Trop Med 2017;10:723–8.

Moving?

Make sure your subscription moves with you!

To notify us of your new address, find your **Clinics Account Number** (located on your mailing label above your name), and contact customer service at:

Email: journalscustomerservice-usa@elsevier.com

800-654-2452 (subscribers in the U.S. & Canada)
314-447-8871 (subscribers outside of the U.S. & Canada)

Fax number: 314-447-8029

Elsevier Health Sciences Division
Subscription Customer Service
3251 Riverport Lane
Maryland Heights, MO 63043

*To ensure uninterrupted delivery of your subscription,
please notify us at least 4 weeks in advance of move.